Culture and Knowledge

Edited by Friedrich G. Wallner

Vol. 22

PETER LANG

Frankfurt am Main · Berlin · Bern · Bruxelles · New York · Oxford · Wien

Fengli Lan

Culture, Philosophy, and Chinese Medicine

Viennese Lectures

兰凤利著

文化哲学与中医学

维也纳大学讲稿

李鼎题

PETER LANG
Internationaler Verlag der Wissenschaften

Bibliographic Information published by the Deutsche Nationalbibliothek
The Deutsche Nationalbibliothek lists this publication in the Deutsche Nationalbibliografie; detailed bibliographic data is available in the internet at http://dnb.d-nb.de.

Supported by the Austrian Ministry
of Science and Research, the Cultural Department
of the Municipal of Vienna and Robert Rogner jr.

Cover illustration:
"Nike von Samothraki"
Courtesy of Kovac-Verlag.

ISSN 1613-902X
ISBN 978-3-631-61981-0

www.peterlang.de

Table of Contents

List of Tables……………………………………………………………………11

List of Illustrations…………………………………………………………13

Author's Foreword…………………………………………………………15

I Overview of Chinese Culture through Chinese Characters

Introduction………………………………………………………………18

1 Etymology: Six Categories of Chinese Graphs……………………………21
1.1 Pictographs: *Xiang Xing* 象形………………………………………23
1.2 Ideographs: *Zhi Shi* 指事……………………………………………24
1.3 Associative Compounds: *Hui Yi* 会意…………………………………25
1.4 Signific-Phonetics: *Xing Sheng* 形声…………………………………27
1.5 Mutually Interpretive: *Zhuang Zhu* 转注………………………………29
1.6 Loan Sinograms: *Jia Jie* 假借…………………………………………29

2 Evolution of the Scripts: From Oracle-Bone Inscription to Regular Script……31
2.1 Oracle-Bone Inscription: *Jia Gu Wen* 甲骨文…………………………31
2.2 Bronze Inscription: *Jin Wen* 金文……………………………………32
2.3 Larger Seal Script: *Da Zhuan* 大篆……………………………………32
2.4 Lesser Seal Script: *Xiao Zhuan* 小篆…………………………………33
2.5 Simplified Lesser Seal Script: *Li Shu* 隶书, Official Script in the Han Dynasty……33
2.6 Cursive Script: *Cao Shu* 草书…………………………………………33
2.7 Regular Script: *Kai Shu* 楷书…………………………………………33
2.8 Running Hand: *Xing Shu* 行书…………………………………………35

3 Classical Chinese Thinking Ways Residing in Chinese Characters……………39
3.1 Man and Universe Uniting and Resembling Each Other: *Tian Ren He Yi*……39
3.2 Imaging Thinking: *Xiang* 象……………………………………………40
3.3 Balanced & Symmetrical Thinking: Yin-Yang 阴阳………………………42
3.4 Squared Shaped Sinograms, Four Directions, and Five Phases………………44
3.5 Being Conservative: Venerating Classics and Worshiping History…………45

4 The Prospect of Chinese Characters……………………………………47
4.1 Combining Signific with Phonetic: The Basic Sinogram-Creating Method…47
4.2 Being Conservative: Venerating Classics and Worshiping History…………48

4.3 Chinese Culture: the Most Advanced and the Leading One of All in the History of China……………………………………..……………………48
4.4 No Access to Other Better Choices…………………………………………..50
4.5 Understanding Chinese Characters: A Historical Outline……………….……51

5 Western Scientific Thinking Ways Implied in Phonetic Writing………………57

6 *Tian Ren He Yi*: The World View of Chinese Culture…………………………59
6.1 Pan Gu 盤古, the Creator of the Universe in Chinese Mythology…………..59
6.2 Some Important Concepts: One, Heaven, Man, Earth, and Three…….……60
6.3 *Tian Ren He Yi:* The World View of Chinese Culture………………………..67

7 *Xiang*: Key to Understand Chinese Culture and Philosophy…………………73
7.1 The Original Meaning of "*Xiang* 象": Elephant……………………………73
7.2 *Xiang*: An All-Embracing Symbol in Chinese Culture and Philosophy…..…74
7.3 Xiang Implies a Vital Methodology of Chinese Philosophy…………………80

8 Worship of Thunder and Lightening: SHEN & RU……………………….…..83
8.1 Understanding SHEN in Classical Chinese Texts……………………………83
8.2 Shape, Pronunciation and Meaning: From "XU 需" to "RU 儒"…………..95

9 Reflections of Philosophy of Chinese Medicine in Chinese Characters……101
9.1 Cultural Connotations of Philosophy of Chinese Medicine………………..102
9.2 *Qi* 气 Explains Ontology of Philosophy of Chinese Medicine……………109
9.3 *Xiang* 象 Implies Methodology of Philosophy of Chinese Medicine………111
9.4 *He* 和 Shows Ultimate Aim of Philosophy of Chinese Medicine…..……112

II Fundamental Concepts of Classical Chinese Philosophy

Introduction……………………..…………………………….………………… 118

1 Intellectual Flowering in Early China: The "Hundred Schools of Thought"…121
1.1 Sima Tan Identified Six Schools of Thought……………………………..…121
1.2 Liu Xin Identified Ten Schools of Thought……...…………………………121
1.3 Lǚ Simian Identified Twelve Schools of Thought…………………………122
1.4 Brief Introduction to Twelve Schools of Thought…………………………..122
1.5 The Master Philosophers and the Hundred Schools…………………….....126

2 Backgrounds of Classical Chinese Philosophy…………………………...….129
2.1 Cultural Background: Rise of "Literati"……………………………………....129
2.2 Economic Background: Agriculture as Foundation of the Country………..130
2.3 Geographical Environment: Relative Isolation………………………….…131

2.4 Social Background: The Crisis in the Zhou (ca. 771-221B.C.) Order.........135
2.5 Logographic Writing Language and Image Thinking..........................135

3 Confucianism and Its Influences on Chinese Medicine..........................137
3.1 Confucius (551-479B.C.) and His Historical Contexts..........................138
3.2 Timeline of Confucianism..143
3.3 The Main Ideas of Confucius..149
3.4 Dispute between Confucianism and Mohism: Literati and Knights...........155
3.5 English Translation and Dissemination of *Lun Yu* in the West...............161
3.6 The Influences of Confucianism on Chinese Medicine..........................164

4 Taoist School and Its Influences on Chinese Medicine..........................173
4.1 Differences between Taoist School and Taoist Religion.........................173
4.2 Development of Taoist School...174
4.3 English Translation and Dissemination of *Lao Tzu* and *Chuang Tzu* in the West...186
4.4 Taoist Philosophy: the Philosophical Foundation of Chinese Medicine......190

5 The Yin-Yang Theory..207
5.1 The Original Meanings of Yin and Yang..208
5.2 Exploring the Origin of Yin-Yang in Chinese Medicine.........................210
5.3 Understanding Yin-Yang in the Way of *Qu Xiang Bi Lei*......................211
5.4 Translation of Yin-Yang in Classical Chinese Medical Texts..................213
5.5 The Application of Yin-Yang Theory in Chinese Medicine.....................216
5.6 Yin-Yang Diagram and Dichotomy..218

6 The Five Phases Theory...221
6.1The Origin and Background of *Wu Xing*...221
6.2 Introduction of the Five Phases into Chinese Medicine.........................223
6.3How to Translate *Wu Xing* into English?...224
6.4 Understanding the Engendering and Restraining Cycles in the Way of *Qu Xiang Bi Lei*...228
6.5Application of Five-Phase Theory in Chinese Medicine.........................228

III The Importance of Metaphors in Chinese Medicine

Introduction.. 238

1 Contemplating "*Zhong Yi*"..241
1.1 Possible meanings of "*Zhong Yi* 中醫"...241
1.2 Chinese Medicine: Being both Classical and Traditional......................244

1.3 Understanding Chinese Medicine as Its History, a Linguistic Medical System, and aPhilosophy 253

2 Cultural Differences between Chinese Medicine and Western Medicine 259

2.1 Chinese Medicine Going Closer to Humanities Rather than Natural Science 260
2.2 Linguistic Differences 261
2.3 Differences in Their Philosophical Foundations 272
2.4 The Incompatible Thinking of Chinese Medicine with Western Medicine 274
2.5 Strangification: Bridging Cultural Differences between Chinese Medicine and Western Medicine 275

3 *Qu Xiang Bi Lei*: The Metaphorizing Process & the Way to Form Metaphors in Chinese Medicine 279
3.1 Metaphor East and West: Similarities and Differences 279
3.2 Imaging – Analogizing – Metaphorizing: Three Key Elements of *Qu Xiang Bi Lei* 283
3.3 Metaphors in Chinese Medicine: Revealing Relationships and an Exact Thinking 296

4 Metaphorizing: The Way to Bridge *The Book of Changes* and Chinese Medicine 307
4.1 *The Book of Changes* and Chinese Medicine Being of the Same Origin: Shamans' Practice 307
4.2 *Qi* and *Xiang*: Fundamental Metaphors to Bridge *The Book of Changes* and Chinese Medicine 309
4.3 Metaphorizing: The Way to Bridge Specific Symbols of *The Book of Changes* and Metaphors of Chinese Medicine 311

5 Metaphorizing: A Vital Way to Understand the Human Being 317
5.1 Essence, *Qi*, *Shen*: From Universe to Man 317
5.2 The Visceral Image: Weaving Yin-Yang, Five Phases, and Social Phenomena with Basic Understanding of Internal Organs Together 321
5.3 The Vessel Theory: From the Rivers in the Universe to the Vessels in Man 329

6 Metaphorizing: A Vital Way to Understand and Modernize Chinese Herbal Medicine 333
6.1 Differences between *Ben Cao* and *Yao* 333

6.2 Properties, Flavors, and Meridian Entry..334
6.3 Metaphorizing: A Vital Way for Genesis of Actions of Materia Medica......334
6.4 Metaphorizing: A Vital Way to Understand Medicine made from a Formula/Prescription (*Yao*)..340
6.5 Metaphorizing: A Vital Way to Modernize Chinese Herbal Medicine........340

7 Number Metaphors for Constructing the Theoretical System of Chinese Medicine..343
7.1 Numbers in Chinese Medicine...343
7.2 One (一 and 壹): The Origin of All things......................................344
7.3 Three Gives Birth to All Things..346
7.4 Five *Zang* Organs and Six *Fu* Organs...348
7.5 Regular Meridians: From Eleven to Twelve.......................................349

8 Metaphorizing: A Vital Way to Develop Chinese Medicine.......................353
8.1 Metaphorizing: A Vital Way to Develop Clinical Explorations of Chinese Medicine..354
8.2 Metaphorizing: A Vital Way to Develop and Modernize Chinese Medicine..356

Epilogue:

Etymology-Based Literal Translation Approach and Strangification: Efficient Methods for Successful Intercultural Communications 361

Bilingual Glossary (Chinese-English)...377

Historical Bibliography...383

List of Tables

1 Examples: Ideographs……………………………………………………………25
2 Examples: "步" and "涉", "陟", "降"……………………………………………..26
3 Creating Signific-Phonetics to Translate Chemical Elements…………………29
4 Naming Usages of the Eight Principles of "永 Yong"…………………………35
5 Different Views of Heart in *Hippocratic Corpus* and *Huang Di Nei Jing*……108
6 Differences of Mo Tzu and his followers from Ordinary Knights-Errant........159
7 A Comparison of Some Quotations from *Lao Tzu* and *Huang Di Nei Jing Su Wen*……………………………………………………………………...198
8 A Comparison of Some Quotations from *Chuang Tzu* and *Huang Di Nei Jing Su Wen*…………………………………………………………………...201
9 Examples of *Yin-Yang*…………………………………………………………...212
10 Pattern Identification According to Yin and Yang…………………………..213
11 Relating the Nature and Man to the Five Phases……………………………224
12 The Gap between Classical Chinese Medicine and Traditional Chinese Medicine……………………………………………………………………..252
13 Differences between Chinese Medicine and Western Medicine…………….259
14 The Incompatible Thinking of Chinese Medicine with Western Medicine…274
15 Translations of "六節藏象論" &"藏象何如" by Different Translators…….362
16 Translations of Some Basic Concepts of Chinese Medicine………………..364
17 A Comparison between Standardized Translation Approved by WHO and Popular Translations in the West……………………………………………..365

List of Illustrations

1 "Jia 家 (Residence, Home) " in *The Great Dictionary of Oracle, Bronze, Seal, and Official Scripts*......19
2 Original Forms of Some Sinograms: Pictographic and Self-Explanatory........23
3 The Sinograms "考" and "老" from Oracle, Bronze, Lesser-Seal to Regular Script......29
4 "永" Illustrates Eight Writing Strokes in Chinese Calligraphy......34
5 Evolution of Chinese Writing Forms From Oracle Inscription to Running Hand......37
6 A Swimming Elephant (Horizontal & Vertical) and "象" in Oracle Script.......40
7 "Xiang 象" from Oracle, Bronze, Lesser Seal, to Regular Script......41
8 A Panorama of The Imperial Palace (Forbidden City) in Beijing......43
9 Square-Shaped Sinograms......45
10 The Bottle Gourd......61
11 Fu Xi & Nü Wa Coupling Figure Unearthed in Xinjiang......63
12 "Tian 天" from Oracle, Bronze, Lesser Seal to Regular Script......64
13 Along the River in Qingming Heyday（Part）......77
14 Xu Guangqi: Configuration of Stars at Night......78
15 "SHEN 神" from Bronze, Lesser Seal to Regular Script......84
16 "SHI 示 (礻)" from Oracle, Bronze, Lesser Seal to Regular Script......85
17 Maps of China and Ancient Greece......132
18 The Statue of Confucius Standing in Tian'anmen Square......145
19 The Sinogram "Yin 阴" from Oracle to Simplified Regular Script......208
20 The Sinogram "Yang 阳" from Oracle to Simplified Regular Script......209
21 Yin-Yang Diagram and Dichotomy......219
22 The Greek System of the Four Elements......226
23 Variant Original Complex Forms of "*Mai* 脉"......291
24 Tongue Reading......297
25 Fu Xi's Eight Trigrams......312

Author's Foreword

This is a stern reality: Information in English accounted for over 80% of the total information stored in the computers of the world; databases owned by the U.S.A. made up over 70% of the globe;[1] the statistics of the United Nations showed that 80% of all the original documents were in English and less than 1% in Chinese; there existed great deficit in the cultural exchange: the works translated from Western languages into Chinese were about 50 to 100 times of the works translated from Chinese into Western languages.[2]

Influences of Chinese culture on the Western culture have still remained very limited although Confucius Institutes have been established internationally and widely by the P.R. China across the world, which aims at promoting dissemination of Chinese language and culture worldwide and in real fact promotes teaching and learning of Chinese language among foreigners.

Does globalization mean westernization, easternization or similarization or even uniformation? No, globalization should be pluralization. Almost everybody has traveling experience. As a traveler, everyone would like to see something, some place, and some people with distinctive, specialized and local features. If everywhere were the same someday in the future, the world would be very boring. This is the same with the culture, philosophy and science of the globe, which should be manifold not unified. The world is manifold, which needs approaches from different cultures to enrich human understanding of the world from as many as possible perspectives.

The research team of a key research project of National Social Science Fund of China - "Strategic Studies on Developing Soft Power of Chinese Culture" (07&ZD037) announced its periodic achievement of "A Survey of Symbols for Chinese Culture" recently. This survey lasted half a year and involved teachers and students from colleges and universities in the country. The survey shows that, among the 270 candidate symbols for Chinese culture, the first ten most representative ones are as follows: 1 Chinese language (Chinese characters), 2 Confucius, 3 Chinese calligraphy, 4 the Great Wall, 5 the Five-Starred Red Flag (the national flag of the People's Republic of China), 6 Chinese medicine, 7 Mao Zedong (the founder of the P. R. China), 8 the Imperial Palace (also known as the Forbidden City, the world's largest royal palace), 9 Deng Xiaoping (the general designer of China's reform and opening-up policy), and 10 Terracotta Warriors and Horses unearthed at the Qin Shi Huang's Imperial Mausoleum in Shaanxi province. Among the 10 most representative cultural symbols, 70% are traditional ones. I think that Chinese characters, Confucius (Confucianism), and Chinese medicine are rich most in cultural connotations, and have general and specific cultural identification feeling among all the Chinese people.

---

1 Yu Keping. Globalization: Westernization or Chinesization [M]. Beijing: Social Sciences Academic Press, 2002: 4-256.

2 Wang Yuechuan. Discovering the East [M]. Beijing: Beijing Library Press, 2003: 29.

Along with the formation of a worldwide aging society and the significant variations in disease spectrum, it has become thus clear that Chinese medicine is a real gem worth to cherish and to carry on in the unending quest for human health and a long life. Chinese medicine is a culture dependent art of healing originating from China, and is deeply rooted into Chinese culture and philosophy. I feel greatly honored to have got this chance to stand on the platform of Vienna University and to reveal the essentials of philosophy of Chinese language, classical Chinese philosophy and Chinese medicine to my students from different cultural backgrounds.

In publishing this book, I welcome the opportunity of expressing my thanks to Prof. Dr. Friedrich Wallner of Faculty of Philosophy, Vienna University, who made it possible for me to come from Shanghai to Vienna as Visiting Professor in the Winter semester of 2010-2011, which resulted in the writing of this book. I am also grateful to my students of Vienna University for their interests, cooperation and encouragement. Also I wish to thank Dr. Norbert Willenpart of Peter Lang for his help in making arrangement for the publication of the book. Besides, I also thank Lu Bin of Shanghai University of TCM for his professional technical assistance in type-setting and making the manuscript ready for publication.

The book is based on my teaching PPT slides and lecture notes, which are composed of three parts with the same titles as the three topics of my lectures and seminars: Overview of Chinese Culture through Chinese Characters (180364), Fundamental Concepts of Classical Chinese Philosophy (180367), and The Importance of Metaphors in Chinese Medicine (180368). They were classified as courses in the fields of linguistic philosophy and intercultural philosophy. It is worth to note that, what present in this book is my specific research outcome from my own work in the last years, esp. from the part of cooperation with Prof. Dr. Friedrich G. Wallner.

In fact, the book is a starting point where I meet myself and the needs of transmitting Chinese culture to the West. I do hope this booklet can bring you a unique experience into culture, philosophy, and Chinese medicine, and help you understand China and Chinese culture much better than before.

I Overview of Chinese Culture through Chinese Characters

“Language is the outcome of a culture. Language of a nation is the general reflection of the culture of the nation; but we can also say that language is a part of the culture … and that culture and language have developed together for thousands of years.”

- Claude Levi Strauss[3]

“The role of language within a culture and the influence of the culture on the meanings of words and idioms are so pervasive that scarcely any text can be adequately understood without careful consideration of its cultural background."

- Eugene A. Nida[4]

Introduction

As regards to the historical development, generally speaking, the remoter the antiquity and the slower the development. The mankind underwent a very long period of uncivilized state, and gradually has entered an age of civilization. Civilization refers to “an advanced state of human society, in which a high level of culture, science, industry, and government has been reached”[5]. One of the most important marks for a civilization is the emergence and application of a written language.

Ancient civilizations all appeared along rivers for water provides essential living conditions for other living creatures such as plants and animals, and thus ensures the survival of human beings. Chinese civilization was born in the Yellow River valley, and has been developing independently for thousands of years. Chinese characters or sinograms[6], the writing forms of Chinese language and one of the most important marks of Chinese civilization, emerged[7] independently around 6,000 years ago, which is identified by the history of Banpo Ruins of Xi’an, Shaanxi Province[8]. The sinogram 家 Jia, which is interpreted as

3 Translated from Chinese translation. Quoted from a secondary source: See He Yumin. 1990: 149.

4 Nida, Eugene A. 1993: 1.

5 Webster’s Encyclopedic Unabridged Dictionary of the English Language (New Revised Edition) [Z]. 199 : 270.

6 For translation of Chinese 汉字 I prefer “sinogram” instead of “Chinese character”, which was originally proposed by Prof. Pan Wenguo (1944-) in his monograph entitled “Sinogram as the Basic Unit and Chinese Language Study” published in 2002. The author advanced that Chinese language study should take Zi or sinogram instead of Ci or word as the basic unit for Chinese language study.

7 Cang Jie 仓颉 (?-?) was said to be the creator of Chinese characters in Chinese legendary. He was said to be an official historian of the Huang Di’s (Yellow Emperor) reign, or a king of the remote antiquity. It is said that he had four eyes on his head, could communicate with gods, and created sinograms by integrating beauties he collected widely from myriad of things. Modern scholars hold that a writing form is a collective creation of human society, that Chinese characters were also a collective creation, which were conceived, created, chosen, refined, and developed by the Chinese people, and that Cang Jie was possibly the earliest most famous figure who did so in the remote antiquity.

8 In 1972, Archaeological Institute of China Academy of Science identified the history of Banpo Ruin as around 6,000 years by C14 determination in its labs.

“residence” in *Shuo Wen Jie Zi* or *The Origin of Chinese Characters*[9] 说文解字 and now is Chinese equivalent for English word “home”, is composed of two parts 宀 (the image of “the roof of a house” in ancient China for house) and 豕 Shi (the image for swine, pig). Residence or Home should be a living place for human beings, but why there was a pig in the house? Could it be said that “residence or home” was also supposed to keep a pig? You will come to understand this sinogram suddenly if you visit the Banpo Ruin. In the matriarchal clan society, the pig had already been raised and kept in human’s residence. It can be seen that the sinogram 家 had been conceived 6,000 years ago; and developed into 家 of the oracle script and bronze script 2,000 years later. See Illus. 1.[10]

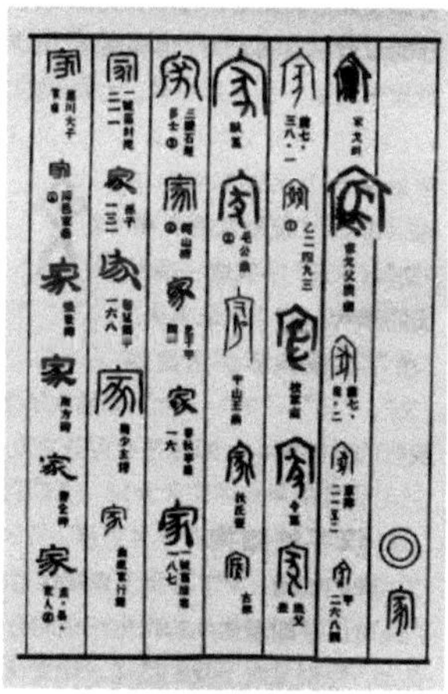

Illus.1 "Jia 家 (Residence, Home) "in *The Great Dictionary of Oracle, Bronze, Seal, and Official Scripts*

Chinese characters, Egyptian hieroglyphics, Sumerian cuneiforms, primitive scripts of ancient Elam, and scripts of Crete, etc. are the oldest writing forms in the world. Chinese characters, like the other oldest writing forms, underwent the

---

9 *Shuo Wen Jie Zi* 说文解字 literally means “explaining pictographs and analyzing composite sinograms”. I prefer to translate the title into *The Origin of Chinese Characters*. It is the first comprehensive systematic dictionary of sinograms arranged by sections with shared components, called radicals (*bùshǒu* 部首, lit. "section headers") and finished in 100 A.D. by Xu Shen 许慎 (A.D.58? – 147?) of the Eastern Han Dynasty. It is also the first dictionary which interprets the original meaning of a sinogram by analyzing its structure and gives the rationale behind it, sometimes the etymology of the sinogram as well. Actually, it is far beyond a dictionary, and moreover it can be interpreted from cultural and philosophical perspectives. It is indeed the case that no monograph on philosophy of Chinese language has ever been available up till today except this book.

10 Zuo Min’an. 2005:7.

period of evolution from pure pictographs to ideographs; but all of the others lost their vitality and were stopped being used during the evolution, some became phonetic writings, some were not recognizable and therefore were replaced by a foreign writing system; Chinese writing form is the only exceptional case, which has been used up till today and becomes the only logographic writing[11] as opposed to phonetic writing. The sinograms contain rich Chinese culture, and reflect Chinese way of understanding the world.

11 Logographic writing or *Xiang Xing* 象形, also known as ideographic or pictographic writing in English. Here logographic writing is a better translation for here it refers to the general writing form of the Chinese characters as a whole as opposed to phonetic writing. *Xiang Xing* 象形 as one of the 6 categories of Chinese characters classified in *The Origin of Chinese Characters* (Shuo Wen Jie Zi, 说文解字) are pictographs. *The Origin of Chinese Characters* classifies all of the Chinese characters into 6 categories (Liu Shu, 六书), i.e. *Xiang Xing* 象形(pictographs), *Zhi Shi* 指事[ideographs (or indicators, self-explanatory sinograms)], *Hui Yi* 会意(associative compounds), *Xing Sheng* 形声[pictophonetic (or signific-phonetic)], *Zhuan Zhu* 转注 (mutually interpretive), and *Jia Jie* 假借(loan sinograms).

The world is too new, and many things have still not got their names. We had to stretch out our fingers to point them out.[12]

- Gabriel García Márquez

1 Etymology: Six Categories of Chinese Graphs

"Chinese etymology is far from a science. Sinologists could debate for decades over the origins of certain characters and never come to a final resolution".[13] But it is well known that Chinese characters are a kind of ideographic writing, where the shape of a Chinese character is directly related to its meaning. Correct analysis of structures of sinograms will be of great help for us to understand their original meanings and extended meanings, and to understand Chinese culture as well.

Liu Shu 六书 or Six Categories of Chinese Graphs are always used to illustrate the structures and creating methods of sinograms. This term first appeared in the section of *Di Guan. Bao Shi*[14] 地官•保氏 of *Zhou Li* 周礼 or *The Rites of Zhou [Dynasty]*; its detailed categories first appeared in *Qi Lüe* 七略 by Liu Qin 刘歆(50?B.C.-23A.D.)[15].

There are different versions on *Liu Shu* 六书 or Six Categories of Chinese Graphs in the history. Hereafter are 3 main figures of the Eastern Han Dynasty (25-220 A.D.), who gave their explanations of *Liu Shu*.

The first is Ban Gu 班固 (32-92)[16]. In the *Treatise on Literature* of *History of the Former Han Dynasty* (Han Shu. Yi Wen Zhi, 汉书•艺文志), it states that "In ancient times children started school at the age of eight. Mr. Bao, an official of Zhou dynasty, was in charge of teaching children of the country. He taught them *Liu Shu* 六书, namely *Xiang Xing* 象形 (pictographs, literally "resembling shapes"), *Xiang Shi* 象事 (ideographs or indicators, literally "resembling things"), *Xiang Yi* 象意 (associative compounds, literally "resembling meanings"), *Xiang Sheng* 象声 (pictophonetics, literally "resembling

12 Translated from Chinese translation. The original reference is the CIEN ANOS DE SOLEDA.D., known as "One Hundred Years of Solitude" in English, originally by Gabriel García Márquez (1927-).

13 Wiseman, Nigel & Zhang Yuhuan. 2003: 16.

14 Bao Shi 保氏, an official to be in charge of teaching in an elementary school (opposed to "Great Learning") and remonstrating with King, as well as teaching children of high officials of Zhou Dynasty (11th C. -256 B.C.).

15 *Qi Lüe* 七略, the first official library catalogue compiled by Liu Qin 刘歆(50?B.C.-23A.D.) in 6-5 B.C based on his father Liu Xiang's 刘向 (77?-6B.C.) work *Bie Lu* 别录, which records the authors, contents, academic values, etc. of the books collected and systematized at that time.

16 Ban Gu 班固 (32-92), had been the national imperial librarian during Ming Emperor's reign 汉明帝 (57-75A.D.), and accomplished the first historical records *Han Shu* 汉书 or *History of the Former Han Dynasty* presented in a series of biographies divided into periods in between 206 B.C. and 23 A.D. His *Han Shu. Yi Wen Zhi* 汉书•艺文志 or *Treatise on Literature* of *History of the Former Han Dynasty*, the first systematic book catalogue extant in China, was compiled on the basis of *Qi Lüe* 七略.

pronunciations"), *Zhuang Zhu* 转注 (mutually interpretive), and *Jia Jie* 假借 (loan sinograms), which are the foundation of creating sinograms[17]".

The second is Zheng Zhong 郑众 (?-83)[18]. His annotation on the section of *Di Guan. Bao Shi* of *The Rites of Zhou [Dynasty]* reads that "*Liu Shu* 六书 refers to *Xiang Xing* 象形(pictographs), *Hui Yi* 会意(associative compounds), *Zhuan Zhu* 转注 (mutually interpretive), *Chu Shi* 处事 [ideographs (or indicators, self-explanatory sinograms)], *Jia Jie* 假借(loan sinograms), and *Xie Sheng* 谐声 [pictophonetics (or signific-phonetics)]".

The third is Xu Shen 许慎 (58?-147?)[19]. In the preface of *The Origin of Chinese Characters* it states that "the first is *Zhi Shi* 指事 [ideographs (or indicators, self-explanatory sinograms)], the second is *Xiang Xing* 象形 (pictographs), the third is *Xing Sheng* 形声[pictophonetics (or signific-phonetics)], the fourth is *Hui Yi* 会意(associative compounds), the fifth is *Zhuan Zhu* 转注 (mutually interpretive), and the sixth is *Jia Jie* 假借(loan sinograms)".

As regards to the names of the Six Categories of Chinese Graphs, most of the scholars adopt the names given by Xu Shen not only because he gave detailed interpretation for the Six Categories of Chinese Graphs but also because he composed the first monograph on studying and analyzing Chinese characters. As regards to the order of the Six Categories of Chinese Graphs, most of the scholars adopt Ban Gu's version because Chinese characters originated from pictures, which is closely related to *Xiang Xing* 象形(pictographs), *Zhi Shi* 指事[ideographs (or indicators, self-explanatory sinograms)], and *Hui Yi* 会意 (associative compounds); *Xing Sheng* 形声[pictophonetics (or signific-phonetics)] have been developed on the basis of pictographs, which also accords with the developing rule of a written language – from pictographic to ideographic, then to phonetic

17 It is worth to note that the Six Categories of Chinese Graphs are the concluded rules on structures of Chinese characters according to their characteristics summarized by ancient scholars. We should not believe that ancient Chinese people created sinograms according to the six rules. Actually, *Xiang Xing* 象形 (pictographs), *Zhi Shi* 指事 [ideographs (or indicators, self-explanatory sinograms)], *Hui Yi* 会意 (associative compounds), and *Xing Sheng* 形声 [pictophonetics (or signific-phonetics)] are ways of creating and developing sinograms, while *Zhuan Zhu* 转注(mutually interpretive) and *Jia Jie* 假借 (loan sinograms) have nothing to do with structures of sinograms, and are ways of using sinograms.

18 Zheng Zhong 郑众 (?-83), an expert in Confucian classics of Eastern Han Dynasty. His works had been lost. Ma Guohan 马国翰 (1794-1857) collected "Zheng Zhong's Annotations of *The Rites of Zhou [Dynasty]*" (6 volumes) 周礼郑司农(众)解诂 and "Zheng Zhong's Syntactic and Semantic Analysis of Examples of *The Spring and Autumn Annals*" (1 volume) 郑众春秋牒例章句.

19 Xu Shen 许慎 (58?-147?), a distinguished expert in Confucian classics, philologist, linguist, and the pioneer of the study of Chinese characters of the Eastern Han Dynasty. He was perfect in critical interpretation of ancient sinograms, and accomplished the writing of *Shuo Wen Jie Zi* 说文解字 or *The Origin of Chinese Characters* (15 volumes) after fifteen years of hard work, which collects 9,353 sinograms arranged according to significs or radicals. It is the first monograph on exploring etymology of sinograms and interpreting original meanings of sinograms by analyzing their original structures, and it is known as the first systematic dictionary with complete collection of sinograms, comprehensive analysis of the shape, pronunciation and meanings as well as scientific arrangement.

writings; *Jia Jie* 假借(loan sinograms) mainly show the relations between pronunciations, which have nothing to do with the meanings of sinograms. Therefore, the generally recognized names and order of the Six Categories of Chinese Graphs are formed after a comparison of the three versions mentioned above: *Xiang Xing* 象形(pictographs), *Zhi Shi* 指事[ideographs (or indicators, self-explanatory sinograms)], *Hui Yi* 会意(associative compounds), *Xing Sheng* 形声[pictophonetics (or signific-phonetics)], *Zhuan Zhu* 转注(mutually interpretive), and *Jia Jie* 假借(loan sinograms). Hereafter is a detailed interpretation of the Six Categories of Chinese Graphs.

1.1 Pictographs: *Xiang Xing* 象形

Xiang Xing 象形 or Pictographs, just as its name implies, means sinograms resembling shapes of concrete things, and depicting shapes of objects. *The Origin of Chinese Characters* defines *Xiang Xing* 象形 or pictographs as sinograms created by "drawing objects with curves by following their natural shapes, like 日 sun and 月 moon".

It is well known that the Chinese writing system was originally pictographic. In their original forms, graphs representing animals and objects were self-explanatory. See Illus. 2.

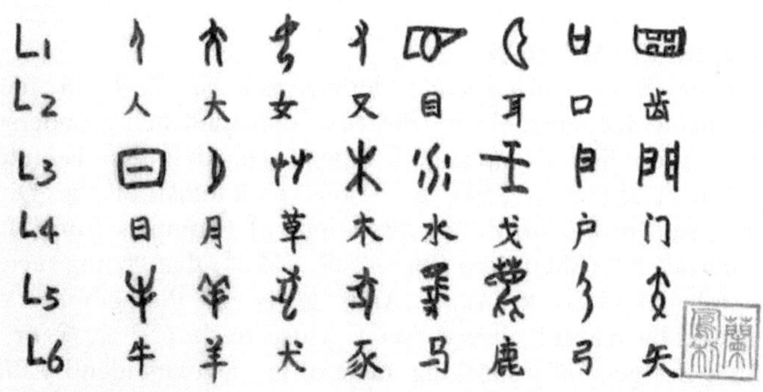

Illus.2 Original Forms of Some Sinograms: Pictographic and Self-Explanatory

In this Illustration, the lines 1, 3, 5 show some pictographs in oracle script, and the sinograms of the lines 2, 4, 6 bear the same meaning as those of the lines 1, 3, 5 respectively but in their regular script. The objects or animals of the sinograms of the line 1 denote (from left to right): human, big (man), female (resembling the side image of a pregnant woman), right (hand), eye, ear, mouth, and teeth; those of the line 3 denote (from left to right): sun, moon (the image of crescent or new moon), grass, wood (tree), water, dagger-axe (a weapon used in ancient China), one-paneled door, two-paneled door; those of the line 5 denote (from left to right): ox, goat, dog, pig, horse, deer, bow, arrow.

The way of being pictographic is still alive. An interesting example is 囧 Jiǒng, which was written as  in oracle script, resembling the image of a window with light in, and so its original meaning is "bright". But in the recent years, it has been given a new meaning, which is much popular than its original meaning now, by Internet users in China by relating the image of the sinogram with a mournful face - 八 for two eyebrows, 口 for a mouth. Then you can imagine the meaning if a person's face looks like this: depressive, sad, helpless, wordless, etc.

As pictographs are created by "drawing objects with curves by following their natural shapes", this way of creating sinograms bears big limitations for writing pictographs was very troublesome and for the same object writings of different persons could be very different. Therefore, compared to the other three ways of creating and developing Chinese characters, this way of *Xiang Xing* 象形 or "drawing objects with curves by following their natural shapes" has been becoming less and less important in the developing course of Chinese characters.

Not all elements of the language could be represented in pictorial form. Other devices had to be used.

1.2 Ideographs: *Zhi Shi* 指事

The Origin of Chinese Characters defines *Zhi Shi* 指事 or Ideographs as sinograms "being recognizable by the first sight and being understandable by careful observation, like 上 up and 下 down". This definition is quite confusing, as Wang Jun 王筠(1784-1854), a famous philologist of the Qing Dynasty (1644-1911), said in his work "Interpretations of Examples from *The Origin of Chinese Characters*" (Shuo Wen Shi Li, 说文释例) that "being recognizable by the first sight is close to *Xiang Xing* 象形 or Pictographs, while being understandable by careful observation is close to *Hui Yi* 会意 or Associative compounds". But generally speaking, most of the scholars identify *Zhi Shi* 指事 or Ideograph as a sinogram with a pictograph as its basic form and an indicating mark to denote its meaning. Some notions could be represented in this vivid fashion. See Table 1, which shows some examples to illustrate this way of creating and developing Chinese characters.

Oracle Script	Regular Script	Denotation	Explanatory Notes
	上 Shang	Up	Both with the horizontal as their first stroke, one dot above the horizontal indicates Up, while one dot below the horizontal indicates Down.
	下 Xia	Down	
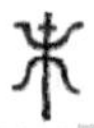	末 Mo	Tip of a Tree	Both with 木 (tree) as their basis, one dot at the top indicates the tip of a tree, while one dot at the foot indicates the root of a tree. A Chinese idiom 本末倒置, which literally means "take the tip for root or take the root for tip", is based on the two sinograms to mean "have the order reversed" or "set the cart before the horse".
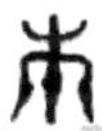	本 Ben	Root of a Tree	
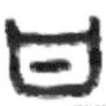	甘 Gan	Sweet	The outer represents a tongue, the stroke in the center stands for the place for feeling tastes, something which can be kept at the middle of the tongue must be sweet.
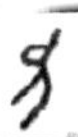	刃 Ren	Edge of a Knife	The stroke on the left indicates the edge of a knife (the part on the right).

Table 1 Examples: Ideographs

1.3 Associative Compounds: *Hui Yi* 会意

The Origin of Chinese Characters defines *Hui Yi* 会意 or Associative Compounds as sinograms formed by "combining pictographs to get a new denotation, like 武 and 信". 武, written as  in oracle script, an associative compound, showing the image of fingers holding a dagger-axe, a weapon of ancient times, means "is going to start a fight, use force", so its original meaning is "valiant". 信, an associative compound, follows 人 (man) and 言 (words), means "honest, sincere" for all of man's words were honest and sincere in ancient times of China.

Another example is 步. In ancient China, raising one foot names 跬 (kui, half step), and then raising the other foot names 步 (one step). *Xun Tzu*[20] states

20 ***Xun Tzu*** is the representative work by Xun Tzu 荀子 (300?-230?B.C.). Xun Tzu was a Chinese Confucian philosopher, thinker, and educator who lived during the Warring States Period and contributed to one of the Hundred Schools of Thought. Xun Tzu believed that man's inborn tendencies need to be curbed through education and ritual, counter to Mencius's view that man is innately good. He believed that ethical norms had been invented to rectify mankind. Xun Tzu was one of the most sophisticated thinkers of his time, and was the teacher of Li Si 李斯 (280?-208 B.C.), a famous politician, writer and calligrapher of Qin Dynasty and Han Fei 韩非 (281-233B.C.), a famous philosopher, thinker, essayist, and political commentator as well as the synthesizer and the representative figure of the Legalist School.

in the chapter of "*Encouraging Learning*" that "You will never reach a place of one thousand miles away if you do not start from one step of walking".

Oracle Script	Regular Script	Categories	Meaning	Explanatory Notes
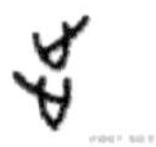	步 Bu	Pictograph	To walk, go on foot; pace, step	Resembling the image of walking with two feet, one front one back.
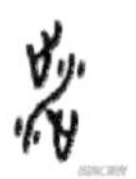	涉 She	Associative compound	To walk through a water, wade or ford a water	Showing the image of walking through a stream; in the middle of the two feet is the image of water.
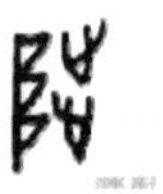	陟 Zhi	Associative compound	To climb, walk up a hill	The left part indicating a hillside, the right part indicating walking with toes upward.
	降 Jiang	Associative compound	To walk down from a hill	The left part indicating a hillside, the right part indicating walking with toes downward.

Table 2 Examples: 步 and 涉 陟 降

Generally speaking, associative compounds can be classified into 3 main subcategories:

① The first is composed by combining different pictographs, which makes up the major part of the associative compounds. For example,

The combination of the 日 Sun and the 月 Moon is 明, meaning “bright or brightness”.

The combination of the 日 Sun, the 月 Moon, and the 空 sky makes 曌, which means “The sun and the moon shine together up in the sky”. Wu Zetian 武则天 (625 – 705), the only female emperor in the history of China, created this sinogram to name herself.

The combination of the 田 Farmland and the 力 Labor gives birth to 男 Male, for males usually labored in the farmland in ancient times.

The combination of the 人 human and the 木 tree produces 休, indicating human is resting against a tree.

The combination of the 女 female and the 子 girl results in 好, its original meaning is beautiful and now its common meaning is good.

② The second is composed by combining the same pictographs. For example,

从, being composed of two 人（human）, one front one behind, means “to follow”.

众, being composed of three 人 (human）, means “many people”.

林, being composed of two 木 (tree), means “forest, woods”.

森, its oracle script written as  , being composed of three 木 (tree), means “full of trees”; “multitudinous, in multitudes”, e.g. in 森罗万象 which means myriads of things, everything under the sun; “dark, gloomy, grim”, e.g. 阴森.

淼, being composed of three 水 (water), means “wide expanse of water being vast”.

③ The third is composed of different non-pictographs by the way of being pictographic. For example,

Being unable to go “up 上” nor go “down 下” is “卡 block”.

The upper “small 小” and the lower “big 大” is “尖 pointed or tapering”.

A “mountain 山” being “high 高” is 嵩 to describe mountains of being high and lofty.[21]

1.4 Signific-Phonetics: *Xing Sheng* 形声

The Origin of Chinese Characters defines *Xing Sheng* 形声 or Signific-Phonetics as sinograms formed by “combining one part of meaning and the other part of pronunciation, like 江 and 河”. 江, written as  in *The Origin of Chinese Characters* (lesser seal script), is composed of 水 water (signific) and 工 (phonetic), originally refers to the Changjiang River or Yangtze River; 河, written as  in *The Origin of Chinese Characters* (lesser seal script), is composed of 水 water (signific) and 可 (phonetic), originally refers to the Huanghe River or the Yellow River. The Yangtze River is the longest river in Asia, while the Yellow River is the second longest river in China (after the Yangtze River), and is honored as "the cradle of Chinese civilization" as its basin is the birthplace of the northern Chinese civilizations and was the most prosperous region in early Chinese history.

As we know that the ways of creating pictographs, ideographs and associative compounds bear certain limitations in creating and developing sinograms for many things, phenomena and abstract concepts can not be expressed in such ways. Take fish as an example. “鱼 Fish”, a pictograph, is a collective term for all different kinds of fish, but different species of fish bear

21 Zuo Min’an. 2005:12.

nearly the same shape or image. How is it possible to create different sinograms to denote thousands of different species of fish by mirroring their shapes? It would be very difficult to identify and distinguish them even if you could create thousands of sinograms by so doing. Therefore, in Chinese there is a pictograph "鱼 fish" as a collective term for all different species of fish; and then different signific-phonetics are created by combining the pictograph "鱼 fish" as the signific part to show its general meaning and different pronunciation parts to denote specific kinds of fish, such as 鳕 Cod, 鲨 Shark, 鲈 Perch, 鳗 Eel, 鲳 Pomfret, 鲱 Herring, 鲑 Salmon, 鲔 Tuna, 鲮 Dace.

The need for creating new signific-phonetics results from either distinguishing the meanings of one sinogram or conveying new concepts. For example, the sinograms "藏府 Zang Fu" bear at least two major meanings: One is "depots and palaces for storing precious things and goods respectively", and the other is "the yin and the yang internal organs respectively of the human body". Later on, in order to distinguish the two meanings from each other, the sinograms "臟腑 Zang Fu" were created by adding "the flesh moon part 月"[22] on the left of "藏府" respectively to denote specifically the internal organs of the human body. Now the simplified writing forms of the two sinograms are 脏腑. As regards to creating new signific-phonetics to convey new concepts, I would like take Chinese translation of chemical elements as an example.

In 1871, John Fryer 傅兰雅 (1839–1928)[23] and his Chinese colleague Xu Shou 徐寿(1818–1884)[24], both of them working for the translation office of the Jiangnan Arsenal, created a principle for the translation of chemical elements according to the way of creating signific-phonetics, where a root signific classifies the element as of the "metal", "air", "stone (metalloid)", or "water" groups, and a single descriptive word or an imitation of the sound of one syllable in the English name of the element gives the pronunciation. See Table 3.

---

22 Sinograms denoting parts of human body usually carry this flesh moon part.

23 John Fryer 傅兰雅 (1839–1928), English, had long been working for the translation office of the Jiangnan Arsenal. His ideal was clearly written down in *Biographical Sketch of Translating Western Works at Jiangnan Arsenal* 江南製造總局翻譯西書事略 that "All I hope is that China spreads out knowledge of science so as to make the East similar developed to the West. Therefore I will do nothing but devote my whole life time to translating Western scientific works into Chinese". It is indeed the case that he translated numerous books on science, technology and some on social sciences into Chinese, and thus did a very important contribution to the transmission and development of Western science in modern China.

24 Xu Shou 徐寿 (1818–1884), a scientist of the late Qing Dynasty, initiated and introduced chemistry to modern China.

Root Classifiers (Significs)	Combinations of Significs and Phonetics			
金 Metal	鈣 Calcium	鋰 Lithium	鎳 Nickel	鈀 Palladium
气 Air (Gas)	氧 Oxygen	氫 Hydrogen	氮 Nitrogen	氟 Fluorine
石 Stone (Metalloid)	砷 Arsenic	硼 Boron	碘 Iodine	硅 Silicon
水 Water	汞 Mercury			

Table 3 Creating Signific-Phonetics to Translate Chemical Elements

The impact of their translations on the fields of chemistry and chemical engineering proved to be enormous.

In the Six Categories of Chinese Graphs stated in *The Origin of Chinese Characters*, the pictographs, ideographs (or indicators, self-explanatory sinograms), associative compounds, and signific-phonetics explain sinograms in terms of their formation. Chinese etymologists speak of two other categories that are based on how the sinograms are used, i.e. "mutually interpretive" and "loan sinograms".

1.5 Mutually Interpretive: *Zhuang Zhu* 转注

The definition of *Zhuang Zhu* 转注 or Mutually Interpretive in *The Origin of Chinese Characters* has been explained in several different ways. The most common interpretation is that "synonymous sinograms with the same radical (signific) being mutually interpretive, like 考 and 老". "老 old age" and "考 originally meant 'long life' or 'aged', later has come to mean 'test'", both share the same radical (signific) "老 old age", and is the only pair of example for *Zhuang Zhu* 转注 or Mutually Interpretive from *The Origin of Chinese Characters*. See Illus. 3.

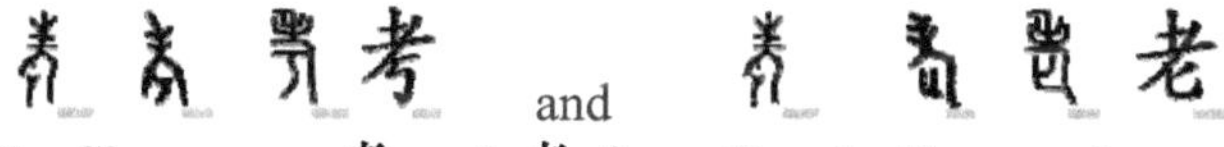

Illus. 3 The Sinograms 考 and 老 from Oracle, Bronze, Lesser-Seal to Regular Script

1.6 Loan Sinograms: *Jia Jie* 假借

The definition of *Jia Jie* 假借 or Loan Sinograms in *The Origin of Chinese Characters* indicates that a colloquial form first appears in spoken language but no written form for something new, and then a sinogram with the same pronunciation as that of the colloquial of the new thing is borrowed to denote this new thing. We can understand *Jia Jie* 假借 or Loan Sinograms as sinograms that are taken from one context and used, mostly for their pronunciations, in an entirely different context. For example,

來: originally a pictograph of "wheat", was later borrowed to denote "come";

午: originally a pictograph of "pestle", was later borrowed to denote the seventh of the 12 Earthly Branches[25]- *Wu*;

我: originally following "戈", a kind of weapon, was later borrowed to denote "I or me";

難: following "隹", originally a collective term for short-tailed birds, was later borrowed to denote "difficult or difficulty";

亦 and 腋: 亦, its oracle script written as , originally ideographic with one dot under each arm of a man, who is standing with both arms spreading out, denotes "axilla, armpit". But later on, it has been borrowed as an adverbial word to mean "also, too". Therefore, a new sinogram of signific-phonetic was created to replace the original meaning of 亦 to denote "axilla, armpit", i.e. 腋;

自 and 鼻: 自, its oracle script written as , originally pictographic, denotes nose. Later on it has been borrowed to mean "oneself". Therefore, a new sinogram of signific-phonetic was created to replace the original meaning of 自 to denote "nose".

Here is worth to note that frequent use of loan sinograms in ancient times somehow results from not enough sinograms in its initial period of the development. Many inscriptions on bones, shells, and ancient bronze objects are loan sinograms, which makes understanding the texts very difficult. Nowadays, it is not advisable to use sinograms in the way of loan sinograms, which in most cases will be identified as wrong written sinograms instead of "loan sinograms".

According to the above analysis of the *Liu Shu* 六书 or the Six Categories of Chinese Graphs, it is thus clear that the Six Categories of Chinese Graphs are the concluded rules on Chinese characters according to their characteristics summarized by ancient scholars. We should not believe that ancient Chinese people created sinograms according to the six rules.

25 The Twelve Earthly Branches used in combination with the Ten Heavenly Stems to designate years, months, days and hours.

[Chinese] calligraphy originated from the nature. 书肇于自然。

- Cai Yong[26]

2 Evolutions of the Scripts: From Oracle-Bone Inscription to Regular Script

The scripts of Chinese characters appear as a fully developed writing system in the late Shang Dynasty (1600-1100B.C.), and have gone through such an evolution process from *Jia Gu Wen*（Oracle-Bone Inscription，甲骨文）to *Jin Wen* (Bronze Inscription, 金文) to *Da Zhuan* [Larger Seal Script of Zhou Dynasty (11th Century – 256 B.C.), 大篆] to *Xiao Zhuan* (Lesser Seal Script adopted in 213 B.C. during the Qin Dynasty for the purpose of standardizing the script, 小篆) to *Li Shu* [Simplified from Lesser Seal Script, official script in the Han Dynasty (206 B.C.– 220 A.D.), 隶书] to Cao Shu (Cursive Script, 草书), *Kai Shu* (Regular Script since the end of Han Dynasty, 楷书), and then *Xing Shu* (Running Hand, 行书).

2.1 Oracle-Bone Inscription: *Jia Gu Wen* 甲骨文

Jia Gu Wen 甲骨文 or Oracle-Bone Inscription, also known as bone and shell script, oracle script, is the oldest writing form extant in China. In the Shang Dynasty, tortoise shells and animal bones were used in divining activities. After divination the time, purpose and result of the divining activity would be carved by knife on tortoise shells. This kind of writing is named *Jia Gu Wen* 甲骨文 or Oracle-Bone Inscription.

In 1899 of the late Qing Dynasty, bones and shells with inscriptions were first found in Xiaotun village, 2 kilometers away from Anyang County, Henan Province, where has been proved to be the capital of the late Shang Dynasty since the 20th king of the Shang Dynasty named Pan Geng 盘庚 according to archaeological studies. The writing was identified by Wang Yirong 王懿荣 (1845-1900)[27] as the writing of Shang Dynasty. Over 100,000 pieces of bones and shells with inscriptions have been unearthed up till now. *Qi Wen Ju Li* 契文举例 or *Examples of Oracle-Bone Inscriptions* (1904) by Sun Yirang 孙詒让 (1848-1908) is the first work on philological studies on Oracle-Bone Inscriptions. In the following over 100 years, about 1/3 of around 4,000 Oracle-Bone Inscriptions have been identified. The vocabulary, grammar, and structures of Chinese characters of the later times are consistent with and identical to those of

---

26 Cai Yong 蔡邕 (133-192), a famous literati and calligrapher of the Eastern Han Dynasty. His daughter Cai Yan 蔡琰(177?- ?), also known as Cai Wenji 蔡文姬, was a famous talented writer of that time.

27 Wang Yirong 王懿荣 (1845-1900) was an expert in the study of inscriptions on ancient bronzes and stone tablets and the discoverer of oracle-bone inscriptions. He died in the fight for defending Beijing against invasion by the Eight-Power Allied Forces, i.e. the aggressive troops sent by Britain, the United States, Germany, France, Tsarist Russia, Japan, Italy, and Austria, in 1900.

Oracle-Bone Inscriptions, which shows Oracle-Bone Inscriptions are a mature writing system.[28]

Besides of Oracle-Bone Inscriptions, there must be writings on bamboo slips because of the existence of 册 and 典 in Oracle-Bone Inscriptions. 册, written as  in oracle script, resembles the image of bamboo slips threaded together with oxhide ropes; 典，written as  in oracle script, resembles the image of a pair of hands holding 册. That's why important works are named as *Jing Dian* 经典 or classic by later generations. But no writings on bamboo slips of the Shang Dynasty have been found up till now maybe because the time is too long to preserve them for over 3,000 years underneath the earth.

2.2 Bronze Inscription: *Jin Wen* 金文

Jin Wen 金文 or Bronze Inscription or Bronze Script refers to the inscriptions on ancient bronze objects, esp. bells and tripods, from the Shang-Zhou Dynasties to Spring-Autumn and Warring States Periods (ca.1600-221B.C.). Its writing style transformed from square-shaped strokes in the Shang Dynasty (ca.1600 - ca.1100 B.C.) and the early stage of the Western Zhou Dynasty (C.1100-771B.C.), which is close to that of the Oracle-Bone Inscriptions, to round-shaped strokes from the middle stage of the Western Zhou Dynasty until the early stage of the Eastern Zhou Dynasty (770-256B.C.), to thin-strong strokes until Spring-Autumn Period (770-476B.C.), and then was thrown into confusion because of wars.

Zhuan Shu 篆书 or Seal Script came out to replace *Jin Wen* 金文 or Bronze Inscription. What is it meant by "Zhuan 篆"? Guo Moruo 郭沫若 (1892-1978)[29] interpreted it as "official". In this sense *Zhuan Shu* 篆书 should be "official script", which can be classified into *Da Zhuan* 大篆 or Larger Seal Script and *Xiao Zhuan* 小篆 or Lesser Seal Script.

2.3 Larger Seal Script: *Da Zhuan* 大篆

In the preface of *Shuo Wen Jie Zi* or *The Origin of Chinese Characters* it states that "Zhou, an official historian of the King Xuan of the Zhou Dynasty (Zhou Xuan Wang), wrote 15 pieces of *Da Zhuan* 大篆 or Larger Seal Script, which is somehow different from ancient writing forms". The King Xuan of Zhou Dynasty revived Zhou Dynasty during his 46 years of reign, which provided a good condition for systematizing and unifying Chinese characters.

Its existing form is *Shi Gu Wen* 石鼓文, inscriptions on drum-shaped stone blocks of the Warring States Period (475-221B.C.). *The Origin of Chinese Characters* includes 233 *Da Zhuan* 大篆 or Larger Seal Scripts, which are very important materials to study *Da Zhuan*.

---

28 Britannica Concise Encyclopedia (Chinese Version), 2010.

29 Guo Moruo 郭沫若 (1892-1978), was a famous Chinese author, poet, historian, archaeologist, and government official from Sichuan, China.

2.4 Lesser Seal Script: *Xiao Zhuan* 小篆

According to records of the preface of *The Origin of Chinese Characters,* Qin Shi Huang(259-210B.C.), the First Emperor of Qin Dynasty, uniformed written sinograms after he unified the country by adopting Li Si 李斯 (280?–208 B.C.) advice: simplifying *Da Zhuan* 大篆 or Larger Seal Script to *Xiao Zhuan* 小篆 or Lesser Seal Script. The main body of *The Origin of Chinese Characters* is mainly written in the typical *Xiao Zhuan* 小篆 or Lesser Seal Script, which is beautiful and composed of regular and neat lines.

2.5 Simplified Lesser Seal Script: *Li Shu* 隶书, Official Script in the Han Dynasty

Li Shu **隶书** was simplified from *Xiao Zhuan* 小篆 or Lesser Seal Script, by Cheng Miao 程邈 (?-?) of Qin Dynasty (221-206 B.C.) according to legendary. But actually this style of writing already appeared on some cultural relics of the Warring States Period (475-221 B.C.). Therefore, Cheng Miao (?-?) 程邈 can be considered as one of the earliest scholars who collected, systematized, and standardized sinograms in this style of writing. *Li Shu* resulted in the formation of *Kai Shu* or regular script, thus promoting the appearance of *Cao Shu* or cursive script and *Xing Shu* or running hand.

The evolution from Lesser Seal Script to *Li Shu* shows the transformation process from round to square in the shapes, from arc to straight lines in the strokes, and from complicated to simplified by cutting out the superfluous as a whole. By so doing, Chinese characters have lost their features as pictures and become more signific. Therefore, *Li Shu* is critical to the evolution of the writing forms of Chinese characters.

2.6 Cursive Script: *Cao Shu* 草书

The preface of *The Origin of Chinese Characters* reads that "*Cao Shu* 草书 started since Han Dynasty (206B.C.-220A.D.) ". This is indeed the case: *Cao Shu* is a kind of writing style parallel to *Li Shu.* This style of writing is usually written in a very fast continuous way, thus, the sinograms in this style of writing usually just bear their rough sketches. But later on some handwritings in *Cao Shu* are not recognizable except their calligraphers for they are written too freely just like dragon flying and phoenix dancing, so such *Cao Shu* is known as the wild scribble or *Kuang Cao* 狂草, an excessively free cursive style in Chinese calligraphy.

2.7 Regular Script: *Kai Shu* 楷书

Kai Shu 楷书 or Regular Script has replaced *Li Shu* or Simplified Lesser Seal Script for over 1,800 years up till today since the Eastern Han Dynasty (25-220A.D.), which evolved from *Li Shu*. Handwritings of *Kai Shu* are straight in strokes, square-shaped in structures, and are easy to write. The shape of *Kai Shu* can be basically displayed by the eight principles of 永 yǒng (means "forever" or "permanence"), which was put forward by Zhang Huaijin 张怀瑾 (?-?), a famous calligrapher of the Tang Dynasty (618-907). And thus the eight principles of 永 yǒng has become the foundation of *Kai Shu* and Chinese calligraphy as well. We could say that the writing strokes of all the Chinese characters are no more than these eight principles. See the Illus. 4 and Table 4[30].

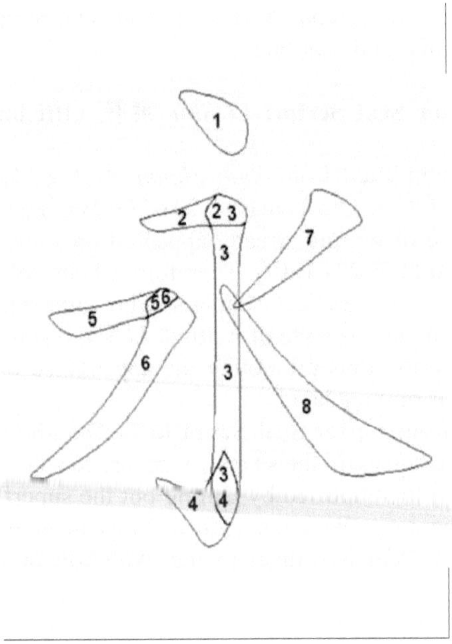

Illus. 4 "永" Illustrates Eight Writing Principles in Chinese Calligraphy

Notes: 1) ㇏ – *Xié* 斜 is sometimes added to the 永's strokes. It's a concave *Shù* falling right, always ended by a *Gōu*, visible on this image;
2) In addition to these eight common strokes in 永, there are at least two dozen strokes of combinations which enter in the composition of CJK[31] strokes and by including the CJK sinograms themselves, all sinograms which consist of ideograms, in contrast to Western phonetic alphabets and characters.

30 http://en.wikipedia.org/wiki/Eight_Principles_of_Yong
31 CJK Unified Ideographs refer to unified ideographs from Chinese, Japanese, and Korean.

List of Yǒng Principles (by Stroke Order)

	Stroke	Name (Pinyin, Chinese, Translation)	CJK Stroke name	Lǐ's name	Additional description
1		*Cè* 側/侧 "Sideway"	*Diǎn* 點/点 "Dot"	*Guài Shí* 怪石 "Strange stone"	Tiny dash, speck.
2		*Lè* 勒 "Bridle"	*Héng* 横 "Horizontal"	*Yù Àn* 玉案 "Jade table"	Rightward stroke.
3		*Nǔ* 弩 "Crossbow"; *Nǔ* 努 "Strive"	*Shù* 竪 "Erect"; *Tiěchǔ* 鐵杵/铁杵 "Iron staff"	*Tiězhù* 鐵柱/铁柱"Iron pillar"	Downward stroke.
4		*Tí* 趯 "Jump"	*Gōu* 鉤 "Hook"	*Xièzhuǎ*, (蟹爪) "Pincer of a crab"	Appended to other strokes, suddenly going down or going left only.
5		*Cè* 策 "Horsewhip"	*Tí* 提 "Raise"; *Tiāo* 挑 "Lifting off"	*Hǔyá* 虎牙 "Tiger's tooth"	Flick up and rightwards.
6		*Lüè* 掠"Passing lightly"	*Wān* 彎/弯 "Bend, curve"	*Xījiǎo* 犀角 "Horn of rhinoceros"	A tapering thinning curve, usually concave left (convex outward right) and with fast speed as if skimming.
7		*Zhuó* 啄 "Pecking"	*Piě* 撇 "Throw away, slant"; *Duǎn Piě* 短撇"Short slant"	*Niǎo Zhuó* 鳥啄/鸟啄"Bird pecking"	Falling leftwards (with slight curve).
8		*Zhé* 磔 "Dismemberment"	*Nà* 捺 "Pressing forcefully"; *Bō* 波 "Wave"	*Jīndāo* 金刀 "Golden knife"	Falling rightwards (fattening at the bottom), where the end point is "as sharp as a knife" (hence the name "Dismemberment").

Table 4 Naming Usages of The Eight Principles of "永 Yong"

2.8 Running Hand: *Xing Shu* 行书

Xing Shu 行书 or Running Hand is the flowing or running *Kai Shu*, formed in the late Eastern Han Dynasty (25-220A.D.) for *Cao Shu* is too free while *Kai Shu* is too restricted, and *Xing Shu* is just in between two of them. Therefore handwritings of *Xing Shu* are somehow continuous in strokes, separate and independent from each other, are faster in writing than that of *Kai Shu*, and are easily recognizable as well.

The Illus. 5 on the next page shows such an evolution process. You can see that the Chinese script has changed greatly from its beginning in oracle-bone inscriptions 甲骨文 through the regular scripts 楷书 of today. But "Despite the great changes in the language, the Chinese script provides access to the literature of the past in a way no other language does. In English, we can barely read the 14th century Middle English of Chaucer[32] without a translation, let alone the 8th century Old English of *Beowulf*[33]; yet knowledge of written Chinese gives us access to the literature of two thousand years ago or earlier. … The great stability of the written language means that the modern student of Chinese medicine has relatively easy access to the literature of the past".[34]

Dr. Wiseman encourages students to study etymology of Chinese characters for a better and deeper understanding of Chinese medicine. He said, "Students learning Chinese for the purpose of understanding Chinese medicine could mistakenly think of etymology as a specialty field of little professional interest to themselves, but investing some time in the study of the roots of characters not only facilitates memorization of those characters, it also helps the student develop a deeper understanding of the patterns of thought and expression that are implicit in the language and therefore the literature of Chinese medicine".[35] Besides of this, etymology investigation of sinograms is a vital approach to reveal classical Chinese thinking ways and presuppositions of Chinese culture.

---

32 Geoffrey Chaucer (1343-1400) was an English author, poet, philosopher, bureaucrat, courtier and diplomat. He is best remembered for his unfinished frame narrative *The Canterbury Tales*, written in London dialect and reflecting his humanism through narrating living conditions of different walks of life of the 14th century. Sometimes called the father of English literature, Chaucer is credited by some scholars as the first author to demonstrate the artistic legitimacy of the vernacular Middle English, rather than French or Latin.

33 Beowulf is the conventional title of an Old English heroic epic poem, commonly cited as one of the most important works of Anglo-Saxon literature. Its composition by an anonymous Anglo-Saxon poet is dated between the 8th and the early 11th century. In the poem, Beowulf, a hero of the Geats, battles three antagonists: Grendel, who has been attacking the resident warriors of the mead hall of Hroðgar (the king of the Danes), Grendel's mother, and an unnamed dragon. After the first two victories, Beowulf goes home to Geatland in Sweden and becomes king of the Geats. The last fight takes place fifty years later. In this final battle, Beowulf is fatally wounded. After his death, his servants bury him in a tumulus in Geatland.

34 Wiseman, Nigel and Zhang Yuhuan. 2003: 6.

35 Wiseman, Nigel and Zhang Yuhuan. 2003: 16.

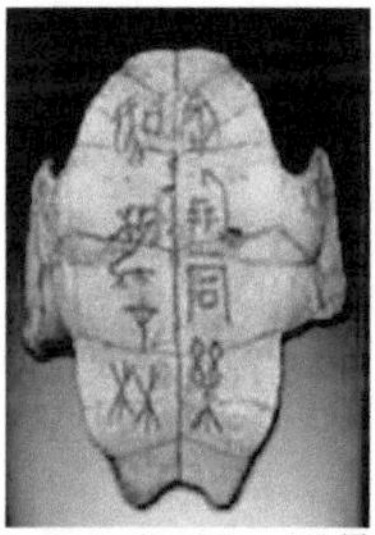

5-1. *Jia Gu Wen* 甲骨文

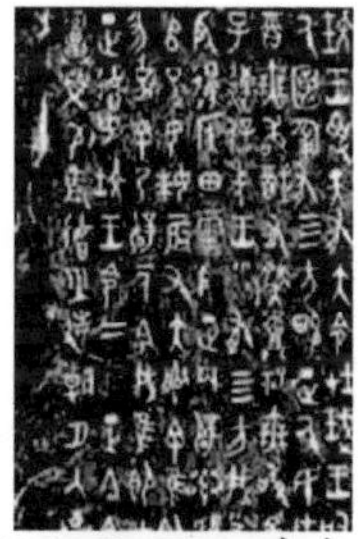

5-2. *Jin Wen* 金文

5-3. *Da Zhuan* 大篆[36]

5-4. *Xiao Zhuan* 小篆[37]

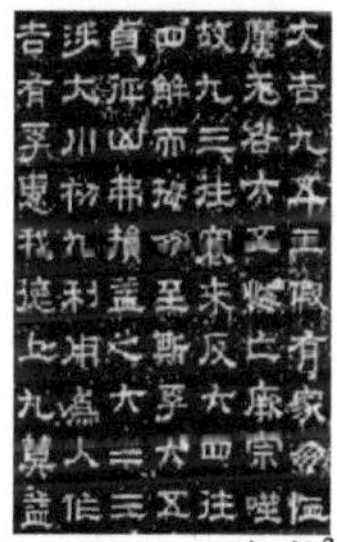

5-5. *Li Shu* 隶书[38]

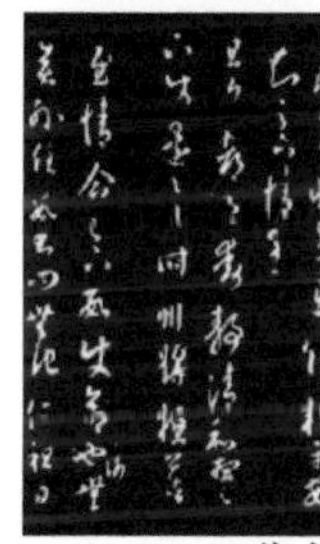

5-6. *Cao Shu* 草书[39]

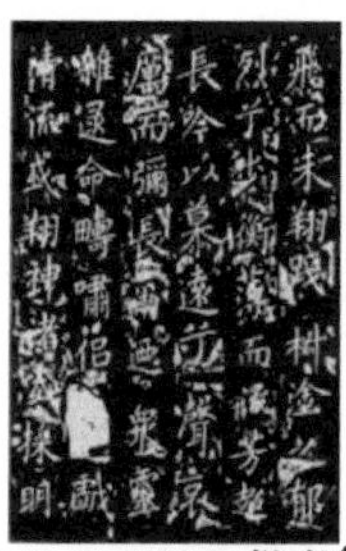

5-7. *Kai Shu* 楷书[40]

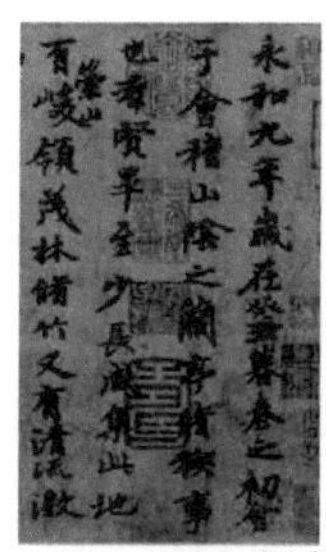

5-8 *Xing Shu* 行书[41]

Illus.5 Evolution of Chinese Writing Forms From Oracle Inscription to Running Hand

---

36 *Shi Gu Wen* 石鼓文, inscriptions on drum-shaped stone blocks of the Warring States Period (475-221B.C.).

37 *Tai Shan Shi Ke* 泰山石刻, inscriptions on a stone of Mount Tai-Shan.

38 *Xi Ping Shi Jing* 熹平石经, inscriptions of the first Official-Issued Confucian Classics on stone tablets in the 4th year of Emperor Xiping's reign (175 A.D.) of the Han Dynasty.

39 *Shi Qi Tie* 十七帖, a representative work of cursive script by a famous calligrapher, Wang Xizhi 王羲之 (303-361).

40 *Luo Shen Fu* 洛神赋, by Wang Xianzhi 王献之 (344-386), calligrapher, the 7th son of Wang Xizhi.

41 *Lan Ting Xu* 兰亭序, a representative work of running hand by Wang Xizhi 王羲之 (303-361).

The writing form keeps the old [thinking] ways. 斯文存古道。

3 Classical Chinese Thinking Ways Residing in Chinese Characters

Chinese characters reflect classical Chinese thinking ways and the way of Chinese people understanding the world.

3.1 Universe and Man Uniting and Resembling Each Other: *Tian Ren He Yi*

Classical Chinese thinking is empirical and synthetical, tends to seize the holistic feature of things based on experiences. Man is vivid and complicated, while universe is vast and boundless. How did the ancient Chinese people understand the complicated man and the vast universe? The answer is to relate man and universe to each other, guided by the idea of *Tian Ren He Yi* or Universe and Man Uniting and Resembling Each Other. Such ideas actually imply in Chinese characters.

Man is a small universe, and universe is a big man. On one hand, sinograms referring to human body's parts, behaviors and characteristics can also denote things in the nature, i.e. one relates to man, while the other relates to the nature. For example, *Shou* 首 originally means head, but also refers to the thing at the top of the handle of a weapon; *Er* 耳 originally means ear, but also refers to any ear-like thing, e.g. the ears of a tripod (鼎); *Xing* 性 originally means Man's nature, but also refers to nature, characteristics of things; *Tian* 天 originally means Man's vertex, but also refers to the sky, the heaven, the God, which reflects a subject-centered universe.

On the other hand, sinograms referring to things in the nature can also denote parts, behaviours and characteristics of man, i.e. one relates to the nature, while the other relates to man. For example, *Qi* 气 originally refers to thin, floating clouds in the nature, but later refers to the invisible basic material constituting man which can be transformed into blood, essence, and body fluid, etc., and the normal functional activities of life which is governed by "*qi*" is known as *Shen* or spirit; *Shen* 神 originally refers to lightening in the nature, but later on refers to the spirit or mind of man; *Jing* 经 originally denotes the longitudinal lines of the textiles, but later on refers to the running routes of the main stems of the meridian system of man; etc.[42]

Tian Ren He Yi leads to frequent introspection, self-examination and observation of the universe, therefore it is a kind of circular reasoning: from man to universe and from universe to man, based on the subject, reflecting the direct communication between and unification of the subject and the object. The subject is the center of the universe, is the one to understand himself and the world

42 See the related chapters for detailed interpretation.

outside him, and so is the norm to understand the myriad of beings. Well-understanding of the subject and the nature means knowing the ways, principles of all the things in the universe.

The Origin of Chinese Characters interprets man as "the most valuable being in between the heaven and the earth". *The Book of Changes* reads that "In the remote antiquity when Fu Xi 伏羲 ruled the country, he raised his head to observe images on the heaven, bowed his head to observe phenomena on the earth, observed images of birds and beasts and those of the earth, took near images from man and far images of other things from the universe, on the basis of which he then started to make the Eight Trigrams to illustrate the phenomena".

3.2 Imaging Thinking: *Xiang* 象

Chinese character is a unity of the shape and the meaning. The shape of a Chinese character is directly related to its meaning, and both integrate into a unity. The formation of a Chinese character, an organic whole of the shape and the meaning, is one-step made following the rule of the nature, reflecting the direct communication between and integration of the subject and the object. The formation also implies a vital thinking way of Chinese culture, i.e. *Xiang* 象 *or* Imaging thinking.

The Origin of Chinese Characters states that "*Xiang* 象, with long nose and teeth, a big mammal in the Southern Yue area, will be pregnant every three years", so you can see that the original meaning of "*xiang*" is elephant. In remote antiquity, the elephant had lived in the Central Plains of China. Later on, the elephant had to migrate south because of the changes in climate, so the people in the Central Plains had few opportunities to see live elephants again. Han Fei, a famous philosopher and the representative of the Legalist School of the late Warring States Period (475-221B.C.), said in the chapter of *Jie Lao Pian* of *Han Fei Tzu* 韩非子·解老篇 that "people seldom see the live elephant, but has gained the skeleton of a dead one, so they can imagine what it is like after investigating the picture or image of its skeleton. Therefore, all in people's imagination is known as '*xiang*'". This quotation also reveals the mystery of the origin of the Chinese compound "*xiang xiang*" 想象 which literally means "thinking or imagining elephant", and now means imaging or imagination, setting off "*xiang* 象"'s "imagining" cultural connotations. The Illus.6 shows how the sinogram 象 was conceived in the way of resembling the real image of an elephant.

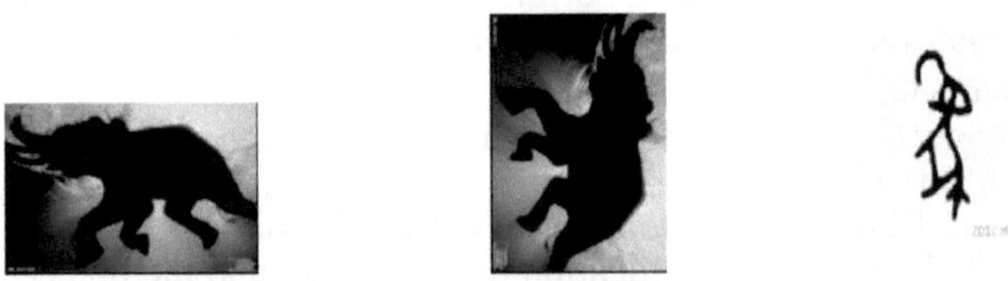

Illus. 6 A Swimming Elephant (Horizontal & Vertical) and 象 in Oracle Script[43]

43 Here is worth to note that I cannot find a skeleton of a dead elephant in a lying position. The former two photos in the Illus. 5 are just used to illustrate the conceiving process of this character 象.

The Illus. 7 shows the evolution process of the sinogram *Xiang* 象 from oracle to regular script. In the meanwhile, we can see that "*xiang*" originally evolved from "seeking similarities" between things from the angle of genetics, as stated in *The Book of Changes* "*Xiang* refers to something being like or resembling this thing". It is well known that Chinese characters are a kind of *Xiang Xing* 象形 writing, literally "resembling shape", or pictographic, ideographic, logographic writing in English. That is to say, sinograms are pictures, images, and surely suggest the imaging thinking of Chinese culture.

Illus. 7 "Xiang 象" from Oracle, Bronze, Lesser-Seal to Regular Script

Actually, it is not easy to completely and exactly express the thinking only with spoken language. *The Book of Changes* reads that "Setting up image to display its connotations to the full… interpreting words for trigram to explain its implications to the full." Wang Bi[44]'s Annotation of *The Book of Changes* states that "Getting connotations lies in forgetting the image; getting the image lies in forgetting the words".

Integration of the subject and the object is a thread running through the classical Chinese culture and science, on the basis of which *Tian Ren He Yi* constitutes the foundation of them. The imaging thinking is a classical thinking way of the Chinese culture, and whose process, methods, and rules make up *Qu Xiang Bi Lei* 取象比类 or Taking Image and Analogizing, the framework of the classical Chinese culture and science.[45]

Chinese characters are the only logographic writing which has been preserved for over 6,000 years. An oracle script still shows the image a sinogram implies. I just give you two examples: 朝 zhao, written as  in oracle script, an associative compound, depicts the image of the sun being in the grass but the moon is still visible, means sunrise, dawn, morning, daybreak; 暮 mu, written as 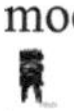 in oracle script, an associative compound, depicts the image of the sun setting into the grass, means sunset, dusk, evening.

Go drive in the early morning and the late afternoon in your countryside, think of the two images the two sinograms embody, and understand the imaging thinking!

---

44 Wang Bi 王弼 (226-249) discarded the traditional way of interpreting *The Book of Changes* such as annotating the *Xiang Shu* 象数 or Image & Numbers, but interpreted it with ideas of *Lao Tzu*, and expounded his philosophical thoughts, and thus became the founder of the metaphysical school of Wei-Jin Periods (221-420).

45 See related chapters for detailed information about *Qu Xiang Bi Lei*.

3.3 Balanced & Symmetrical Thinking: Yin-Yang 阴阳

Classical Chinese thinking is a holistic approach, stressing coupling into pairs and even numbers, e.g.,

① Inscriptions on tortoise shell are symmetrical. See Illus. 5-1.

② *Dui Zhang* 对仗 (in poetry, prose) or Antithesis refers to a matching of both sound and sense in two lines, sentences, etc. usually with the matching words in the same part of the speech. For example,

才饮长江水，Just drank the water from the Yangtzu River,
又食武昌鱼。Again ate the fish from Wuchang City.

(Mao Zedong, Swimming, June 1956)

③ *Dui Lian* 对联 or Antithetical Couplet, usually written on scrolls, refers to a pair of scrolls containing a poetic couplet. The following couplet is designed for the Spring Festival of 2010 in China, the traditional Chinese new year of 2010: 2009 is the year of ox, and 2010 is the year of tiger.

牛奔福地普天献瑞 An ox runs to the happy land & propitious signs come to the whole world

虎卧华堂满院生辉 A tiger lies in the magnificent hall & lustre radiances go to the whole courtyard

with a horizontal scroll bearing an inscription (横批, Heng Pi): 辞旧迎春 Ring out the old year and ring in the new spring.

④ The Forbidden City or the Imperial Palace in Beijing is a place you should not miss if you visit China. You will see that the palace was built in a balanced and symmetrical way with the middle line as the axis if you go to a high point and have a panorama of it. See Illus. 8.

Lǚ Shi Chun Qiu or *Lǚ's Spring and Autumn Annals* reads that "King of the ancient times selected the center of the land under the heaven to set up the country, and selected the center of the country to build his palace". The Forbidden City has been the heart of the city Beijing, and Beijing has been the center of the Country China since it was built in 1420 as the Imperial Palace for the Emperor Zhu Di 朱棣 (1360-1424) according to *The Rites of Zhou [Dynasty]* (*Zhou Li. Kao Gong Ji* 周礼．考工记), which embodies and implies the classical Chinese values and ideals of "Zhong 中 (Middle, Spine, Center, Heart), Zheng 正 (Upright, Just), An 安 (Peace, Safety, In Good Health), and He 和 (Harmony)" for each individual, each family, and the whole country.

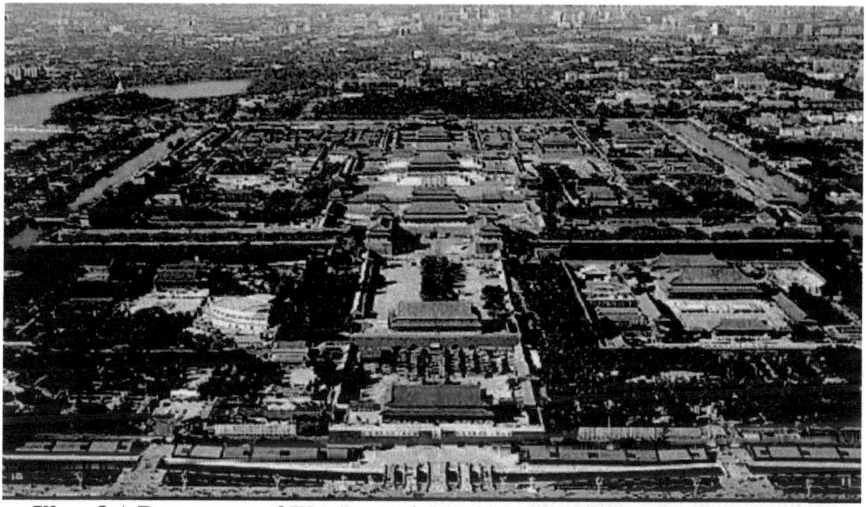

Illus. 8 A Panorama of The Imperial Palace (Forbidden City) in Beijing

Now let's go to Chinese characters, most of which are symmetrical. Most of Chinese Characters are composed of 2 parts, esp. the signific-phonetics.

Chinese characters are a kind of meaning-pronunciation signific-phonetic writing system. ... The evolution history of Chinese characters is actually the history of the development of signific-phonetics, i.e. the history of gradual increasing of the proportion and gradual gaining advantages of signific-phonetics in the whole system of sinograms.[46]

This is indeed the case. According to a statistics, the number of signific-phonetics has been growing faster and faster as time goes by:

Only about 2% of the existent oracle scripts (ca.1600-ca.1100B.C.) are signific-phonetics; *The Origin of Chinese Characters* 说文解字 (finished in 100A.D.) of the Eastern Han Dynasty includes 9,353 sinograms, among which 7, 679 are signific-phonetics, accounting for nearly 80% of the sum; *Comprehensive History. Outline of Six Categories of Chinese Graphs* 通志•六书略 (finished in 1147)[47] of the Song Dynasty includes 24,235 sinograms, among which 21,343 are signific-phonetics, accounting for nearly 88% of the sum; The *Kangxi Dictionary* 康熙字典 (finished in 1716)[48] of the Qing Dynasty includes 47,035 sinograms,

46 Liang Donghan. 1984: 54.

47 *Tong Zhi* or *Comprehensive History* 通志, a comprehensive history presented in a series of biographies, was written by Zheng Qiao 郑樵 (1104-1162), a historian and bibliographer of the Song Dynasty (960-1279).

48 *The Kangxi Dictionary* 康熙字典 was the standard Chinese dictionary during the 18th and 19th centuries. The Kangxi Emperor of the Qing Dynasty ordered its compilation in 1710. It was named after the Emperor's era name, and eventually published in 1716.

among which 42,300 are signific-phonetics, accounting for nearly 90% of the sum.[49] In the official popular simplified forms of sinograms in mainland China, the number of signific-phonetics is still the absolute overwhelming majority of the sum. Actually, the method of combining significs with phonetics has been the most productive method of creating sinograms for thousands of years.

Signific-phonetics, in fact, function to systematize sinograms according to significs, e.g.,

鱼 Fish: 鳕 Cod, 鲨 Shark, 鲈 Perch, 鳗 Eel, 鲳 Pomfret, 鲱 Herring, 鲑 Salmon, 鲔鱼 Tuna, 鲮鱼 Dace, etc., where different species of fish carry the radical "fish 鱼";

木 Tree: 樟 Camphora, 枫 Maple, 椴 Linden, etc., where different kinds of trees carry the radical "wood/tree 木";

疒 Illness: 病 Disease, 疟 Malaria, 痢 Dysentery, etc., where different kinds of illnesses carry the radical "illness 疒";

示 offering sacrifices to gods or ancestors[50]: 神 God, 社 offering sacrifice to God of Earth, etc., where sinograms related to SHEN's (God's) things usually carry the radical "示", simplified as "礻".

Balanced & symmetrical thinking is an aspect of yin-yang thinking, where yin and yang counterbalance each other.

3.4 Squared Shaped Sinograms, Four Directions, and Five Phases

The theory of five-phases in fact evolved from the five directions, which is closely related to the specific geographical and climatic conditions of ancient China: climactic extremes (hot summers, freezing winters) and relative isolation (bounded by Pacific, Himalayas, deserts) from other cultures. The ancient Chinese people did not know there are still such places on the earth as the two poles being freezing cold and the equator zones terribly hot all the year round, otherwise they would not have figured out the theory of five phases. This shows that specific geographical and climatic conditions give birth to different cultures, and different cultures give rise to different ways of understanding and cognizing the world, thus result in the formation of different sciences.[51]

---

49 Zuo Min'an. 2005:13.

50 *The Origin of Chinese Characters* interprets 示 as "The heaven hangs down images to show man good or ill luck, following 二. The three falls stand for the sun, the moon and the stars. Observing the images in the sky to detect the current changes. 示 indicates SHEN's things. All with 示 part follow such a connotation".

51 Here science refers to the science in a broad sense. Constructive Realism developed by Prof. Friedrich Wallner understands the basis of science as a process of selecting and excluding certain aspects of the analyzed object guided by theory, and considers a scientific system as an artificial constructed “microworld”, a world that selects and reduces qualities of the object in certain aspects. Therefore, the possibilties of perceiving the world are manifold, and there are many possible ways of selection and reduction, and many corresponding resolutions, and thus many scientific approaches possible.

The Illus.9 shows two sinograms 景 and 幽 in Tian & Mi 田&米 - shaped squares: from upper to lower: regular script, running hand, and cursive script. *Huai Nan Tzu* states that "The heaven is round and the earth is square". In ancient Chinese people's eyes, the concept of "five directions" was actually implied in a square for the Center is the No. 5 besides of the commonly understood four directions: East, South, West, South. Besides, a square implies an integration of time and direction (space): Spring-East, Summer-South, Autumn-West, Winter-North, Late Summer-Center.

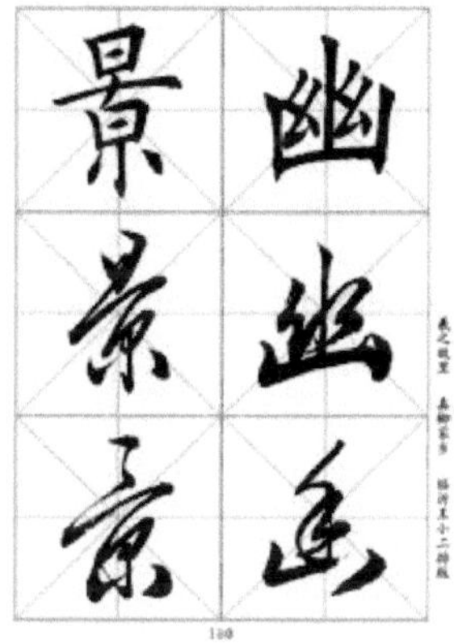

Illus. 9 Squared-Shaped Sinograms

3.5 Being Conservative: Venerating Classics and Worshiping History

Classical Chinese historical thinking is non-critical, being lack of creativity and reform, and always rethinking in the same framework established in the former times. Chinese people hold their ancestors in great veneration, and then worship the wise men and their creations in the history. Chinese medicine is also known as the arts of "Qi Huang" for Qi Bo and Huang Di, known as the Yellow Emperor in the West, have been regarded as creators of Chinese medicine; "Shen Nong, the Divine Husbandman, tasted one hundred herbs", thus became the founder of the Chinese herbal theory; *The Book of Changes* was said to be the work of three sages - "Fu Xi, Wen King of Zhou Dynasty (Zhou Wen Wang), and Confucius" through three eras, and it also records many creations by great men in the remote antiquity such as ① "Fu Xi made knotted cords and used them for nets and baskets in hunting and fishing", ② "Shen Nong split a piece of wood for a plowshare and bent a piece of wood for the plow handle, and taught the whole world the advantage of laying open the earth with a plough", "he held a market, caused the people of the earth to come together and collected the wares of the earth. They exchanged these with one another, then returned home, and each thing found its place. . ." ③ "Huang Di, Yao, and Shun allowed the upper and the lower garments to hang down, and the world was in order",[52] and so and so forth.[53] And interpreting and annotating ancient books esp. classical texts has always been one major part of scholar work up till today in China.

It is the same with Chinese characters. The history of sinograms, the sinograms themselves, and their creator in Chinese legends - Cang Jie 仓颉 have

52 Wilhelm, Baynes. 1997: 329-331.
53 Whether these records are true or not is not the point here.

been paid homage to for thousands of years in Chinese culture. The version that "Cang Jie created Chinese characters" came out already as early as the Warring States Period (475-221B.C.).

To sum up, classical Chinese thinking ways, including *Tian Ren He Yi* or Universe and Man Uniting and Resembling Each Other, imaging thinking, balanced & symmetrical thinking: yin-yang, five phases, and the thinking of venerating classics and worshiping history, all reside in the Chinese characters.

Reviewing its past you can know its present; observing its past and present you can judge its future.

- Mao Zedong[54]

4 The Prospect of Chinese Characters

Chinese characters, Egyptian hieroglyphics, Sumerian cuneiforms[55], primitive scripts of ancient Elam[56], and the scripts of Crete[57], etc. are the oldest writing forms in the world. Chinese characters, like the other oldest writing forms, underwent the period of evolution from pure pictographs to ideographs; but all of the others lost their vitality and were stopped being used during the evolution, some became phonetic writings, some were not recognizable and therefore were replaced by a foreign writing system; Chinese writing form is the only exceptional case, which has been used up till today and becomes the only logographic writing in use as opposed to phonetic writing in the world. Why did they become a memory in the history? Why do Chinese characters have so great vitality? Here I would like to answer these two questions.

4.1 Combining Signific with Phonetic: The Basic Sinogram-Creating Method

Chinese characters have become a kind of meaning-pronunciation signific-phonetic writing system since *The Origin of Chinese Characters* (Shuo Wen Jie Zi, 说文解字) came out in 100 A.D.. The 6,000 years of evolution history of Chinese characters is actually the history of the development of signific-phonetics, i.e. the history of gradual increasing of the proportion and gradual gaining advantages of signific-phonetics in the whole system of sinograms.

As we have mentioned before, the ratio of signific-phonetics in the sum total of sinograms of different times grows from about 2% in the existent oracle scripts (ca.1600- ca.1100 B.C.), to nearly 80% in the *The Origin of Chinese Characters* (说文解字, 100), to 88% in the *Comprehensive History. Outline of Six Categories of Chinese Graphs* (通志•六书略, 1147), and then to nearly 90% in the *Kangxi Dictionary* (康熙字典, 1716).

54 See Chen Jin 陈晋. Mao Zedong's Five True Remarks on Studying Histoty. Nov. 8th 2010, *Ren Min Ri Bao* or *People's Daily*.

55 Sumer (or Šumer) was the earliest known civilization of the ancient Near East, located in the lower Mesopotamia (modern Iraq) from the time of the earliest records in the mid 4th millennium B.C. until the rise of Babylonia in the late 3rd millennium B.C.. The term "Sumerian" applies to all speakers of the Sumerian language.

56 Elam was an ancient civilization located in what is now southwest Iran. Situated just to the east of Mesopotamia, Elam was part of the early urbanization during the Chalcolithic period (Copper Age). The emergence of written records from around 3000 B.C. also parallels Mesopotamian history. The Elamite language has no established affinities with any other, and seems to be a language isolate such as Sumerian.

57 Crete (Greek: Κρήτη) is the largest and most populous of the Greek islands and the fifth largest island in the Mediterranean Sea. Crete was the center of the Minoan civilization (ca. 2700–1420 B.C.), the first civilization in Europe and the first European country with a palace at Knossos.

Generally speaking, writing forms undergo such a process from pictographic to ideographic to phonetic if we review the evolution of writing forms of other cultures, esp. that of the other pictographic writing forms in the early period of civilization. I think the gradual increasing of the proportion and gradual gaining advantages of signific-phonetics in the whole system of Chinese characters is an ideal compromise in between the phonetic and the ideographic.

The signific-phonetics are easily created to meet the needs of recording the development in different aspects of the history[58], and are easily understood, learned, and memorized. Besides they function very well in systematizing the sinograms with the same signific.

4.2 Being Conservative: Venerating Classics and Worshiping History

Classical Chinese historical thinking is non-critical, being lack of creativity and reform, and always rethinking in the same framework established in the former times. Chinese people hold their ancestors in great veneration, then worship the wise men and their creations in the history, and therefore the history of sinograms, the sinograms themselves, and their creator in Chinese legends - Cang Jie 仓颉 have been paid homage to for thousands of years in Chinese culture.

Under such a cultural background, nobody dares to doubt sinograms, to criticize them, deny them, or to reform them radically from logographic to phonetic. Therefore, the development and evolution of Chinese characters just underwent a process from complicated to simplified, from pictographic (oracle script period) to signific-phonetic in the framework established at the time of *The Origin of Chinese Characters*, which came out in 100A.D..

4.3 Chinese Culture: the Most Advanced and the Leading One of All in the History of China

China has been a long-term united country in its history. The Han 汉 people has always been the absolute majority of all ethnic groups: In 1949, the Han people accounted for 99% of the whole population in China; in 2010, the percentage was 92%.[59] Chinese characters, language, and culture had always been the most advanced and the leading one of all in the history of China, even compared to Europe, until the 15th century. Even during the Liao (916-1125), Jin (1115-1234), Yuan (1271-1368), Qing (1644-1911) dynasties when the Non-Han governors dominated the country, the governors learned to write Chinese Characters, studied

58 See 1.4 Signific-Phonetics: *Xing Sheng* 形声.

59 The government of China has implemented the family planning policy since 1973, which transformed into one of the basic national policies in 1982, and has been one of the national laws since 2001. It regulates that a family of the Han people is only allowed to have one child, while a family of minority ethnic groups (one side or both sides of the couple) is allowed to have two children. This is why the percentage of the Han people has dropped so dramatically in 60 years.

Chinese language and Chinese Culture, made Chinese be an or the official language of their reigns, and ruled the country in Chinese ways.

Over one half of the basic inventions the modern world civilization relies on are from China, esp. the papermaking, gunpowder, compass, and movable type of printing. China had the lead in science and technology 1,000 years earlier than the other parts of the world until the 15th century.[60] Joseph Needham held the similar point of view. Until the 15th century, China was the leading power for technology and innovation of the world. Its economy was the world's most efficient until the end of the 18th century. Here below are some facts:

The oldest wood block-manuscript found in China is *Jin Gang Jing* 金刚经 or *Vajracchedika-sutra*, the extant earliest work printed by wood block printing method in the world and a very influential Buddhist classic in China, from Dunhuang manuscripts[61], which was printed in 868 (the 9th year of Xian Tong 咸通, Tang Dynasty).

Based on rich experiences in wood block-printing of the former times, Bi Sheng's 毕昇 (970?-1051) invented movable-type printing[62] in the years of 1041-1048, which is 400 years before Gutenberg[63] (1400-1468).

China had mastered the skill of smelting iron at latest in the 6th century B.C., including iron founding and iron smelting. Around the year 1000 China produced 114,000 tons of raw-iron, an amount that England did not produce until the end of the 18th century.

Long before Europe, the Chinese used waterpower for irrigation and to move textile-machines.

---

60 Translated from Chinese. The original reference would be *The Genius of China: 3,000 Years of Science, Discovery and Invention* by Robert Temple.

61 The Dunhuang manuscripts were discovered by the Taoist monk Wang Yuanlu 王圆箓 (1850?~1931) in the Mogao Caves of Dunhuang, China in the early 20th century. Dating from the 5th to early 11th centuries, the manuscripts include works ranging from history, mathematics, medicine, Buddhism, Taoism, Nestorianism, and even Judaism to folk songs and dance. They are written primarily in Chinese, but also include Tibetan, Pali, Sogdian, and previously unknown languages, such as Khotanese. The documents were later sold to Western explorers by Wang Yuanlu, notably Aurel Stein 斯坦因 (1862-1943) and Paul Pelliot 伯希和 (1878-1945). Russian and Japanese explorers also acquired some. But largely due to Luo Zhenyu's 罗振玉 (1866-1944) efforts, the remaining manuscripts were preserved in China. Those purchased by Western scholars are now kept in institutions all over the world, such as the National Library of China, British Library, and the Bibliothèque nationale de France. They are all being digitized by the International Dunhuang Project, and can be accessed free online.

62 The specific procedures and methods of Bi Sheng's 毕昇 movable-type printing are recorded in details in *Dream Pool Essays* (*Meng Xi Bi Tan,* 梦溪笔谈) by Shen Kuo 沈括 (1031-1095), a polymathic scientist in China, of his same time.

63 Johannes Gensfleisch zur Laden zum Gutenberg (1398-1468) was a German goldsmith, printer and publisher who introduced modern book printing. His invention of mechanical movable-type printing started the Printing Revolution and is widely regarded as the most important event of the modern period. It played a key role in the development of the Renaissance, the Reformation and the Scientific Revolution and laid the material basis for the modern knowledge-based economy and the spread of learning to the masses. Gutenberg was regarded as the first European to use movable-type printing, in around 1439, and the global inventor of the printing press. But actually, compared to the invention of Chinese movable-type printing, he is much later.

In ancient China, the sluice gate, the canal lock, and flash lock had been known since at least the 1st century B.C. (as sources then alluded that they were not new innovations), during the ancient Han Dynasty (202 B.C.–220 A.D.). In the year 984 the engineer Qiao Weiyue developed the tide lock for ships, and thus improved the trade-system which already was highly developed, on 50,000 kilometers canal the Song dynasty transported tea, noble metals, textiles, porcelain, salt, sugar, bricks, even ivory, sulfur, mercury, paper and loads of grain. *Song Shi* or *The History of the Song Dynasty* 宋史 (compiled in 1345) stated that in 984.

In 1024 the first banknote which was printed in three colors, 600 years before paper-money first turned up in Europe.[64]

...

Chinese science and culture had been so advanced in the world, so it is unnecessary for Chinese people to consider to radically change the sinograms and the language. It is also clear and true that nobody will disseminate its language if the culture lags so much behind the others.

4.4 No Access to Other Better Choices

Actually, Chinese culture is a kind of inclusive culture, which can be seen from the intercultural activities happened in the history of China, esp. transmission of Buddhism and Christian & Catholic religions in China. One reason that the writing form of Chinese language remains to be logographic is there is no access to other better choices. China had been long-term isolated by seas on its east and the Himalayas in its west from the outside world, the other advanced languages, and the other advanced cultures for thousands of years until the Opium Wars in 19th century[65] when they broke the door of China with their hard warships, powerful artilleries and big guns, the ancient Chinese people did not know there is still phonetic writing or other better choices available in the world.

While the people of ancient Greece had to always travel from islands to islands to make a living by prosperous trading, thus frequently met different cultures, customs, and languages, and then they had got chances to take a better choice. But all in all, the classical Chinese thinking, together with Chinese culture and China's specific natural, geographical and social conditions, decides the writing form of Chinese characters being logographic.

64 The first proper European banknotes were issued by Stockholms Banco, a predecessor of the Bank of Sweden, in 1660, although the bank ran out of coins to redeem its notes in 1664 and ceased operating in that year.

65 The 1st: was waged in the years of 1840-1842 by the United Kingdom; the 2nd: in the years of 1856-1860 by the United Kingdom and France, supported by Russia and the United States of America.

4.5 Understanding Chinese Characters: A Historical Outline

The fact is that Chinese characters have the longest life span and the most users in the world since its emergence about 6,000 years ago. Actually, the long course of the development of sinograms can be classified into three stages: worship, negation, and reconsideration.

The worship stage started since the sinograms had been preliminary systematic. The sinograms were considered mysterious and dignified, thus had been the object the people adored in the feudal times until the 20th century. For example, Cang Jie 仓颉 was said to be the creator of Chinese characters in Chinese legends. He was said to be an official historian of the Huang Di's (the Yellow Emperor) reign, or a king of the remote antiquity. It is said that he had four eyes on his head, could communicate with gods, and created sinograms by integrating beauties he collected widely from myriad of things. *Huai Nan Tzu* 淮南子 states that "In the former times whenever Cang Jie was writing, millets would fall down from the heaven and ghost would cry in the night". In ancient China, the right of standardizing sinograms was attributed to Kings or Emperors. Zi Si 子思 (481?-402B.C.), the only grandson of Confucius, said that "Only the sons of Heaven (Kings or Emperors) have the right to discuss rites, make rules and regulations, and standardize written sinograms"[66], which has somehow born important significance. For example, Qin Shi Huang (259-210 B.C.), the First Emperor of Qin Dynasty, uniformed written sinograms after he unified the country by adopting Li Si's advice of simplifying Larger Seal Scripts to Lesser Seal Scripts. Xu Shen 许慎 (58?-147?) said that "Written sinograms are the foundation of classical books and the start of emperor's decrees. The ancestors use them to hand down what they knew to later generations, while the descendants use them to understand their ancestors". Dai Zhen 戴震(1724 - 1777)[67] held that "sinograms are the access to gain the language, and the language is the way to understand wills of the ancient sages and men of virtue".

Along with the decline of the feudal dynasties, invasions of China by foreign armies, dissemination of Western culture and science in China, and rise of comparative studies on differences between Chinese Culture and Western culture at the end of Qing Dynasty (1644-1911), the mystery and dignity of Chinese characters did not exist any more, and the negation stage started since then. Some scholars doubted whether Chinese characters promoted or blocked the development of Chinese culture and science. Chinese characters were just like

---

66 These are the words Zi Si quoted his grandfather's, while Zhu Xi 朱熹 (1130-1200), the founder of the Neo-Confucianism, believed that these were originally from Zi Si. Zi Si supposedly wrote *The Doctrine of Mean* 中庸.

67 Dai Zhen 戴震 (1724-1777), a notable versatile Chinese scholar of the Qing Dynasty, made great contributions to mathematics, geography, phonology and philosophy. His philosophical and philological critiques of Neo-Confucianism continue to be influential.

women with small bound feet and men with long plaits, becoming a symbol of China falling behind others in culture, science, and national power. Hegal (1770-1831) held such a point of view that Chinese characters were not complete and perfect, and were a big blockage for development of science.[68] According to the statistics of a book entitled *Introduction to Reforms of Chinese Characters* (1961) by Zhou Youguang 周有光 (1906-)[69], there were as much as 28 plans on how to reform Chinese characters put forward by individual persons in the last 20 years of Qing Dynasty. You can see the right of reformulating Chinese characters already moved to the common people. All the Chinese people at that time, no matter whom he was - reformer, democrat, or communist, held the similar idea that reform of Chinese characters was a way to make the country stronger.

Lu Ganzhang 卢戆章 (1854-1928) read the *Bible* and started to learn Western scientific knowledge, and then signed with feeling that "Prosperous and powerful countries are all established on natural science, while how much advanced of the level of natural science is all based on how much the common people are fond of learning and understand the knowledge. Why is it so easy for their people to be fond of learning and understand the knowledge? Because their languages are a kind of phonetic writing. ... Nowadays, most of the languages of the world except China are composed of 20 to 30 alphabets", and that "Chinese characters may be the most difficult one in the world".

Tan Sitong 谭嗣同 (1865-1898)[70] advocated to change Chinese characters from logographic to phonetic writing in order to "integrate all kinds of the local knowledge on the earth into one".

Qian Xuantong 钱玄同 (1887-1939), a Chinese linguist and a thinker, advocated to abolish Chinese characters. He listed "crimes" of Chinese characters in his *Revolution of Chinese Characters* (1923) that "I dare to declare that education can not be popularized, national language can not be unified, the literature can not be fully developed, the common public new truths, new learning, and new knowledge of the whole world can never be conveniently and freely

---

68 Georg Wilhelm Friedrich Hegel (1770-1831), a German philosopher, one of the creators of German Idealism. The viewpoint here is originally from Chinese translation of his work "Philosophy of History".

69 Zhou Youguang 周有光 (1906-), a Chinese linguist and philologist who is often credited as the "father of Hanyu Pinyin", the official romanization for Mandarin Chinese issued in 1958 in the People's Republic of China. Zhou enrolled in Saint John's University in Shanghai in 1923, where he majored in economics and took supplementary coursework in linguistics. He is proficient in four languages: Chinese, English, French, and Japanese. He was mainly engaged in economic and financial work in his first half life time, and had been a professor in economics. He turned to linguistic and philological studies and has devoted himself to it since 1955. After 1980, Zhou worked with Liu Zunqi and Chen Weizang on translating a Chinese edition of Encyclopedia Britannica, earning him the nickname "Encyclopedia Zhou". Zhou has continued writing and publishing since the creation of Pinyin; for example, in 2003 he published the book entitled *The Historical Evolution of Chinese Language and Script.*

70 Tan Sitong 谭嗣同 (1865-1898), an eminent Chinese revolutionist in the late Qing Dynasty who was in support of liberal reform, was executed in public on September 28, 1898, along with five others. They were dubbed the "Six gentlemen of the Hundred Days' Reform" 戊戌六君子.

written out in the national language if Chinese characters are not revolutionized. What is the reason? Because Chinese characters are difficult to know, to memorize, and to write; because the dead Chinese characters are not adequate enough to express the vivid national language; because Chinese characters are not an efficient instrument to show their pronunciations; because the difficulties created by Chinese characters, the original texts of the new learning and new truths are difficult to import into the national language", and that "The worst is that Chinese characters do not fit into the modern culture of the world". He still said that "If you do not want China to perish, wish Chinese nation become a nation with civilization of the 20th century, the root solution is to terminate Confucianist and Taoist studies; and to abolish the Chinese characters, which record Confucianist teachings and Taoist heresies, will be the root solution of the root".[71]

Lu Xun 鲁迅 (1881-1936)[72] also advocated to Latinize Chinese characters for he thought "The square-shaped Chinese characters are really a good tool to fool the common people. It is not possible not only for the toiling mass to learn and master the characters, but even for the privileged with money and right, there are still quite a lot among them who can not master the characters even after ten or twenty years of learning. ... Chinese characters are just like tuberculosis in the body of the Chinese labouring people, bacteria are latent inside. The only outcome is to die if the bacteria are not eliminated from the body".[73]

The scholars who denied Chinese characters took the absolute overwhelming predominance during this stage. Zhang Taiyan 章太炎, also known as Zhang Binglin 章炳麟 (1868- 1936)[74], was brave enough to publish an essay entitled "*Refutation Against the Proposal 'China Adopting World Language As Its New Language*'", where he said whether a culture is advanced or not bears no positive relationship with whether its writing is phonetic or not, and believed that the logographic writing of Chinese characters is decided by the feature that each sinogram has only one syllable. His points of view are still right even up till today. Whether Chinese characters are Romanized or not should be an academic

---

71 From the article entitled "Problems of Chinese Characters in China in the Future", published in La Jeunesse (The New Youth Magazine) , No.4 of the Vol.4 in 1918.

72 Lu Xun 鲁迅 (1881-1936) is one of the major Chinese writers of the 20th century. Considered to be the founder of modern Chinese literature, he wrote in the vernacular (baihua, 白話) as well as classical Chinese. Lu Xun's works became known to English readers through numerous translations, beginning in 1960 with *Selected Stories of Lu Hsun* translated by Yang Hsien-yi and Gladys Yang, and more recently in 2009 when Penguin Classics published a complete anthology of his fiction entitled *The Real Story of Ah-Q and Other Tales of China: The Complete Fiction of Lu Xun*, of which Jeffrey Wasserstrom said "could be considered the most significant Penguin Classic ever published."

73 From his essay "On New Scripts" in 1934.

74 Zhang Taiyan 章太炎 (1868- 1936) was a Chinese philologist, textual critic and anti-Manchu revolutionary. His philological works include *Wen Shi* 文始 or "The Origin of Writing", the first systematic work on Chinese etymology.

question, not a political question nor a debate between the old and the new.

What will happen if Chinese characters are Romanized? An American Chinese linguist Chao Yuen Ren 赵元任 (1892-1982)[75] had written a story in classical Chinese with restrictions on pronunciation in 1930, which is composed of 92 sinograms, and all of which are pronounced as "shi" in Mandarin Chinese. In fact, classical Chinese is a kind of written language and is very different from spoken Chinese.[76] It makes sense if you read the original Chinese text, but it will be really ridiculous if the Chinese characters of the original text are Romanized. Here is the original text:

《施氏食狮史》
石室诗士施氏，嗜狮，誓食十狮。
施氏时时适市视狮。
十时，适十狮适市。
是时，适施氏适市。
氏视是十狮，恃矢势，使是十狮逝世。
氏拾是十狮尸，适石室。
石室湿，氏使侍拭石室。
石室拭，氏始食是十狮尸。
食时，始识是十狮尸，实十石狮尸。
试释是事。

Here below is the Romanized text (the number "十 shí" is written as Arabic "10"):

Shī Shì shí shī shǐ:
Shí shì shīshì Shī Shì, shì shī, shì shí 10 shī.
Shì shí shí shì shì shì shī.
10 shí, shì 10 shī shì shì.
Shì shí, shì Shī Shì shì shì.
Shì shì shì 10 shī, shì shì shì, shī shì 10 shī shì shì.
Shì shí shì 10 shī shī, shì shí shì.
Shíshì shī, Shì shǐ shì shì shí shì.
Shí shì shì, Shì shí shì shí shì 10 shī.
Shí shí, shǐ shì shì 10 shī, shí 10 shī shī.
Shì shì shì shì.

Here below is the meaning in English:

---

75 Chao Yuen Ren 赵元任 (1892- 1982), Zhao Yuanren in Pinyin, was a Chinese American linguist and amateur composer. He made important contributions to the modern study of Chinese phonology and grammar.
76 Different words that have the same sound when spoken aloud will have different written forms, comparable to *deer* and *dear* in English. This story also implies another fact that there are more synonyms in classical Chinese than in the vernacular.

Lion-Eating Poet in the Stone Den

In a stone den was a poet called *Shi*, who was a lion addict, and had resolved to eat ten.

He often went to the market to look for lions.

At ten o'clock, ten lions had just arrived at the market.

At that time, Shi had just arrived at the market.

He saw those ten lions, and using his trusty arrows, caused the ten lions to die.

He brought the corpses of the ten lions to the stone den.

The stone den was damp. He asked his servants to wipe it.

After the stone den was wiped, he tried to eat those ten lions.

When he ate, he realized that these ten lions were in fact ten stone lion corpses.

Try to explain this matter.

Here below is a translation with all significant words starting with "s/c" by Nicolas M. Williams, who tried to keep both the specific feature in its form and the meaning of the story:

Songster Smith of the stone cell, savoring swine, swore to sup on seven swine.

Sometimes Smith, striding to the city, saw some swine.

At seven, seven swine scampered to the city.

Smith serendipitously saw the seven swine, so Smith sent spears to slay the seven swine.

Smith snatched the seven swine stiffs, and sped to Smith's stone cell.

Smith's stone cell seemingly slippery, Smith suggested servants sweep the stone cell.

The stone cell swept, Smith set to swallowing the seven swine.

Straightaway Smith saw, sadly, the seven swine stiffs were simply seven stone swine stiffs.

Seek to solve such a story![77]

The negation stage of Chinese characters was also a crucial time for China. Many scholars put the blame of Opium wars, the country being ignorant and backward, etc. on Chinese characters and Chinese culture. They ignored the fact that China had been the leading country in culture, science and civilization for so long time in the world in the history. For example, Chang'an, the national capital of the Tang Dynasty (618-907), had been one of the most prosperous cultural, economic and financial centers in the world at that time. At that time, many foreigners came to China from different parts of the world to learn Chinese culture, to disseminate their own, and to be engaged in cultural and diplomatic exchanges,

77 Williams, Nicholas M. Translation of Homonyms [J]. Chinese Translators Journal, 2011, 32 (2): 90-92.

and to do business, etc.; meanwhile the government also sent many envoys to other countries to learn from others and to be engaged in culture and diplomatic exchanges as well.

Then, following the Revolution in 1911, the Chinese Bourgeois Democratic Revolution led by Dr. Sun Yat-Sen 孙中山 (1866-1925) which overthrew the Qing Dynasty, and the New Culture Movement around the time of the May 4th in 1919, the Anti-Japanese War (1937-1945) and the civil war between the Communist Party and Kuomingtang (1945-1949) broke out one after the other. Until 1952, the Government Administration Council of P. R. China set up a Committee for Study and Reform of Chinese Characters, where "Pinyin Scheme Group" drafted several schemes as the phonetic system of Chinese characters in the following several years. "The Chinese Phonetic System" (Hanyu Pinyin Fangan, 汉语拼音方案) was officially released in 1958, and it was acknowledged as the international standard of phonetic Chinese by International Organization for Standardization (IOS) in 1982. Studies on coding, processing, and inputting Chinese characters into computers started in the 1970s, which has been gradually becoming more and more mature and convenient esp. since the 1990s. As regards to Chinese characters, it is a new stage, which I would like to name as the third stage, the revival stage.

How long still will Chinese characters last? A proverb reads that "reviewing the past to know the future". The two well-known facts are that the number of the people who speak Chinese language and write Chinese characters has been the most in the world for centuries; and that the effort to establish a world language – Esperanto since 1887, which is based on the common word roots of European languages and has simple grammars, seems to be a failure. I think Chinese characters will live as long as the Chinese culture.

Alphabets and linguistic rules, two essential steps to form phonetic writing, are the parents of various tools and logic, the foundation of Western science.

- The Author

5 Western Scientific Thinking Ways Implied in Phonetic Writing[78]

Phonetic writing, as opposed to logographic writing, is the most common writing in the world. English, German, French, Spanish, Portuguese, etc. are all phonetic writings, but are different languages composed by the same Latin alphabets. Let's take English as the case in point.

The shape of an English word is directly related to its pronunciation, but has nothing to do with the meaning or the external image of the concrete thing it denotes. That is to say, in phonetic writing, the shape is separate and independent from the meaning, and the meaning comes from man-made prescript outside the shape, which indicates that the formation of a word of the phonetic writing is composed of two steps: first, building its shape, i.e. spelling of alphabets; second, defining its meaning according to linguistic rules or grammar. The understanding of the meaning(s) of a word is based on the sense of hearing, thus jumping out the thinking frame of the visual sense of the concrete image of a thing, then providing a bigger possibility for logic thinking based on the abstraction, finally forming thinking traditions of abstract inference, conceptual thinking, categorization, and trying to make an objective judgment about the world.

This is really indeed the case. The formation of phonetic writing reflects its two important characteristics: tool - alphabets, and abstraction - linguistic rules. Every tool is made to have a certain function according to human beings' specific aim or intention, thus becoming a medium of connection between human beings and the nature, and so interrupting the natural direct communication between them. Tool plays a vital role in the Western culture, esp. in the Western natural science, where it is standardized and systematized, and the experimental research approach characterized by the use of various tools is set up. Actually, the alphabets are the mother of various tools. The thinking way corresponding to the experimental research approach is abstraction. The rule of abstraction is logic, while linguistic rules or grammar are an embryonic form of logic.[79]

The emergence of tool reflects the relationship between the subject and the object, i.e., the separation and opposition of them - man remakes the nature. The abstraction pays more attention to being analytical, logical, and restricts imagination. The tool and abstraction become the foundation of the Western culture and science and of the natural science (including the Western medicine) in

78 Lan Fengli. Globalization of Chinese Medicine: Cultural Differences of Chinese Medicine and Western Medicine. In Wallner Friedrich G., Lan Fengli, Jandl Martin J. (eds). 2010: 24-44.

79 Wang Zhenhua. Theoretical Difference between TCM and Western Medicine on the Basis of Linguistics: Modernization of TCM. China Journal of Traditional Chinese Medicine. 2001: 16 (6): 5.

particular. The Western natural science manifests in two opposite ways or two edges, which have been realized by more and more people as time goes by. The two edges lie in that environmental pollution and ecological imbalance, the repay of the nature to the human beings, always accompany the process of human conquering and remaking the nature. As regards to the Western medicine, the two edges lie in that severe side effects, drug resistance, and effect being temporary always accompany the notable therapeutic effects.

To sum up, logographic writing and phonetic writing represent correlative thinking of Eastern tradition and causal thinking of Western tradition respectively, which together make a complete world like Yin and Yang: they depend on and complement to each other, to some extent oppose to each other. In a globalized world and in a time of globalization, they communicate each other by intercultural activities such as translation and intercultural philosophy. They together make the common world more colorful with their particular features.

The chapters 4 and 5 show that classical Chinese thinking ways and Western thinking ways reside respectively in logographic writing and phonetic Writing. There are no ranking but different cultures in this world. I would like to end this part with a quotation from *The Analects of Confucius* that "The men with honor aim at harmony but not at uniformity; while the mean men aim at uniformity but not at harmony". *He* 和 or Harmony in Chinese culture suggests both different and harmonious at the same time.

In the remote antiquity when Fu Xi 伏羲 ruled the country, he raised his head to observe images on the heaven, bowed his head to observe phenomena on the earth, observed images of birds and beasts and those of the earth, took near images from man and far images of other things from the universe, on the basis of which he then started to make the Eight Trigrams to illustrate the phenomena. Until Shen Nong's 神农 time, tying knots was used to keep records of things; And then things became complicated and numerous, and cheating things started to happen. [Until Huang Di's time,] the historian official Cang Jie 仓颉 created sinograms enlightened by differentiable footprints of birds and beasts.

- Xu Shen[80]

6 *Tian Ren He Yi*: The World View of Chinese Culture

How the universe is created? How the man is created? Why does the man come to this world? Mythology, philosophy and science have always been trying to answer the above questions. Actually, mythology, philosophy and science of a particular culture share common cultural presuppositions.

The source of civilization is hidden in the Chaos[81]. … In order to reveal the source, people not only need to carefully study the unearthed teeth, skulls, and pieces of porcelain, but also need to seek clues from myths and legends of the remote antiquity. Myths are the soul of a nationality. If a nationality does not have myths, its history is just like to originate from a puppet without thinking. It is because of moving myths that it is possible for us to track down our ancestors' footmarks to see their behaviors and their ways of thinking.[82]

6.1 Pan Gu 盘古, the Creator of the Universe in Chinese Mythology

Pan Gu first appeared in Xu Zheng's *San Wu Li Ji* 三五历纪 and *Wu Yun Li Nian Ji* 五运历年纪, both of which are lost. But the related contents are preserved in later works such as *Tai Ping Yu Lan* 太平御览(977-983) and *Yi Shi* 绎史.[83]

Pan 盘, a signific-phonetic, is a household utensil, and its shape is usually round.[84] In ancients' eyes, the heaven was also round, as recorded by Xu Zheng 徐整 of the Three-Kingdom Period (220-280) that "The chaotic universe is just like an egg"[85]. Pan 盘 follows 般, written as  in oracle script and in lesser seal script, which indicates both meaning and pronunciation, and means

80 See the *Preface* of *The Origin of Chinese Characters* by Xu Shen 许慎 (?58-147?A.D.).

81 Chaos refers to the primeval state of the universe according to folklore.

82 Xiao Jiansheng. 2009: 13.

83 The author is Ma Xiao 马骕 (1621-1673) of the early Qing Dynasty. *Yi Shi* 绎史 has altogether 160 volumes, and 5 sections, namely Remote Antiquity, Three Eras, Spring-Autumn Period, Warring States Period, and External Records.

84 He Jiuying, Hu Shuangbao, Zhang Meng. 1995: 195-196.

85 See *Tai Ping Yu Lan* 太平御览 (977-983), which quotes *San Wu Li Ji* 三五历纪.

"rotate", as stated in *The Origin of Chinese Characters* "Resembling the image of rotating a boat. Following 舟 boat and 殳. 殳 means to make it rotate." Gu 古 means ancient, remote antiquity, which was formerly hu 瓠, the bottle gourd.

Pan Gu is not a historical figure but a god created by ancient Chinese people for "Pan Gu grew 1 Zhang (about 3.3 meters) per day as the heaven ascended 1 Zhang per day and the earth thickened 1 Zhang per day for 18,000 years" (*San Wu Li Ji,* 三五历纪). And how did Pan Gu separate the heaven and the earth? He separated the heaven and the earth by rotating the chaotic qi into lucid yang and turbid yin, which is just like the *Tai Ji* Diagram (or the Yin-Yang Diagram). That was the beginning of the world. Then he died, and all parts of his dead body transformed into various beings in the universe, such as "his breathing into wind & cloud, his voice into thunders, the left eye into the Sun, the right eye into the moon, his head, feet, upper limbs and trunk into the Five Mountains, the blood in the vessels into water in the rivers, the tendons into roads, his flesh into soil, his hair of the head into stars, the body hair into grasses and trees, his bones and teeth into metals in the soil, his essence and marrow into pearls and jades, his sweat into rain, and his spirit into birds, beasts, fishes, and insects, etc" according to the records in *San Wu Li Ji* 三五历纪.

Two important ideas can be inferred although there are some contradictory parts about this myth:

① *Tian Ren He Yi* or Universe and Man Uniting and Resembling Each Other: Heaven, Earth and Man (Pan Gu, God[86]) constitute with the same ingredient - *Qi* in the same way, thus uniting and resembling each other, abbreviated as "*Tian Ren He Yi* or Universe and Man Uniting and Resembling Each Other", the world view of Chinese culture;

② *Qu Xiang Bi Lei* or Taking Image and Analogizing, a vital methodology of Chinese culture and science.

6.2 Some Important Concepts: One, Heaven, Man, Earth, and Three[87]

6.2.1 One (一 and 壹): The Origin of All Things

"One (*yi* 一) is the original great beginning. Tao is based on one (*yi* 一), and then is to separate the heaven from the earth and to create all the things".

- *The Origin of Chinese Characters*

"The movements under the heaven start from one (*yi* 一)."

- *The Book of Changes*

86 God or Shen is the metaphor of creating. See Lan Fengli. Understanding SHEN in Classical Chinese Texts. In Lan Fengli, Wallner Friedrich G., Wobovnik Claudia. 2011: 11-27 .

87 Lan Fengli. Influence of *Huang Di's Inner Classic* on *The Origin of Chinese Characters* [J]. Chinese Journal of Medical History. 2006, 36(4): 201-205.

"At the great beginning there was Non-being, [but] no Being nor Name. That was where one (*yi* 一) started, but still no physical appearance."

- *Chuang Tzu. Chapter of Heaven and Earth*

"Where do the rules start to be established? They start to be established at the great oneness. The great oneness is the root of all the beings and the bottom of all the phenomena."

- *Arts of Painting. The Great Oneness of Visual Arts*[88]

One is far beyond the number one. In philosophers' eyes, one is the origin of all the things. *The Origin of Chinese Characters* starts from "*yi* 一", ends with "*hai* 亥", the last of the twelve earthly branches. The interpretation of "*yi* 一" in *The Origin of Chinese Characters* completely carries on the concepts in the myth of creating the world, thus conceiving the system of the concepts of the genesis of the universe in Chinese philosophy. "*Yi* 一" is far beyond the number one, and is the opposite of the multiple as the myriad of things in the universe, and is the exact mysterious being or state before the beginning of the world.[89]

In Chinese, both 一 and 壹 means one. Actually, 壹 is derived from 一. Yi 壹, written as  in lesser seal script, resembles the image of a pot with a lid. *The Origin of Chinese Characters* interprets it as "undivided. Following 壶 (Pot)". *The Book of Songs · July* reads that "To pick up bottle gourds in August"八月断壶, where Mao's interpretation reads that "*Hu* 壶 refers to the bottle gourd". The bottle gourd stands for the creation myth of the world: the upper became the heaven and the lower became the earth. See the Illus. 10.

In Chinese legends, the bottle gourd had functioned as a vessel to save people from flooding like Noah's ark. There are unearthed bottle gourds and bottle gourd-shaped potteries from some early ruins of 7,000 years ago in China. You see, in ancient Chinese people's eyes, the bottle gourd was a symbol for uterus, and so for the female as well. The bottle gourd can be divided into two, which has been an essential utensil for a family, functioning as a spoon or a container. It has long been an original mascot for Chinese people, a symbol of good fortune, happiness, and official salary.

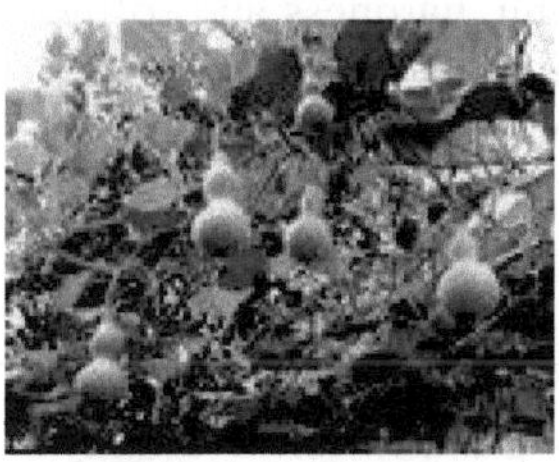

Illus. 10 The Bottle Gourd

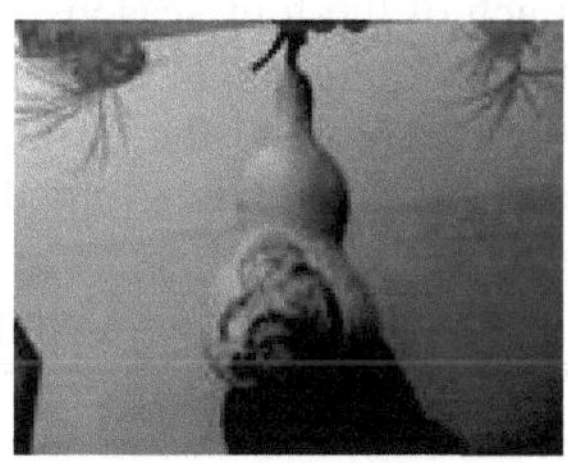

88 The author is Shi Tao 石涛 (1630-1724), a great artist in Chinese painting. As Kaptchuk said that "The arts in China were nourished by the same naturalist and Taoist sensibility that fed Chinese philosophy and medicine". See Kaptchuk, Ted J. 2000: 17.
89 Ye Shuxian, Tian Daxian. 1998:3.

Giradort, Norman J., an American sinologist, believed that the bottle gourd was the sub-type of cosmological egg. He said that Bottle gourd and egg, chaos and nothing, hermaphroditic giant, and incestuous primordial couple can all be understood as the mythological symbol of "the fullness of being", which stresses the primordial unity of the sexes.[90]

The Fu Xi & Nü Wa Coupling Figure has many different versions, from stone figures of the Han Dynasty (206B.C.-220A.D.) to paintings on silk, or paper of later dynasties, esp. until the Northern Dynasties (386-581). Paintings on silk or paper tend to be easily destroyed and decomposed, so are difficult to be found. But a large number of them are available in Turpan[91], Xinjiang. The Illus. 11 is one of those paintings. Fu Xi and Nü Wa in this painting have high noses and deep eyes, just like persons of mixed blood. Wen Yiduo 闻一多 (1899-1946), a Chinese poet and scholar, did a textual research on Fu Xi. He believed that Fu Xi and Nü Wa, two names but one person, were personified bottle gourds, among which the only difference was the gender.[92]

Pan Gu separated the heaven from the earth. "The chaotic universe is just like an egg". And one was the chaotic universe and the egg as well. *The Book of Changes* reads that "Therefore there is in the Changes the Great Primal Beginning. This generates the two primary forces (Yin and Yang). The two primary forces generate the four images (the four seasons). The four images generate the eight trigrams". Here in this quotation one is the *Tai Ji*, the Great Primal Beginning.

Actually, Tao and One can be mutually interpretive. In fact, Tao bears two qualities, i.e., nothing and being. Nothing means without shape or image, i.e., the chaotic universe; Being means with shape and image, i.e. the one. So *Lao Tzu* reads that "Tao gives birth to one", which means that which has physical appearance is generated by that which has no physical appearance.

Qian Zuo Du of *The Book of Changes* 易.乾凿度 reads that "Confucius states that 'Changes start from *Tai Ji*. *Tai Ji* gives birth to two, i.e. yin and yang, so to generate the heaven and the earth. In between the heaven and the earth there are the seasons of Spring, Summer, Autumn, and Winter, i.e. the four seasons. Each of the four seasons has the qualities of yin and yang, hardness and softness; therefore, the eight trigrams are generated. The eight trigrams establish the Tao of the Heaven and the Earth, so the images of thunder, wind, water, fire, mountain and swamp are determined'".

---

90 Translated from Chinese. See the original reference *Myth and Meaning in Early Taoism*. Berkeley and Los Angeles: University of California Press, 1983.

91 Turpan has long been the centre of a fertile oasis and an important trade centre. It was historically located along the Silk Road's northern route, thus being international and intercultural. It was originally one kingdom called Gushi 故師 which the Chinese conquered in 107 B.C.. During the Han era the city changed hands several times between the Xiongnu and the Han, interspersed with short periods of independence.

92 See the first volume of *The Complete Works of Wen Yiduo*.

This figure shows the image of the earliest ancestors in Chinese mythology. In this figure, Nü Wa holds a pair of compasses, which a witch in the remote antiquity used to study celestial phenomena and to communicate the heaven with the earth. Fu Xi holds a carpenter's square, which was used to measure the land. The compasses and the square also imply that the heaven was round-shaped and the earth squared-shaped. They hug each other face to face and with their snake-shaped tails twining together. There is a sun above their heads and a moon below their tails. There are many stars and constellations around them.

It is amazing that the shape of their twining tails is the same as that of DNA with double helix, which contains the genetic instructions used in the development and functioning of all known living organisms.

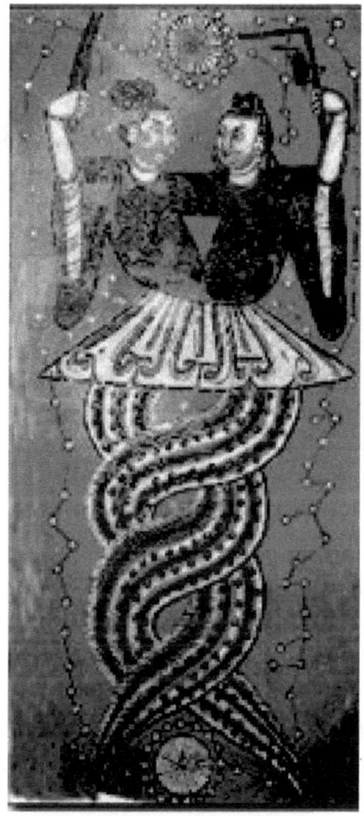

Illus. 11 Fu Xi & Nü Wa Coupling Figure Unearthed in Xinjiang

To sum up, "*yi* 一" is the first beginning of the numbers; "*yi* 壹" represents the image of the bottle gourd, means "undivided". One is far beyond the number one. Philosophers' interpretation of One is the origin of all things. All in all, One is *Tai Ji* or the Great Primal Beginning, the foundation of Tao, and the mystical state before the Genesis of the world.

The Origin of Chinese Characters starts with "*yi* 一" and ends with "*hai* 亥" for "*yi* 一" refers to *Tai Ji* or the Great Primal Beginning, the foundation of Tao, and the mystical state before the Genesis of the world; while "*hai* 亥" is interpreted as "the image of a pregnant woman, delivering a baby, then starting again from *yi* 一", then transforming again into everything in the universe. Such an arrangement also suggests the circular reasoning of Chinese philosophy.

6.2.2 Heaven: Tian 天

Tian is usually translated into Heaven, but actually not the same. *The Origin of Chinese Characters* interprets "Tian 天" as "Vertex, Supreme; following 一 and 大". "Yi 一" is usually translated into one, but as we know it is far beyond the number one, referring to *Tai Ji* or the Great Primal Beginning, the foundation of Tao, and the mystical state before the Genesis of the world". "Da 大" is usually translated into big or great, being composed of "yi 一" and "ren 人 or Man". See Illus.12.

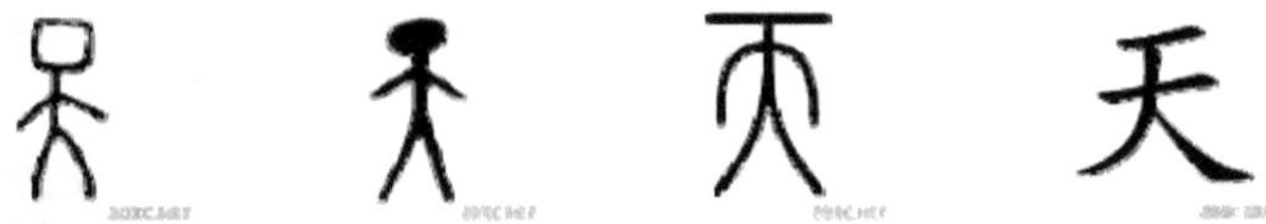

Illus.12 "Tian 天" from Oracle, Bronze, Lesser Seal to Regular Script

Tian 天 means Man's vertex, Sky, Heaven, and God. According to the interpretations of "tian 天" and "yi 一" in *The Origin of Chinese Characters*, *Tian* 天 bears 3 cultural connotations in the ancient China: 1) the mystical *tian*, the master of the universe, like God; 2) the natural *tian*, including all of the natural phenomena, opposed to man-made; 3) the existing Heaven or sky, opposed to the earth.

6.2.3 Man: Ren 人

The Origin of Chinese Characters states that "Man is the most valuable being in between the heaven and the earth".

Huang Di's Inner Classic states that "Of all things under the heaven, nothing is more precious than man. Man is dependent on the nourishment and fortification of the heaven and the earth, water and food, and the essence of the universe to grow and prosper according to the laws and changes of the seasons"; and that "Man is born on the earth, hanging his life to the heaven. The union of the heaven qi and the earth qi gives birth to Man. Man can adapt himself to the seasons for the Heaven and the Earth are his parents".

That is to say, the man, the heaven, and the earth share the common constituent - *Qi*.

6.2.4 Earth: Di 地

The Origin of Chinese Characters states that "Primordial *Qi* (Yuan Qi, 元气) is essential for separating the Heaven from the Earth; the Heaven is light and lucid, and the Earth is heavy and turbid; the Earth functions to carry all the things".

This interpretation tells us three pieces of information: the essential factor to separate the heaven and the earth - Primordial *Qi*; the qualities of the heaven and the earth – the heaven being light and lucid and the earth being heavy and turbid; and the function of the earth – to carry all the things.

6.2.5 Three: San, 三

6.2.5.1 The original meaning of "San 三": Three and Many

The kids in the kindergarten all know the truth of 1+2=3. But actually, "San 三" can be three, or multiple, even ad infinitum, and uncountable. The story of

Confucius studying *The Book of Changes* is cited in *The Historical Records* by Sima Qian[93] that Confucius read *The Book of Changes* in his old age so frequently that the leather ropes fixing the pages (actually the bamboo slips) were fractured three (three=many) times 韦编三绝, which indicated he studied *The Book of Changes* very diligently.

In the remote antiquity, three was the largest number. For example, sinograms composed by three same parts means many:

淼： (of wide expanse of water) vast
森：full of trees
晶：many stars
磊：many stones
众：many people
首：written as 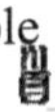 in lesser seal script, a lot of hair on the head

Three in European Languages has the similar connotation[94]:
Thrice (English), Ter (Latin): three; many.
Tres (three, Latin) relates to Tran (beyond).
Très (very, extreme, French) relates to Trois (three).

Actually, using three or times of three for many are very common in Chinese language. For example,

三人成虎：Three (many) people spreading reports of a tiger make you believe there is one around. That is to say, a lie, if repeated often enough, will be accepted as truth.

三折肱而为良医：After having broken his upper arms for three (many) times, he becomes a good surgeon. That is to say, experience is a good teacher.

后宫佳丽三千人：Three thousand concubines of a monarch, which indicates that a monarch could have as many concubines as he liked.

The poem hereafter uses "three thousand feet" as an artistic exaggeration to describe the magnificent sight of the cataract on Mount Lu.

望庐山瀑布	Cataract on Mount Lu
日照香炉生紫烟，	The sunlit Censer perk exhales a wreath of cloud;
遥望瀑布挂前川。	Like an upended stream the cataract sounds loud.
飞流直下三千尺，	Its torrent dashes down three thousand feet from high;

93 Sima Qian 司马迁 (145 or 135? – ca. 86 B.C.), was a prefect historian of the Han Dynasty. He is regarded as the father of Chinese historiography because of his highly praised work, *The Historical Records* (Shi Ji, 史记), a general history of China covering more than two thousand years from Huang Di, the Yellow Emperor, to Emperor Han Wu Di. His definitive work laid the foundation for later Chinese historiography.

94 Translated from Chinese. The original reference is *NUMBER: The Language of Science (A Critical Survey Written for the Cultured non Mathematician)* by Tobias Dantzig (1884-1956).

疑是银河落九天。 As if the Silver River fell from azure sky.

(Originally composed by Li Bai[95], Translated by Xu Yuanchong)

6.2.5.2 Three Gives Birth to All Things

Lao Tzu reads that “Tao begets the one, the one begets the two, the two begets the three, and the three gives birth to all things (in the universe)”. Tao and One can be mutually interpretive. In fact, Tao bears two qualities, i.e., nothing and being. Nothing means without shape or image, i.e., the chaotic universe; Being means with shape and image, i.e. the one. So “Tao gives birth to one” means that which has physical appearance is generated by that which has no physical appearance. Two refers to the heaven and the earth, and yin and yang; "the two begets the three" can be understood as the union of the heaven *qi* and the earth *qi* makes man. And then three, i.e. the heaven, the earth and the man, is the first complete unit of the creation of the world. Therefore three is the foundation for the birth, growth and development of all things in the universe.

Zuo's Spring Autumn Annals (Zuo Zhuan 左传, or Zuo Shi Chun Qiu 左氏春秋)[96] states that “Three is the number of the heaven, the earth and the man”. *The Origin of Chinese Characters* explains “three” as “the Tao (way) of Heaven, Earth and Man”. *The Historical Records* reads that “The numbers start at one, end with ten, and complete with three”. *The Book of Changes* names the heaven, the earth, and the man as “Three *Cai*”. “才 Cai” is written as  in oracle script, pictographic, in which the upper horizontal line stands for the soil, the part below it resembles the image of the tender shoot just sprouting from the seed but not coming up out of the ground, and so its original meaning is (of trees and grasses, or plant) newborn.

6.2.5.3 The Importance of “the Central and Harmonious *Qi*”

Let's now go back to *Lao Tzu. the 42nd Chapter.*

"Tao begets the one,
The one begets the two,
The two begets the three,
And the three gives birth to all things (in the universe).

95 Li Bai 李白 (701 – 762), also known in the West by various other transliterations as Li Po, has been regarded as one of the greatest poets in China's Tang Dynasty, which is often called China's "golden age" of poetry. Thirty-four of his poems are included in the popular anthology *Three Hundred Tang Poems*. As regards to Chinese cultural influence, Li Bai's poetry has been much esteemed from his lifetime through the present day. Indeed, in China he has been known as the best of the Romantic Poets. In the West his influences include many translations, adaptations, and much inspiration.

96 It is the earliest Chinese work of narrative history and covers the period from 722 to 468 B.C.. It is one of the most important sources for understanding the history of the Spring and Autumn Period. Together with the *Gong Yang Zhuan* 公羊传 and *Guliang Zhuan* 谷梁传, the work forms one of the surviving “Three Commentaries on the Spring and Autumn Annals”.

All things in the universe bear yin and embrace yang,
where the central and harmonious *qi* makes them in harmony."

The relationship of "the central and harmonious *qi*" and "the Three Newborns" is just like that of "the soil" and "the five phases", where the soil is in the Center of the other four phases, i.e. Wood-East, Fire-South, Metal-West, and Water-North. If without the middle there would be neither Left Wing nor Right Wing; if without the central and harmonious *qi* there would be neither Yin qi nor Yang *qi*. Take the structure of an atom as an example. Its outer is the electrons (-), while its inner is composed of the protons (+) and neutrons. If without the neutrons, an atom could not be kept as a stable entity. It is clear that the central and harmonious *qi* bears the same importance as the neutrons. And Heaven – Earth - Man make up a holistic system, among which they are independent and closely related to each other and the Man is the dominator.

6.3 *Tian Ren He Yi:* The World View of Chinese Culture

6.3.1 *Chuang Tzu*: Heaven and Earth Were Parents of All Things in the Universe

The idea of *Tian Ren He Yi* or Universe and Man Uniting and Resembling Each Other was first put forward by *Chuang Tzu*, which states that "The heaven and the earth were parents of all things in the universe".

6.3.2 *The Book of Changes:* Viewpoint of Unity with Three Dimensions

"In ancient times the holy sages made *The Book of Changes* to follow the order of their nature and their fate. Therefore they determined the Tao of the heaven and named it yin and yang, determined the Tao of the earth and named it hardness and softness, and determined the Tao of man and named it benevolence and upright. They combined these three fundamental powers and doubled them; hence in *The Book of Changes* a sign is always formed by six lines." (*Shuo Gua*, 说卦)

The above quotation shows the viewpoint of unity with three dimensions in *The Book of Changes:*

Tao of Heaven: yin and yang to make all things begin;
Tao of Earth: hardness and softness to give birth to all things;
Tao of Man: benevolence and upright to complete all things.

And "the Three Cai" or "the Three Newborns" are actually the symbol for the idea of "Universe and Man Uniting and Resembling Each Other".

Viewpoint of unity with three dimensions also exists in Greek mythology. For example, there were three Goddesses for fate: One responsible for spinning the life line for a newborn baby, one determining the length of the life line, and one cutting off the life line when one was dying; three Goddesses for Opportunities to be in charge of good fate and opportunity; three Goddesses for Revenge to be in charge of punishing those who bore false witness, murdered family members, and maltreated non-natives respectively; and three Goddesses for Beauty and Wisdom, i.e. Zeus's three daughters - Aglaia for brightness and handsome, Euphrosyne for happiness and cheerfulness, and Thalia for vigour and youth;[97] etc.

Viewpoint of unity with three dimensions is also available in Christian Belief. Comparative mythologists believed that the relationship among the Father, the Holy Ghost (Spirit), and the son of God reflects the triangle relationship among Heaven Father, Earth Mother, and Man's Son.

Difference between the viewpoint of unity with three dimensions of Christian belief and Chinese philosophy reflects one major cultural difference between the two cultures. Christian belief focuses on the value of the belief of "One God", and thus its culture is a kind of God-based culture. While Chinese philosophy stresses the invaluable position of man 人, written as 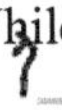 in oracle script, who stands upright with one's two legs in between the heaven and the earth, thus forming a situation of tripartite confrontation, like the three legs of a tripod, and therefore Chinese culture is a kind of Man-based culture. This has been very popular in almost every aspect of Chinese culture, including ancient bureaucratic establishment, and Chinese medicine.

6.3.3 Dong Zhongshu[98]: Man Mirroring Heaven

Dong Zhongshu's proposal of "Proscribing all non-Confucian schools of thought and espousing Confucianism as the orthodox state ideology" was adopted by Emperor Han Wu Di 汉武帝 (live in between 156-87 B.C.; reign in between 141-87 B.C.). His thought integrated Yin Yang cosmology into a Confucian ethical framework.

He is also considered the originator of the doctrine of "Interactions between Heaven and Man", which mainly manifests in two parts: Chinese political philosophy and Chinese natural philosophy. From the standpoint of Chinese political philosophy, his proposal lays down rules for deciding the legitimacy of a monarch as well as providing a set of checks and balances for reining a monarch. Such a proposal legitimated the emperors' autocratic government for thousands of years since Emperor Han Wu Di in China.

97 Translated from Chinese.

98 Dong Zhongshu 董仲舒 (179-104 B.C.) was a Han Dynasty scholar who is traditionally associated with the promotion of Confucianism as the official ideology of the Chinese imperial state. His thought integrated Yin Yang cosmology into a Confucian ethical framework. He is also considered the originator of the doctrine of Interactions between Heaven and Man 天人感应. There are two works that are attributed to Dong Zhongshu, one of which is the *Countermeasures for Recommending Able and Virtuous Men* (Ju Xian Liang Dui Ce, 举贤良对策) in three chapters, preserved under "*The History of the Former Han Dynasty*" (Han Shu, 汉书); the other of which that has survived to the present is the *Luxuriant Dew of the Spring and Autumn Annals* (Chun Qiu Fan Lu, 春秋繁露) in 82 chapters.

While based on his natural philosophy, Chinese medicine, and Chinese astronomy etc. came into being[99] and *Huang Di's Inner Classic* has still functioned as the highest authority on Chinese medicine since then. He said "To unite Heaven and Man into one by the way of analogizing" (From the chapter of *Yin Yang Yi* 阴阳义 of *Chun Qiu Fan Lu*).

Chun Qiu Fan Lu further states in the chapter of *Man Mirroring Heaven* (*Ren Fu Tian Shu*, 人副天数) that

"The virtue of Heaven is to bestow, the virtue of Earth is to transform, and the virtue of Man is to be righteous. … The essence of Heaven and Earth is to generate beings, among which Man is the most honored. … In the universe only Man can be analogized to the Heaven and the Earth. Man has 360 joints, analogizing the number of the Heaven; Man's body, bone and flesh analogize the thickness of the Earth. Ears and eyes on the head can listen and look, metaphorizing the sun and the moon; The orifices and vessels of the body are just like rivers and gorges, Happiness, anger, grief and joy of the heart (the gamut of human feeling) are similar to spirits (SHEN Qi). Man's body is so high, thus analogizes the Heaven. … Therefore, Man's head is round, thus metaphorizing the appearance of the Heaven for the Heaven is also round; hair metaphorizes the stars; the ears and the eyes are bright, thus metaphorizing the sun and the moon; the exhalation and inhalation of the mouth and nose metaphorize the *qi* of the wind; the heart in the chest understands, thus metaphorizing the spirits and the gods; the emptiness or repletion of the organs in the abdomen symbolizes various things; various things is closest to the Earth, therefore the part below the lumbar is the Earth; the images of the Heaven and the Earth are demarcated by the lumbar; the part above the neck is the place of the spirit and dignity, thus showing the dignity of the Heaven; the part below the neck, some rich and thick, some poor and thin, analogizes the soil; the feet are square-shaped, analogizing the shape of the Earth. … The symbols of the Heaven and Yin-Yang are complete in the body; the body is just like the Heaven, so its numbers accord with the numbers of the heaven; therefore the will of the Heaven (or God's will) makes them interrelate and interact with each other. The Heaven takes its numbers of a year to make a man; therefore, man has 366 small joints to accord with the days of a year, 12 big vessels to accord with the months of a year, 5 *zang* organs to accord with the five phases, and 4 limbs to accord with the four seasons; opening eyes and closing eyes accord with the days and the nights; hardness and softness accord with the winter and the summer; grief and joy accord with yin and yang; the heart calculates to accord with moral standard or law; the behaviors observe moral principles to accord with the relationship between the Heaven and the Earth. A

---

99 Wei Zhengtong. 2003: 321-324.

man was born with all of the above mentioned, among which those countable take numbers of the Heaven and the Earth and those uncountable analogize and metaphorize the Heaven and the Earth. Anyway, man mirrors the Heaven".

Dong Zhongshu's thoughts on "Interactions between Heaven and Man"and "Man Mirroring Heaven" have been very influential to Chinese medicine. You may refer to the chapters of *Yin Yang Xi Ri Yue* or *Yin-Yang Relating to the Sun & the Moon* and *Xie Ke* or *Pathogens* of *Ling Shu* or *Miraculous Pivot* and *Qi Xue* or *Acupoints* of *Su Wen* or *Basic Questions* of *Huang Di's Inner Classic*. By the way, *Huang Di's Inner Classic* can also be regarded as a philosophical classic, esp. in the fields of interpreting the nature, beings and life with *qi*, yin-yang and five phases, it is second to none although it is a well-known classic on Chinese medicine.[100]

There are also some critical viewpoints on Dong Zhongshu's Interactions between Heaven and Man. Li Yangbo 李阳波 (1947-1991) commented that it is very difficult for the human society to mirror the nature and the universe, but the components of the society such as plants, animals and human beings themselves as well as their growth, maturity, aging and death, can not escape from the rules dominated by the Heaven. Therefore, he advocated that the social part of Dong Zhongshu's "Interactions between Heaven and Man" should be discarded and the biological part should be preserved in Chinese medicine for man and universe did not unit and resemble each other in the social structure, but only in physiological states, and believed that Chinese medicine is a system of transforming the relationships of *Shu Shu* 术数 among the heaven, the earth and the man, so he preferred the formulation: Perspective of "Universe and Living Beings" or Perspective of "Heaven and Man" instead of *Tian Ren He Yi*.[101] But I still support that "Man Mirroring Universe", in which the universe contains the nature and the society.

As regards to how man mirrors the social structure, a chapter entitled *Ling Lan Mi Dian Lun* or *Discourse on Hidden Canons in the Numinous Orchid Chambers*[102] from *Huang Di's Inner Classic Basic Questions* reads that

Huang Di asked Qi Bo, "Could you please tell me the functions and the relationships of the twelve *zang fu* organs and their meridians?"

Qi Bo replied, "Your question is very precise and I will try to answer you as precisely as you asked. The heart is the sovereign of all the other organs and represents the consciousness of one's being. It is responsible for intelligence, wisdom, and spiritual transformation. The lung is the advisor. It helps the heart in regulating the body's *qi*. The liver is the general, courageous and smart. The

100 Ma Boying. 1994: 247.

101 Narrated by Li Yangbo, Systematized by Liu Lihong, et al. *Opening the Door of Chinese Medicine: Introduction to Doctrine of Periods and Qi*. Beijing: China Press of TCM, 2004.

102 The numinous orchid chambers are said to be Huang Di's library.

gallbladder is a judge for its power of discernment. The pericardium is the court jester who makes the king laugh, bringing forth joy. The stomach and spleen are the officials in charge of granaries, where all the food and essences are stored. They digest, absorb, and extract the food and nutrients. The large intestine is an official in charge of transmission, and it is responsible for transportation of all turbidity. All waste products go through this organ. The small intestine receives the food that has been digested by the spleen and stomach and further extracts, absorbs, and distributes it throughout the body, all the while separating the pure from the turbid. The kidneys are the organ that give strength; they store the vitality and mobilize the four extremities. They also aid the memory, willpower, and coordination. The *san jiao*, or the triple *jiao*, holds the office of the sluices; it manifests as the waterways. The bladder serves as a reservoir; it is the place where the water converges and where, after being transformed by the *qi*, it is eliminated. So these twelve *zang fu* organs must work together harmoniously, just like a kingdom.

"However, the decision-making is the king's job. If the spirit is clear, all the functions of the other organs will be normal. It is in this way that one's life is preserved and perpetuated, just as a country becomes prosperous when all its people are fulfilling their duties. If the spirit is disturbed and unclear, the other organs will not function properly. This creates damage. The pathways and roads along which the *qi* flows will become blocked and health will suffer. The citizens of the kingdom will also suffer. These are the relationships of a kingdom."

You can see that this chapter discusses the importance of harmony of the internal environment of the human being from social and psychological aspects by metaphorizing the rules of administering a country, which is guided by "Man Mirroring Universe" - it reflects some social problems by discussing physiological functions of organs on one hand, and improves understanding of the biological being by metaphorizing the rules of administering a country, social and psychological phenomena on the other. Thus it actually implies the biological-psychological-social medical mode.

Medical mode has evolved in the course of development of medical practice, which mainly reflects basic thinking and main methods when observing and dealing with medical problems. Medical modes have always existed and varied constantly with changes in thoughts of philosophy of medicine of different times. It's generally believed that the development of medical modes has gone through the following stages from god, natural philosophy, mechanism, biological to physiological – psychological – social medical mode. With the considerable progress in social medicine and medical psychology, the academic circle has come to know that practice of the traditional biological medical mode is just one-sided pursuit of well-being of human beings. The significant variations in disease spectrum also objectively require the transition of the medical mode to a comprehensive one, i.e. physiological – psychological – social medical mode, which regards the occurrence and development of diseases as the outcome of changes not only in biological and psychological states but also in social adaptability.[103]

A good social, political environment, the nature in an ecological balance and a man who knows the importance of living harmony with the universe are of vital significance not only in cultivating man's health in both mental and physical aspects but also in establishing a better world for all the living beings.

6.3.4 Connotations of *Tian Ren He Yi*

Tian Ren He Yi bears the following connotations: Man Mirroring Universe, i.e. regarding universe as man, and man as universe; Harmony of Man and Universe, i.e. Man and Universe following the laws of the nature. *The Classic of Rites · The Doctrine of Mean* states that "Sincerity is the way of the heaven; Sincerity is the way of man". That is to say, sincerity makes Man and Heaven unite. My understanding of "sincerity" is to be true to its original, to follow the way of the nature.

Lao Tzu. The 69th Chapter reads that

"Tao is great,
Heaven is great,
Earth is great,
Man is also great.
There are four great things in the country,
Man is one of them.
Man abides by the earth,
Earth abides by the heaven,
Heaven abides by Tao,
Tao abides by the nature".

103 Sun Baozhi. 2003: 26, 29.

The whole land under the heaven[104] is all *Xiang*. *Bi Xing* or Analogizing and Metaphorizing of *Shi* or *The Classic of Poetry*, political affairs of *Shu* or *The Classic of Documents*, fame, position and status of *Chun Qiu* or *The Spring and Autumn Annals*, ceremonial rites of *Li* or *The Classic of Rites*, and melodies of *Yue* or *The Classic of Music* are nothing but *Xiang*. But *Yi* or *The Book of Changes* gets all the principles together.

-Wang Fuzhi[105]

7 *Xiang*: Key to Understand Chinese Culture and Philosophy

Compared to Western culture and philosophy, Chinese culture and philosophy stresses *Xiang,* relationships, and functions rather than causality (whys) and morphological structures, underlines circular reasoning instead of linear reasoning, focuses on understanding an entity from a holistic point of view (holism, integration, unity) rather than understanding it by breaking it down into its constituent parts (reductionism, separation, part), values changing process rather than the unchanged features, and emphasizes perceptual understanding rather than quantified measurement. All in all, *Xiang* is the key to understand Chinese culture and philosophy. Taking image and analogizing is a vital methodology of classical Chinese philosophy and of classical Chinese medicine.

7.1 The Original Meaning of "*Xiang* 象": Elephant

The Origin of Chinese Characters states that "*Xiang* 象, with long nose and teeth, a big mammal in the Southern Yue area, will be pregnant every three years", so you can see that the original meaning of "*xiang*" is elephant. In remote antiquity, elephants had lived in the Central Plains of China. Later on, elephants had to migrate south because of the changes in climate, so the people in the Central Plains had few opportunities to see live elephants again. Han Fei 韩非(281?-233 B.C.), a famous philosopher and the representative of the Legalist School of the late Warring States Period (475-221B.C.), said in the chapter of *Jie Lao Pian* of *Han Fei Tzu* 韩非子·解老篇 that "people seldom see the live elephant, but has gained the skeleton of a dead one, so they can imagine what it is like after investigating the picture or image of its skeleton. Therefore, all in people's imagination is known as '*xiang*'". This quotation also reveals the mystery of the origin of the Chinese compound "*xiang xiang*" (想象, literally "thinking or imagining elephant", means imaging or imagination), setting off *xiang's* "imagining" cultural connotations. See the Illus.5, which shows how the sinogram 象 was conceived in the way of resembling the real image of an elephant. The Illus. 6 shows the evolution process of the sinogram *Xiang* 象.

104 Here the whole land under the heaven refers to the world.

105 Wang Fuzhi 王夫之 (1619-1692), a famous thinker and philosopher of the late Ming and early Qing dynasties. This quotation is from his *Zhou Yi Wai Zhuan* or *External Interpretation of The Book of Changes*.

7.2 *Xiang*: An All-Embracing Symbol in Chinese Culture and Philosophy

In the meanwhile, you can see that "*xiang*" originally evolved from "seeking similarities" between things from the angle of genetics, as stated in *The Book of Changes* that "*Xiang* refers to something being like or resembling this thing". In the chapter of *the Fifteenth Year of Xi Gong's Reign* of *Zuo's Spring and Autumn Annals* it states that "Tortoise is *X*iang"; *The Book of Changes* states that "Change is *X*iang".

In Chinese traditional culture, all of the sceneries, the stars, even man's pulses, tongues and viscera are termed together with *xiang* like "jing (scenery) xiang 景象", "xing (star) xiang 星象", "mai (pulse) xiang 脉象", "she (tongue) xiang 舌象" and "zang (visceral) xiang 藏象"; Dao or Tao 道, the primitive motive force of the origin of everything in the universe, is also known as *xiang*, the big *xiang*. *Xiang* has a very strong adhesive power, and is a vital part of a series of compounds, including everything from the concrete *xiang* of objects which can be felt and the metaphysical subtle *xiang* which is difficult to grasp, thus possessing both perceptual and rational ingredients, and also indicating relationships.

7.2.1 Observing Phenomena and Making Instruments to Explain the Origin of Chinese Culture

The Book of Changes applies the method of observing phenomena and making instruments (guan xiang zhi qi, 观象制器) to explain the origin of Chinese culture. Observing phenomena and making instruments is the core of the rational ideas in *The Book of Changes*, i.e., following (modelling) examples of phenomena and all things in the nature to invent & make instruments in accordance with the image thinking, which is somehow similar to bionics in modern scientific setting.

In the chapter of *History of Civilization* of *The Book of Changes*, it reads that

"In the remote antiquity when Fu Xi 伏羲 ruled the country, he raised his head to observe images on the heaven, bowed his head to observe phenomena on the earth, observed images of birds and beasts and those of the earth, took near images from man and took far images of other things from the universe, on the basis of which he then started to make the Eight Trigrams to illustrate the phenomena.

"He made knotted cords and used them for nets and baskets in hunting and fishing. He probably took this from the hexagram of THE CLINGING (Li, 离)[106].

"When Bao Xi's clan was gone, there sprang up the clan of the Shen Nong (Divine Husbandman). He split a piece of wood for a plowshare and bent a piece of wood for the plow handle, and taught the whole world the advantage of laying

106 A net consists of meshes, empty within and surrounded by threads without. Hexagram Li represents a combination of meshes of this sort.

open the earth with a plow. He probably took this from the hexagram of INCREASE (Yi, 益).

"When the sun stood at midday, he held a market. He caused the people of the earth to come together and collected the wares of the earth. They exchanged these with one another, and then returned home, and each thing found its place. Probably he took this from the hexagram of BITING THROUGH(Shi Ke, 噬嗑)[107].

"When the clan of the Shen Nong (Divine Husbandman) was gone, there sprang up the clans of the Huang Di (Yellow Emperor), of Yao, and of Shun. They brought continuity into their alterations, so that the people did not grow weary. They were divine in the transformations they wrought, so that the people were content. When one change had run its course, they altered. Through alteration they achieved continuity. Through continuity they achieved duration. Therefore: "They were blessed by heaven. Good fortune. Nothing that does not further.

"The Huang Di (Yellow Emperor), Yao, and Shun allowed the upper and lower garments to hang down, and the world was in order. They probably took this from the hexagrams of THE CREATIVE (Qian 乾) and THE RECEPTIVE (Kun 坤).

..."

The chapter of *History of Civilization* shows how all the appurtenances of civilization came into existence as reproductions of ideal, archetypal (typical) images. In a certain sense this idea contains a truth. Every invention comes into being as an image in the mind of the inventor before it makes its appearance in the phenomenal world as a tool, a finished thing. The 64 hexagrams present, in a mysterious way, images paralleling nature, which can be understood as relationships represented by the hexagrams the inventions took shape in the mind of their originators.[108]

7.2.2 Pictographic Writing: the Foundation of Chinese Characters

It is well known that the Chinese writing system was originally pictographic. In their original forms, graphs representing animals and objects were self-explanatory. But not all elements of the language could be represented in pictorial form. Other devices had to be used. "The Six Categories of Chinese Graphs" were put forward to show the way of creating and developing Chinese characters.

As regards to the names and the order of the Six Categories of Chinese Graphs, most of the scholars adopt the names given by Xu Shen, the order of Ban Gu's version because Chinese characters originated from pictures, which is

107 Hexagram Shi Ke means food & merchandise.
108 Wilhelm, Baynes. 1997: 328-336.

closely related to *Xiang Xing* or pictographs, *Zhi Shi* or ideographs, and *Hui Yi* or associative compounds; *Xing Sheng* or pictophonetics have been developed on the basis of pictographs, which also accords with the developing rule of a written language - from ideographic to phonetic writings. *Zhuan Zhu* or mutually interpretive and *Jia Jie* or loan sinograms are two ways of using sinograms.

Therefore, it is no doubt that pictographic writing is the foundation of Chinese characters.

7.2.3 Literature: Word-Image-Idea

Word-Image-Idea in literature was inspired by philosophy of Pre-Qin days before 221B.C. and metaphysics of Wei-Jin Dynasties (220-420). *Chuang Tzu* states that "What can be sensed cannot be explained in words". *The Book of Changes* states that "What one wants to say cannot be fully written out; and words cannot express all one intends to say. … Therefore, the sages establish *Xiang* or image to express all what they intend to say" and that "Setting up image to display its connotations to the full … interpreting words for trigram to explain its implications to the full." Wang Bi's Annotation of *The Book of Changes* states that "Getting connotations lies in forgetting the image; getting the image lies in forgetting the words".

The text of the literature is composed of organization of the language, a system of images, and world of implications. Take Du Mu[109]'s poem "Spring Comes to South of the Yangtze River" as an example.

江南春	Spring Comes to South of The Yangtze River
千里莺啼绿映红，	Red against green, and a huge troupe of warblers singing;
水村山郭酒旗风。	Hillside, riverside hamlets, with blue flags fluttering.
南朝四百八十寺，	The Southern Dynasties had four hundred eighty Building temples;
多少楼台烟雨中。	How many towers and terraces are wrapped in misty drizzles?

After reading this poem (word or language), you must have a beautiful scenic painting in your mind (image). Now come the implications (ideas). The last two lines - 'The Southern Dynasties had four hundred eighty Building temples; How many towers and terraces are wrapped in misty drizzles?' actually suggest Emperors of the Southern Dynasties[110] indulged in Buddhism and building temples, which wasted money and manpower, rather than improving the common people's life quality.

109 Du Mu 杜牧 (803–852) was a leading Chinese poet of the late Tang Dynasty.

110 The Southern Dynasties refer to the six dynasties installed between the downfall of the Han Dynasty in 200 A.D. and the reunification of China in 589 A.D. Nanjing was the capital of the successive dynasties.

7.2.4 Chinese Aesthetic Tradition: Beautiful Image

Classical Chinese painting, usually in a scroll and done with special soft brush and unique pigments in China, stresses beautiful image and beautiful artistic conception even it depicts the real life. It seems to be quite different from classical Western oil painting, which takes sketching as its foundation and generally emphasizes so much the reality in both contents and styles.[111]

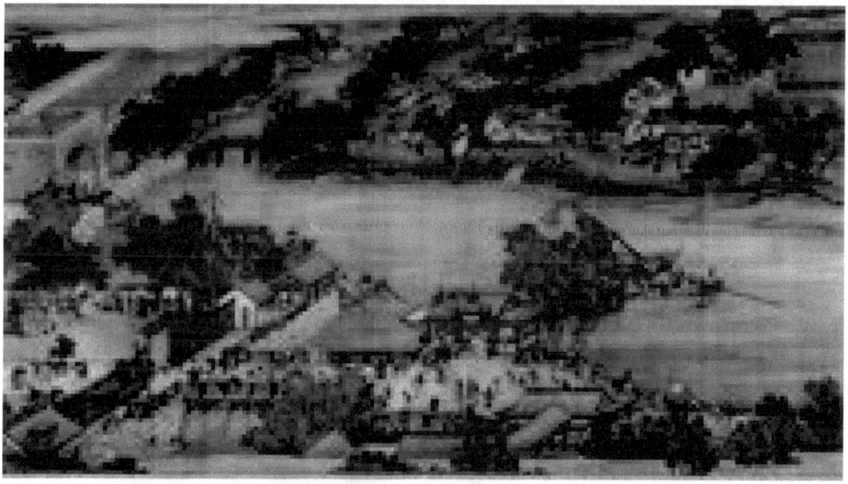

Illus. 13 Along the River in Qingming Heyday（Part）

The Illus. 13 is a part of the painting "Along the River in Qingming Heyday", which is well-known in Chinese as the work of an artist, Zhang Zeduan. The painting captures the daily life of people of the Song Dynasty at the capital, Bianjing (today's Kaifeng). The title was given by the emperor Song Huisong (1082-1135) to indicate that his reign was clear and bright. The entire piece was painted in hand scroll format and the content reveals the lifestyle of all stratum of the society from the rich to the poor as well as different economic activities in rural areas and the city. It offers glimpse of the costumes and architecture during that period. As an artistic creation, the piece has been well revered and over the centuries, court artists of subsequent dynasties have reproduced several versions.

7.2.5 Observing Phenomena and Issuing an Official Calendar

Observing phenomena and issuing an official calendar (guan xiang shou shi, 观象授时) was the approach to traditional Chinese astronomy and calendar system.

111 Here I do not want to discuss the different schools of traditional Chinese painting and Western oil painting, just refer to both kinds of paintings in general.

The Spring Equinox, the Autumn Equinox, the Summer Solstice, and the Winter Solstice were clearly identified by this way in around 4300 B.C.. The earliest and quite complete record on observing phenomena to issue an official calendar seems to be from the chapter of *Yao's Standards* of *The Book of Documents*. Yao, a legendary monarch in ancient China, employed able and virtuous personages from the Xi's and He's clans, who respected and followed the natural principles, observed the movement of the sun, the moon and stars and mastered the rules, finally issued an official calendar to the people so as to serve the agriculture. China issued official calendars by this way until the late Ming dynasty. The Illus. 14 is a statue Xu Guangqi 徐光启 (1562-1633) observing astronomical phenomena named "Configuration of Stars at Night" in Guangqi Park at Xujiahui, Shanghai.

In 1629 (the second year in the reign of Emperor Chongzhen), Xu Guangqi led the reform of calendar. In 1632, the Chongzhen Calendar was basically completed. The work laid the foundation for the early modern Chinese calendar because of its combination of eastern and western, ancient and contemporary astronomic research results. (The Memorial Park for Xu Guangqi, Shanghai)

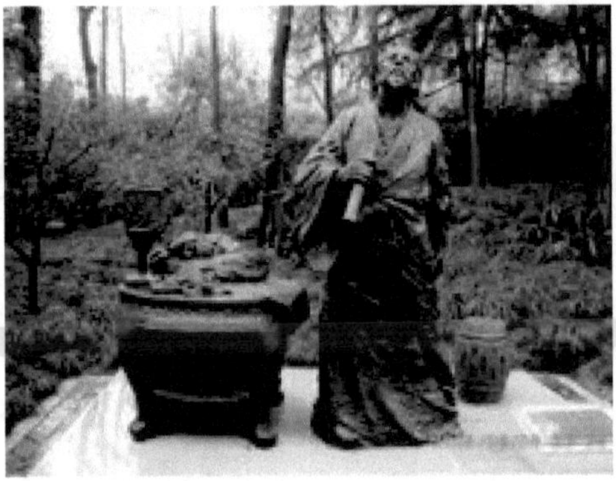

Illus. 14 Xu Guangqi: Configuration of Stars at Night

Xu Guangqi was a Chinese bureaucrat, agricultural scientist, astronomer, and mathematician in the Ming Dynasty. Xu was a colleague and collaborator of the Italian Jesuits Matteo Ricci 利玛窦(1552-1610) and Sabatino de Ursis 熊三拔 (1575–1620) and they translated several classical Western texts into Chinese, including parts of *Euclid's Elements* (collaborated with Matteo Ricci) and *Hydraulic Machinery of the West* (collaborated with Sabatino de Ursis). He was also the author of the *Nong Zheng Quan Shu* 农政全书 or *A Complete Works on Agriculture*, one of the first comprehensive treatises on the subject of agriculture, and *Chongzheng Calendar* 崇祯历书, etc. He was one of the "Three Pillars of Chinese Catholicism". Matteo Ricci is the founder of the Catholic missions of

China. He was expert in the Four Books and Five Classics[112], and advocated to integrate the doctrines of Confucius and Mencius with Catholic religion, which can explain his success in transmitting catholic religion in China. It is worth to note that one of the earliest introductions of Chinese Medicine to the West is from *Ricci Matteo's Reading Notes:*

Medical skills and methods in China were very different from those we were accustomed to. The pulse-taking methods were the same as ours, and they were quite successful in treating diseases. Generally speaking, the medicinal substances they used were very simple such as grasses, roots, stalks and the like. In fact, the Chinese art of healing was all contained in the laws and rules they observed when using the herbal substances. There were no public medical schools here in China. Every one who wanted to be a practitioner should be taught by another one who was proficient in the way of healing. It was possible to get a degree in medicine by passing a test held by Imperial Hospital in Nanjing and Beijing, the two capitals of the Ming Dynasty. But it was just a form, could not bring any benefit to those with it. A practitioner with a medical degree was not more authoritative nor respected than one without the degree because anyone was allowed to practice medicine no matter he was good at the art of healing or not. [113]

7.2.6 Chinese Medicine: An Image Medicine

There is a major misunderstanding that Chinese philosophy mainly discusses society, politics, and ethics, but neglects the nature. Actually, agriculture, astronomy, geography, mathematics, and medicine of the ancient China were very advanced, and even more advanced than that of the West esp. before the 15th century. That is to say, Chinese philosophy of the nature and life in probing into the relationship between the Universe and Man produced all of the Chinese traditional natural science, which worked very well before or even has worked quite well until today. For example, Du Jiang Yan 都江堰, the water control and irrigation dam, which has been listed in the World Inheritance Name List and was designed and built in accordance with the classical scientific ideas, has been working so well in preventing serious flooding for over 2,000 years, and even survives the Sichuan Earthquake in 2008; While cracks appeared in a modern big dam made of concrete mixer just after the earthquake in 2008, which was designed and built nowadays according to the modern science. So, it's clear that Classical Chinese sciences have their own unique values.

---

112 "Four Books and Five Classics" are a collective term for the classics of Confucianism, in which Four Books refer to *The Analects of Confucius, Mencius, The Great Learning,* and *The Doctrine of Mean*; Five Classics refer to *Shi, Shu, Li, Yi*, and *Chun Qiu*, namely *The Book of Songs (or The Classic of Poetry), The Book of Documents (or The Classic of Documents), The Book of Rites (or The Classic of Rites), The Book of Changes (or The Classic of Changes), and Zuo's Spring Autumn Annals.*

113 Translated from Chinese. Originally by Ricci Matteo. Translated by He Gaoji, Wang Zunzhong, Li Shen. 1983: 34.

Today, only Chinese medicine survives ever after facing the serious challenges from Western medicine, and almost all of the other Chinese classical natural science like agriculture, astronomy, geography, and mathematics etc. have declined and are totally replaced by the corresponding Western natural science. It is a great pity. But the fact also indicates philosophy of Chinese science fits much better to the living system than to the other systems, and the living system is the only one which is always in a state of constant changing and transforming.

Undoubtedly, Chinese medicine works quite well in treating many illnesses, which usually cannot be successfully treated by Western medicine. That's why so great interests arouse in studying Chinese medicine among researchers of different fields of study at both home and abroad. Generally speaking, most of them try to find out the scientific evidence on mechanism of Chinese medicine mainly by doing lab experiments and clinical trials (such as RCT) as the same way in researching Western medicine, but actually it is a wrong approach.

In fact Chinese medicine is the product of the integration of understanding of the human being and culture, and therefore is an image medicine, which accords with the Tao of Chinese Natural Philosophy. For example, its fundamental theories such as *Qi*, Yin-Yang, Five Phases, Visceral Image Theory, Vessel Theory, and Herbal Theory are all formed by mirroring similarities between Universe and Man; In its clinical practice, diagnosis is made according to patient's outward manifestations, including tongue Image, pulse image, and so on, and finally is given as a certain "Pattern Image"; its development is based on image observation, and the ability of relating the image in the nature to man.

7.3 *Xiang* Implies a Vital Methodology of Chinese Philosophy

Integration of the subject and the object is a thread running through the classical Chinese culture and science, on the basis of which *Tian Ren He Yi* constitutes the foundation of them. The imaging thinking is a classical thinking way of the Chinese culture, and whose process, methods, and rules make up *Qu Xiang Bi Lei* 取象比类 or Taking Image and Analogizing, the framework of the classical Chinese culture and science.

Hereafter are four concepts indicating the progressive process of *Qu Xiang* or Taking Image:

① *Wu Xiang* 物象: the appearance, phenomena the object manifests itself outside, the existing or being form of the object itself;

② *Zhi Jue Xing Xiang* or "Perceptual Image" 知觉形象: the intuition image the subject produces when the *wu xiang* 物象 acts on man's sense organs;

③ *Biao Xiang* or "External Image" 表象: the internalized *Wu Xiang* 物象, or the trace of the perceptual image left in man's memory, the image of the object taken, stored and reflected by man's brain after feeling, perceiving the *wu xiang* many times;

④ *Yi Xiang* or "Imagery Image or Image in Imagination or Image" 意象: the result of generalizing and abstracting the image information of the common features of the objects of the same category, the rational image generalized from the external image, the unity of the external image of the object and the subject's deep understanding of it. *Yi Xiang* is the cell of the image thinking, running through the thinking process from the beginning to the end.

The whole process of *Qu Xiang* or Taking Image lies in observing, understanding and taking "*xiang*", and manifests in transformation and flow of "*xiang*".

Bi Lei or Analogizing compares, finds, and catches similarities between two different kinds of things, then migrate and infer the knowledge of one to the other.

The Book of Changes classifies *Qu Xiang Bi Lei* into four Steps: ① Observing object or phenomenon (*guan wu* 观物): directly observing an object or a phenomenon; ② Taking image (*qu xiang* 取象): summarizing and refining the image of the object or phenomenon after repeatedly observing and feeling it; ③ Comparing and analogizing (*bi lei* 比类): comparing the things which need to know with the "image (*xiang* 象)" just taken; ④ Understanding the Way or Rule (*ti dao* 体道): finding the rules through the above comparing and analogizing. *Qu Xiang Bi Lei* results in the formation of metaphors, and such metaphors show the process of *Qu Xiang Bi Lei* and the relationship of the involved things or objects or phenomena or images. Therefore, *Qu Xiang Bi Lei* is an immanent methodology which is given by the activity.

To sum up, *Xiang*, an all-embracing Chinese cultural and philosophical symbol, runs through almost every aspect of Chinese culture, such as its origin – Observing Phenomena and Making Instruments, its logographic writing - with pictographs as its foundation, literature – being composed of Word, Image and Idea, arts of painting – stressing the beauty of image rather than the reality, Calendar - Observing Phenomena and Issuing an Official Calendar, medicine – based on understanding of the dynamic living being instead of the dead body, and also implies a vital methodology of classical Chinese sciences - *Qu Xiang Bi Lei* or Taking Image and Analogizing. Therefore, we can say that classical Chinese culture is a kind of *Xiang* culture, classical Chinese science a kind of *Xiang* science, and classical Chinese medicine a kind of *Xiang* medicine.

Thunder and lightening were true backgrounds of Gods.

- Xu Shan[114]

Gods and Ghosts are metaphors; SHEN or God is the metaphor of creating, while GUI or Ghost is the metaphor of vanishing.

- The Author

As regards to return and restoration of traditional "*Li* 礼" and deep-going understanding of "*Ren* 仁" in the human nature, Confucius fully deserves the first RU in the history of Chinese culture to serve as a link between past and future.

- The Author

8 Worship of Thunder and Lightening: SHEN & RU

8.1 Understanding SHEN in Classical Chinese Texts

The topic SHEN reminds me a poem - *Auguries of Innocence* by William Blake (1757-1827):

"To see a world in a grain of sand,
And a heaven in a wild flower,
Hold infinity in the palm of your hand,
And eternity in an hour".

I think SHEN is the very "grain of sand", "the wild flower", "the infinity", and "the eternity" in Chinese culture and Chinese medicine as well. In the chapter on *Moving Essence and Changing Qi* of *Huang Di's Inner Classic • Basic Questions,* it reads that "A patient with SHEN is apt to recover from illness, while a patient losing SHEN has a poor prognosis". Then what is it meant by SHEN? Actually, SHEN is a half religious and half scientific concept in Chinese culture, and bears many meanings, which are shown differently in different authoritative dictionaries or books. For example, *Dictionary of Commonly Used Characters in Archaic Chinese* explains SHEN as "god or supernatural being; the law in the nature; spirit; magic, superb, excellent";[115] *A Concise Dictionary of Chinese Medicine* interprets SHEN as "a collective term for life activities of man in a

114 For a better understanding of this formulation, you may further investigate the origin and evolution of the writing forms of the following sinograms: Lei 雷, Shen 神, Ling 灵, Long 龙, Gui 鬼, Di 帝, and Wang 王. See Xu Shan. Worship of Thunder God: Exploration into the Origin of Chinese Culture [M]. Shanghai: Shanghai Joint Publishing House, 1992.

115 Dictionary of Commonly Used Characters in Archaic Chinese [Z]. 1998: 254.

broad sense” and “thinking and awareness activities in a narrow sense”;[116] *The Fundamental Theories of Chinese Medicine*, the national textbook of the fifth edition on fundamental theories for higher education of Chinese medicine in China, reads that “SHEN bears 3 meanings in the Chinese medical theory: the first, the transformations, the changes, and the functions of the materials in the nature; the second, all of the activities of man’s life; the third, thinking and awareness of man”.[117] So first, let’s start understanding SHEN on the basis of its etymological investigation.

8.1.1 Understanding the Original Meaning of SHEN Based on an Etymological Investigation

One principal way of knowing the Universe in classical China is *Qu Xiang Bi Lei*, or Taking Image and Analogizing. The universe has been constantly changing in most of the time with certain regular rules such as the alternate change of the four seasons and the corresponding changes in the nature: growing, developing, transforming, harvesting, storing. Generally speaking, people can live a calm and peaceful life under such conditions. But there are still sometimes radical changes in the nature such as thunder, lightening, violent storm, sudden downpour, flooding, earthquake, and so on, which are characterized by sudden onset, unpredictable changing, and very powerful. Facing such radical changes in the nature, ancient Chinese people were deeply shocked, felt helpless, but held in awe and veneration toward such mysterious and unpredictable phenomena.

The Book of Changes reads that "The Supreme Being (Di, 帝) came out from Zhen (震 Thunder, East)"; "The myriads of beings (in the universe) came out from Zhen (震 Thunder, East)"; "Arouse with thunderclap, and moisten with wind and rain"; "The great virtue of the heaven and the earth is to give birth"; "SHEN is to create the myriads of beings (in the universe)". *Huang Di's Inner Classic· Basic Questions* states that "Thunder Qi connects with the heart"[118] and that "Heart stores Shen"[119] for both thunder and heart are attributed to fire.

The sinogram for SHEN 神 has undergone the following evolution process:

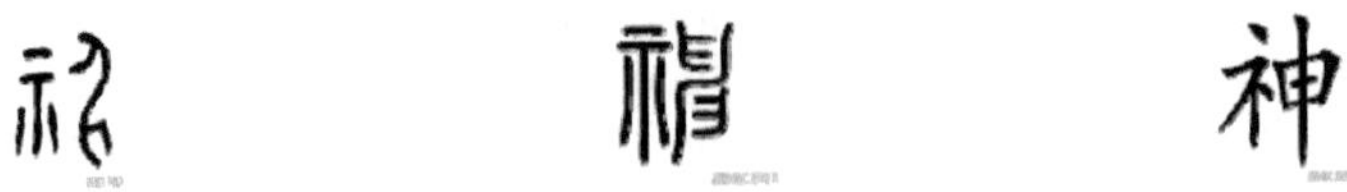

Illus. 15 “SHEN 神” from Bronze, Lesser Seal to Regular Script

116 Li Jingwei, Ou Yongxin, Yu Ying’ao, et al. 2001: 775.
117 Yin Huihe. 1984: 3.
118 See chapter 5 "Great Discourse on Images Corresponding to Yin and Yang from Macrocosm to Microcosm" (Yin Yang Ying Xiang Da Lun, 阴阳应象大论).
119 See chapter 23 "Elucidating the Five Qi" (Xuan Ming Wu Qi, 宣明五气).

The sinogram 神, an associative compound, is composed of two parts: "示" and "申". The ancient form of the right part "申" is the image of lightning in the sky, and is actually the ancient writing form of "電"(the upper is the rain radical 雨, the lower is 电, indicating the meaning); the ancient Chinese people named lightning as "SHEN 申" for they believed that the lightning was so changeable, unpredictable, invincible, knew no bounds, and therefore mysterious, and was governed by or the embodiment of "SHEN or Gods". *The Origin of Chinese Characters* explains that "申 refers to 神". The left part "示" is also an associative compound, and is made up of "二" (the ancient form of "上", means "upper" or "heaven"), and the three falls ("111"), representing the sun, the moon and the stars. The ancient form of "示" was written as "T", representing the image of a sacrificial altar. The part "示" is a radical, and the meanings of the sinograms with "示" are usually related to offering sacrifices to gods or ancestors, or to rites. *The Origin of Chinese Characters* explains "示" as "The heaven hangs down images to show man good or ill luck, following 二. The three falls stand for the sun, the moon and the stars. Observing the images in the sky[120] to detect the current changes. 示 indicates SHEN's things. All with 示 part follow such a connotation." Thus, we can figure out the ancient Chinese people's mysterious feeling about the future world and their great reverence for the gods.

Illus.16 "SHI 示 (礻)" from Oracle, Bronze, Lesser Seal to Regular Script

The Origin of Chinese Characters interprets SHEN as "Tian (Heaven) SHEN who induces all things of creation". Xu Xuan 徐铉 (916-991)[121] interprets "SHEN 申 as induce 引", and further explains that "The heaven governs downbearing qi to induce all things of creation". Here you can also see how difficult to translate or interpret archaic quotations from classical Chinese texts: The SHEN in the compound TIAN SHEN 天神 of this quotation may imply both "lightening" and "god". Yang Bojun 杨伯峻 (1909-1992) explained SHEN in *Zuo's Spring Autumn Annals* as bearing two specific meanings:[122] One refers to the spirits of all things on the earth including the heaven, the earth, the mountains, the rivers, and so and so forth, e.g. "The people are the governor of SHEN (the spirits)"; The other refers to the spirits of famous men or of those who had performed exceptionally meritorious services after they died, e.g. "In former

---

120 天文 is usually translated into astronomy, but I think here it is better translated into the images in the sky.

121 The most important Northern Song scholars on the study of *The Origin of Chinese Characters* were the Xu brothers, Xu Xuàn 徐鉉 (916-991) and Xu Kǎi 徐鍇 (920-974).

122 Yang Bojun, Xu Ti. 1985: 559.

times, Yao[123] killed Gun[124] in the Yushan[125] mountain, and Gun's SHEN (Spirit) transformed into a yellow bear, which went into a deep pool of the mountain". *The Book of Changes* states that "The unpredictable changes of Yin-Yang are named SHEN". Here SHEN refers to the unpredictable, mysterious and wonderful changes.

To sum up, SHEN originally refers to the lightening in the nature, and then was first metaphorized to mean the God who created the world, and then was extended to mean the spirits of the nature, the spirits of dead famous or great men (gods and ghosts), and the unpredictable wonderful changes.

Here is worth to mention "*Gui* 鬼", which is explained in *The Origin of Chinese Characters* as 'what the people return to is named *Gui*, following the part of human and metaphorizing the image of the head of the dead'. Duan Yucai 段玉裁 (1735-1875)[126] further explains that SHEN is yang while GUI is yin. *Gui* originally refers to the spirits of the dead, and is usually translated into ghost. Actually ghost is not a satisfied translation for it is still different from *Gui* in Chinese culture, and here ghost is used only in a metaphorical way.

8.1.2 Understanding SHEN in Classical Chinese Texts

8.1.2.1 Gods and Ghosts

As it is shown in the first part, the ancient Chinese people believed that the various changeable and unpredictable phenomena in the nature were the results of SHEN's (Gods') actions for they were unable to understand them. Then all of the records on gods and ghosts after that can be generally classified into three categories before Buddhism traveled to China:[127] the first referred to those who were grateful to somebody and sought ways to return their kindness, e.g. the story of paying a debt of gratitude; the second those who revenged, e.g. Du Bo shot the King Xuan of the Zhou Dynasty (Zhou Xuan Wang) who killed him for no reason three years before (From *Guo Yu•Zhou Yu* or *Records of States•Records of*

123 Yao 尧 was a Chinese ruler, one of the Three Sovereigns (Fu Xi 伏羲, Nu Wa 女娲, and Shen Nong 神农) and the Five Emperors (Huang Di 黄帝, Zhuan Xu 颛顼, Di Ku 帝喾, Yao 尧, and Shun 舜), which were mythological rulers and culture heroes of China during the period from ca. 2852 B.C. to 2205 B.C., which is the time preceding the Xia Dynasty.

124 Gun 鲧 was Yu's father. Yu the Great 大禹, was the legendary founder of the Xia Dynasty (ca.2100-1600 B.C.), who is best remembered for teaching the people flood control techniques to tame China's rivers and lakes.

125 Yushan 羽山 refers to the northwest of the Donghai County, Jiangsu Province of nowadays (see Page 274 of *Dictionary of Zuo's Spring Autumn Annals*).

126 Duan Yùcái 段玉裁 (1735-1815), due to the quality of his research in *The Origin of Chinese Characters*, stands above all the other scholars in this field of study. His annotated edition of *The Origin of Chinese Characters* is the most commonly used one today.

127 Ren Jiyu. 1985: 11-18.

the Zhou State); the third those spirits of dead people who had been called back by some divining activities. It is thus clear that SHEN in the above three categories is more or less the same as "ghosts" or "the spirits of the dead", manifesting in the appearance of personified SHEN.

What was Confucius's attitude about "gods and ghosts"? He said that "(I would like to) keep gods and ghosts at a respectful distance" (*The Analects of Confucius*). Gods and ghosts of his time still referred to the spirits of our ancestors, which were mainly supposed to support us and rectify our virtues and behaviors, and therefore stood for a kind of good will. He said that "How popular the virtue (of letting justice prevail) which gods and ghosts performed is" (*The Doctrine of Mean*)! And then how about his attitude on "SHEN"? In *The Analects of Confucius*, there is only one place stating SHEN alone in the chapter of *Ba Yi* 八佾 that "(We should) regard our ancestors as being here when offering sacrifices to them, and regard SHEN as being here when offering sacrifices to SHEN. Confucius remarks 'Offering sacrifices to them (by others) is the same as not offering sacrifices at all if I do not participate in the ceremony personally'", which shows that here SHEN is another kind of "being" different from the spirits of our ancestors, i.e. gods, and is of the same importance as the ceremony proper. So Confucius's attitude about SHEN can be summarized as "to admit SHEN's existence but do not want to discuss it".

Chuang Tzu talks about "perfect man", "supernatural (SHEN) man" and "wise man", which actually refer to ideal men who have achieved Tao and therefore have reached the highest states. In this sense, those supernatural (SHEN) men are still not different from gods, e.g. Lie Yu Kou 列御寇 could fly in the wind. And it even records such supernatural (SHEN) men who "could not rely on the five grains to survive, just inhale the wind and drink the dew, fly in the clouds, drive a flying dragon, and swim beyond the four seas", which actually are the same as gods. You can see the deep influence of the ancient Chinese people's original belief on "SHEN" on *Chuang Tzu*. But such an influence had been gradually declining until the later stage of Spring Autumn Period (770-476B.C.). *Zuo's Spring Autumn Annals* states in *The 32nd Year of Zhuanggong's Reign* that "The common people's will should be followed when a country is going to prosper; while SHEN's will should be observed when a country is going to decline. SHEN refers to those who are intelligent, honest, upright, concentrated and constant".

Most of the philosophers of the later generations interpret SHEN in the sense of gods and ghosts as bending or stretching changes of *Qi* or Essential *Qi*. *The Book of Changes* states that "Essential *Qi* (*shen* or gods) gathers to form the shape, while wandering ethereal soul or *Qi* (*gui* or ghosts) results in changes and transformations. And therefore (you) can know the conditions of gods and ghosts." *Guan Tzu* states in the chapter of *Nei Ye* 内业 or *Inner Working* that "*Qi* generates all things of creation, including the five grains on the earth and the stars in the sky (heaven); and that *Qi* in between the heaven and the earth is 'gods and ghosts'; and that one who can guard *Qi* in the chest is a wise man. That's why *Qi* is so termed as *Qi*"[128]. That is to say, even the gods and the ghosts are just *Qi*!

Wang Chong 王充 (27-100A.D.)[129] said that "Gods and ghosts are the names of yin and yang. Yin *Qi* going against the form to return is named ghosts (gui, 鬼), while Yang *Qi* resulting in the generation of the form is named gods (shen, 神)" (*Lun Heng•Lun Si* 论衡•论死 or *Critical Essays•On Death*).

Zhu Xi 朱熹 (1130-1200)[130] said that "Gods (shen, 神) are (those being) stretching, while ghosts (gui, 鬼) are (those being) bending"(*Zhu Zi Yu Lei* 朱子语类 or *Excerpt of Analects of Zhu Xi*[131]).

Wang Fuzhi 王夫之 (1619-1692)[132] further explains that "The *Qi* of the Heaven stretches itself to men and forms and perform its transformations is named gods (shen, 神); while *Qi* bends and returns instead when man's life activities terminate is named ghosts (gui, 鬼) (*Zhang Zi Zheng Meng Zhu•Shen Hua Pian* 张子正蒙注•神化篇 or *Annotations on Zheng Meng by Zhang Tzu•SHEN's Transformations*). To sum up, Gods and Ghosts are metaphors; SHEN or God is the metaphor of creating, while GUI or Ghost is the metaphor of vanishing.

Anyway, SHEN in this sense, i.e. gods and ghosts, has been gradually declining, but never disappears and still runs through Chinese people's mind, and works as the foundation for all of its other connotations. Interpreting SHEN's original meaning - gods and ghosts as bending or stretching changes of *Qi* or Essential *Qi* gives rise to SHEN's second basic meaning: spirit/mind.

8.1.2.2 Spirit/Mind

The second basic meaning of SHEN is spirit/mind, which is always opposed to form, shape, or body. *Chuang Tzu* makes a clear division between spirit and form,

---

128 The translation here accords with Ong Bendick's interpretation in his M.A. Thesis. 2004: 69.

129 Wang Chong 王充 (27–100 A.D.) was a Chinese philosopher during the Han Dynasty (202B.C.-220 A.D.), who developed a rational, secular, naturalistic, and mechanistic account of the world and of human beings.

130 Zhu Xi, or Chu His, 朱熹 (1130-1200), was a Confucian scholar of Song Dynasty, and became the leading figure and the most influential rationalist of Neo-Confucianism in China. His contribution to Chinese philosophy includes his assigning special significance to *The Analects of Confucius*, *The Mencius, The Great Learning,* and *The Doctrine of Mean* (the Four Books), his emphasis on the investigation of things (ge wu), and the synthesis of all fundamental Confucian concepts.

131 *Zhu Zi Yu Lei* 朱子语类 or *Excerpt of Analects of Zhu Xi* is a collection of questions and answers between Zhu Xi and his disciples compiled by Li Jingde 黎靖德 in 1263, printed and publised in 1270.

132 Wang Fuzhi 王夫之 (1619–1692) was a Chinese philosopher of the late Ming (1368—1644), early Qing (1644-1911) dynasties. Wang was a follower of Confucius, but he believed that the Neo-Confucian philosophy which dominated China at the time had distorted Confucius's teachings. He therefore wrote his own commentaries on the Confucian classics, and gradually developed his own philosophical system. He wrote on many topics, including metaphysics, epistemology, moral philosophy, poetry, and politics.

stresses spirit but underestimates form. It states that "The Marquise (of Wei Wu Hou 魏武侯) asked, 'How do you send your best wishes to me'? Xu Wugui answered, "I send my best wishes to your body and spirit (SHEN)' ", and that "The essence and the spirit result from Tao, and the form generates from the essence", which attributes the spirit to the form and finally to Tao. *Chuang Tzu* also puts forwards that the activities of SHEN (spirit) should accord with the Tao of the heaven or the Way of the nature, which is shown in the statement "The Tian (Heaven) will follow when SHEN (spirit) moves".

Xun Tzu also states that "As long as the body forms the spirit will ensue to store the good, the ill, happiness, anger, grief and joy", but does not discuss this statement in details. *Huang Di's Inner Classic•Miraculous Pivot* talks about it in details in the chapter *Tian Nian* or *On the Natural Span*:

Huang Di asked Qi Bo, "I would like to know how a man is conceived, how *qi* builds and makes the foundations (roots), what establishes and makes the parapets (protective screens), what is lost in death, and what is gained in life".

Qi Bo answered, "The mother makes the foundations (roots), and the father makes the parapets (protective screens). Losing the spirit (SHEN) is death, while gaining the spirit (SHEN) is life" (SHEN).

Huang Di asked, "What is the spirit (SHEN)"?

Qi Bo answered, "When blood and qi are harmonized, when the nutrient qi and protective qi are dredged, when the five *zang* organs are formed and matured, when the spirit *qi* (SHEN QI) houses the heart, and when the ethereal soul and corporeal soul are complete, then forms the spirit (SHEN)[133]".

The above quotation shows that the essence, *qi*, and blood are the substantial basis of SHEN (spirit). *Huang Di's Inner Classic* forwards that "To maintain a wellbeing of body and spirit" 形与神俱 is the very point to preserve, cultivate and promote health, which reads in the first chapter of *Basic Questions* that "The people of the remote antiquity practiced Tao by following the rules of yin-yang, harmonizing themselves with the universe by performing some exercises such as *Dao-Yin*[134], having a balanced diet, arising and retiring at regular hours, avoiding overstressing their body and mind, therefore they maintained a wellbeing of body and spirit, and lived over one hundred years which was beyond their natural life span".

As regards to the relationship between the body and the spirit, there are two famous metaphors in classical philosophical texts. One is the metaphor of candle and its flame, in which candle metaphorizes the body and its flame the spirit.[135]

133 Judged from the context (What is the spirit or SHEN), I think here *Ren* or Man is a mistake, which should be SHEN or spirit.

134 *Dao-Yin* 导引 refers to an exercise of combining stretching, massaging, breathing, and meditation to cultivate health.

135 See *Xin Lun • Xing Shen* 新论•形神 by Huan Tan 桓谭 (23 B.C.- 50 A.D.), the first treatise on body and spirit in the history of Chinese philosophy.

The flame (the spirit) will immediately disappear as long as the candle (the body) burns out and does not exist, which shows that the spirit exists on the body. The other is the metaphor of a sword and its sharpness, which was put forward by Fan Zhen 范缜(ca. 450-515)[136]. He said, "The body is the substantial foundation of the spirit, and the spirit is the function of the body. … The relationship between the spirit and its substantial foundation is just like that between the sword and its sharpness; the relationship between the body and its function is just like that between the sword and its sharpness. However, there is neither sword without its sharpness nor sharpness without the sword. As there is no sharpness without a blade, it is impossible for a spirit to exist without its body. "

8.1.2.3 Marvelous Changes

Marvelous changes, the third meaning of SHEN, can still be traced back to *Chuang Tzu*. It describes a kind of superb, excellent skill due to marvelous changes through telling some stories. It reads in the chapter of *Da Sheng* or *Thorough Understanding of Life* that "A carpenter named Zi Qing 梓庆 cut wood into *Ju*, a musical instrument. The people who saw it were so surprised that they all believed the *Ju* was just like to be made by ghosts and gods". The Chinese idiom *Gui Fu Shen Gong* 鬼斧神工 comes from this quotation, which means that something is done by gods and ghosts, implying uncanny workmanship which cannot be reached by man. In the same chapter it also states that " I (Yan Yuan 颜渊, one of the Confucius students) crossed a deep river by a ferryboat before, and the man drove the boat like a god," where another Chinese idiom *Cao Zhou Ruo Shen* 操舟若神 comes from. This Chinese idiom literally means driving a boat like a god, now is used to indicate superb skill which has gained through long term hard practice and deep understanding of the rules. You see that SHEN here mainly means superb skill due to marvelous changes, which still relates to gods, ghosts, and spirit.

Besides of *Chuang Tzu, Mencius* also states that "What is worth to love is Good (Shan, 善); what you really possess is True (Xin, 信); that you enrich yourself with Good (Shan) is Beauty (Mei, 美); what is both rich and brilliant is Great (Da, 大); what is great and can be set as an example is Holy (Sheng, 圣); what is holy and too wonderful to be known is SHEN (神)", where SHEN can be clearly interpreted as "wonderful, marvelous, and unpredictable changes".

Xun Tzu also reads that "All of the stars move and rotate in turn, the sun and the moon shine alternately, the four seasons alternate and make the time advance, yin and yang are in great transformations, and wind and rain are bestowed to all things of creation. All things of creation generate from harmony, and mature from

136 Fan Zhen 范缜 (ca. 450-515) was a Chinese philosopher of the Southern Dynasty, remembered today for his treatise *Shén Miè Lùn* 神灭论 or *On the Annihilation of the Spirit.*

nourishment. The process of creating all of the beings is unseen, what can be seen is the result of such a process, which is the so-called SHEN", where SHEN refers to the marvelous, wonderful changes of the nature.

The Book of Changes shows the evolution from religious belief to philosophical thoughts of the ancient Chinese people in both the content and the writing form. Therefore SHEN in *The Book of Changes* bears its all major connotations, such as Heaven God, gods and ghosts, spirits, marvelous changes, etc. The famous quotation that "The unpredictable changes of Yin-Yang are named SHEN" has the following three implications:[137] ① One clue should be reasoned out in order to know and understand the world for the world is so changeable and complicated; ② Intrinsic rules lie in the ever-changing phenomena although the changes and transformations of yin and yang are so subtle and difficult to be known. That is the way to know the world when you grasp the essentials; ③ The rhythms of the changes and transformations are sometimes so sudden and swift that people even have no time to respond them, as stated that "Only SHEN is so swift without hurry, arrives without the need of traveling". Therefore, *The Book of Changes* teaches people to have the awareness of hardness, i.e. "take preventive measures against possible troubles". In Chinese medicine, SHEN-Cultivating is one of the major methods to preserve and promote health. It is thus clear that SHEN in *The Book of Changes* can be understood as the rules and laws of the changes and transformations of all things of creation.

In fact, SHEN bears many meanings. Here I just introduce its three major connotations in classical Chinese texts, which actually all relates to its original meaning, i.e. the god who created all things in the universe. In reality, the three major connotations themselves are not clearly and completely cut from each other, but show an evolving relationship.

8.1.3 SHEN and Psychotherapy in Chinese Medicine

Huang Di's Inner Classic Basic Questions states in the chapter of *Further Discourse on the Five Zang Organs* that "It is not necessary to explain him the medical theory if a patient is superstitious in gods and ghosts; it is not necessary to show him the needling skills if a patient dislikes needling stones; if a patient refuses any treatment, then no matter what the practitioner does, the patient will not get well. This is evidence that healing actually comes from within.", which shows that *Huang Di's Inner Classic* is not superstitious in gods and ghosts, reflecting its rational or scientific approach.

I agree with the point of view that Chinese medicine is evolved from shaman's practice, which can be shown in the original forms of the sinogram 医

137 Li Shunlian. The Connotations of "SHEN" in *The Book of Changes* [J]. Journal of South-Central University for Nationalities (Humanities and Social Sciences). 2003, 23 (5): 66-70.

(medicine or medical practitioner): 毉 and 醫. The sinogram 毉, appearing in *Guan Zi* and *Guang Ya*, is composed of 医 (yi, medicine or medical practitioner) and 巫 (wu, shaman or shamans' practice), thus showing the close relationship between them. *The Origin of Chinese Characters* explains 醫 as "The shamans who specialize in treating illnesses. The upper part means bad postures. Their treating behaviors were driven by wine (酉→酒), therefore following the wine part 酉. Wine was applied to treat illnesses. According to the records of *The Book of Rites* there existed medicinal wine in the Zhou Dynasty (11th century-256 B.C.), and the Shaman Peng 巫彭 was one of the first medical practitioners of the remote antiquity." [138] Actually, Chinese medical practice of nowadays includes Chinese herbal medicine, acupuncture and its related techniques, and consulting like Shaman's practice. In modern times practitioners of Chinese medicine are the only profession which is so close to the ghosts, by which I mean Chinese medicine has been used for treating mental diseases for thousands of years.

Miraculous Pivot reads in the chapter of *Pathogenic Wind* that

Huang Di said, "The causes of which Your Master has said today, all diseased people can know that themselves. But for those who have not encountered any pathogenic influence or have any worry or fear in the mind but suddenly fall ill, what are the reasons for this? Are those only caused by ghosts?"

Qi Bo answered, "The old pathogenic influences retain inside and do not arise. Under the condition that the mind dislikes and admires something, the blood and *qi* are disordered inside and the healthy *qi* and the old pathogenic influences battle together. But the manifestations appear in a very subtle way, which are usually ignored by the patients themselves. That's why those illnesses seem to be caused by ghosts".

Huang Di asked, "But those illnesses can be cured by *Zhu*[139]. What is the reason?"

Qi Bo answered, "In former times, shamans knew what overcome various illnesses, and also knew beforehand where those illnesses came from. Therefore, those illnesses can be terminated by *Zhu*".

From the above questions and answers we can get two points: ① In the ancient times gods and ghosts had been regarded as causes of some illnesses; ② Some illnesses could be cured by *Zhu*, or *Zhu You*, including praying, chanting

138 Lan Fengli. Metaphorizing: The Way to Bridge *The Book of Changes* and Chinese Medicine. In Wallner F.G., Schmidsberger F., Wimmer F.M. (eds). 2010: 178.

139 *Zhu* 祝, or *Zhu You* 祝由, is an old medical practice in China including praying, chanting incantations, holding ceremonies, and shamanism.

incantations, holding ceremonies, and shamanism. The department of *Zhu You* was one of medical departments in ancient China.[140]

As regards to the idea that ghosts could cause illnesses, Xu Dachun 徐大椿 (1693-1771), a famous physician of the Qing Dynasty, discussed it in details in his work *Yi Xuen Yuan Liu Lun* 医学源流论 or *The Origin and Development of [Chinese] Medicine*[141]. The chapter *Bing You Gui Shen Lun* or *On Causation of Illnesses by Ghosts* reads that "If a person's essence and spirit are complete and strong, then no external pathogens dare invade the person. … There is a viewpoint that some illnesses are caused by ghosts. Ignorant and stupid people believe that ghosts can really cause illnesses; while sensible and reasonable people think illnesses manifest their way of development, certainly have nothing to do with ghosts. In reality both are equally wrong. Ghosts are just like pathogenic wind, cold, summer-heat, and dampness. When one's defensive *qi* is in deficiency, he is susceptible to be invaded by cold; when one's nutrient *qi* is in deficiency, he is susceptible to be invaded by heat; when one's spirit *qi* (SHEN QI) is in deficiency, he is susceptible to be invaded by ghosts (or to get mental diseases); because man's spirit is attributed to yang, when yang is in decline, ghosts will break through at this weak point. … *Nan Jing* or *The Classic of Difficult Issues* states that 'one whose yang prostrates sees ghosts'. Therefore, there are some acupoints named after ghosts, such as Ghost Bed, Ghost Room, etc.[142] These acupoints rely on man's spirit *qi* (SHEN QI) to replenish it. … Therefore, invigorate yang to treat cold; nourish yin to treat heat; then replenish spirit (SHEN) to treat ghosts (or mental diseases). … There are also some illnesses caused by phlegm, anxiety, or fright, which should be treated from their root causes. Therefore, sensible and reasonable people will inevitably make a thorough inquiry into everything, and thus have no doubts but evidences. …

---

140 The Imperial Hospitals of the Yuan (1271-1368) and Ming Dynasties (1368-1644) classified medicine into 13 departments, i.e. departments of internal medicine for adults, internal medicine for children, gynecology and obstetrics, skin and external diseases, acupuncture and moxibustion, eye diseases, mouth & teeth diseases, throat diseases, cold attack, bone-setting, wounds by metal weapons, massage, and *Zhu You* (大方脉、小方脉、妇人、疮疡、针灸、眼、口齿、咽喉、伤寒、接骨、金镞、按摩、祝由) in the Ming Dynasty. The Imperial hospital of the Tang Dynasty (618-907) classified medicine into 4 major departments: medicine (including 4 sub-departments, i.e. internal medicine and pediatrics, external medicine, ears, eyes, mouth and teeth, and cupping), acupuncture, massage, and *Zhu You* (医科、针科、按摩科和咒禁科).

141 *Yi Xuen Yuan Liu Lun* or *The Origin and Development of [Chinese] Medicine* 医学源流论 (1757): A collection of 99 essays on Chinese medicine by Xu Dachun 徐大椿 (1693-1771). It has 2 volumes: Vol. 1 one on the vessels, *zang fu* organs, pulse, illnesses, prescriptions and medicinals, and Vol. 2 on therapeutic methods, commentaries on medical books, clinical medicine and other topics. The book presents a lot of author's original creative ideas on Chinese medicine.

142 *Zhen Jiu Da Quan* or *A Complete Book on Acupuncture and Moxibustion* 针灸大全 (1439) by Xu Feng 徐凤 of the Ming Dynasty records *Sun Simiao's Thirteen Ghost Acupoints in Rhyme*, which is also included into national textbooks of nowadays for higher education to train modern acupuncturists in China. See Liang Fanrong. Acupuncture and Moxibustion. Beijing: China Press of Traditional Chinese Medicine, 2005: 415. The 13 ghost acupoints are supposed to treat mania, depression, mental and psychosomatic diseases.

Besides, there are some other illnesses resulting from offending ghosts, which can be cured by praying. Moreover, there are many other reasons for ghosts to offend man, such as ghosts who had been done bad deeds when they were still humans, which may relate to the patient himself or his ancestors by an offence through negligence or deep-seated hatred. … Indisputable proofs exist for such things, which seem as if the Confucians did not accept this. But there are many examples recorded in both Confucian classics and historical books, such as Gong Zi Peng Sheng 公子彭生 and Bo You 伯有. I myself have also witnessed some such cases with my own eyes. Such ghosts can be expelled neither by medicinal herbs, needling stones, nor by praying".

Here is worth to quote another statement from *Huang Di's Inner Classic Basic Questions • On Regulating Meridians* that "Spirit (SHEN) in excess results in continuous laughing; while Spirit (SHEN) in deficiency leads to being grief".

To sum up, Xu Dachun believed that mental diseases are caused by deficiency of SHEN Qi (or spirit *qi*), that the principle of treating mental diseases is to replenish SHEN Qi, and that acupuncture (esp. acupoints named after ghost), Chinese herbal medicine, praying and consulting can be used to treat mental diseases.

In the chapter on *Moving Essence and Changing Qi* of *Huang Di's Inner Classic Basic Questions,* it reads that

Huang Di asked, "I have heard that in ancient times, when practitioners treated diseases, they just moved the essence and changed the *qi* by *Zhu You*. While nowadays, when practitioners treat diseases, they employ medicinal herbs to treat the interior and use needling stones to treat the exterior, and as a result, some diseases are cured while others are not cured. Why is this?"

Qi Bo answered, "People of the remote antiquity lived among animals, moved and became active to fend off the cold in winter, and stayed in shade places to escape the heat in summer. Internally, their minds were calm and peaceful without any desire or admiration; externally, their bodies were not over-stressed without any suffering. That's a time without any greed or fame or gain, which prevented the pathogens from invading. Therefore, they did not need either medicinal herb to treat their interior or needling stone to treat their exterior. When they contracted diseases, *Zhu You* could move the essence and thus cure diseases. However, people of nowadays are different from those of the remote antiquity. Internally, their minds are affected by worries and sufferings; externally, their bodies are harmed by hard work and heavy labor. Besides, they do not follow the rules of the four seasons, oppose the needs against cold and summer-heat, therefore, they are susceptible to the invasion of pathogenic wind. The pathogens are present from the morning till the evening; internally, they reach the five *zang* organs, the bones and the marrows; externally, they harm the orifices, the muscles and the skins. Therefore, minor diseases will inevitably develop into serious ones; serious diseases will certainly lead to death. That's why *Zhu You* can not terminate a disease any more".

Based on the above classical texts, some related points can be summed up as follows: ① Chinese medicine is not superstitious in ghosts and gods, which are usually used as metaphors, reflecting its rational or scientific approach; ② Deficiency or excess of Man's spirit *qi* (SHEN QI) is one of the major causes of mental diseases; ③ *Zhou You* had been a kind of medical practice from the remote antiquity until at least Ming Dynasty. But its indications were very different in different times. Since there are medical records in written forms, *Zhu You* had been mainly supposed to treat mental diseases; ④ The 13 acupoints named after Ghost have been used up till today to treat mania, depression, mental and psychosomatic diseases; ⑤Patient's self-confidence in healing his illness is of vital significance for his recovery.

8.2 Shape, Pronunciation and Meaning: From "Xu 需" to "Ru 儒"

8.2.1 Philosophical School of Confucius: Why Not "Kong 孔" School Nor "Ren 仁" School But "Ru 儒" School

Confucianism, the philosophical school of Confucius, exerts far-reaching, deep-going, and great influences on almost every aspect of Chinese culture. Here Confucianism suggests that it seems to be named after the founder Confucius. But actually, the original Chinese for Confucianism is "Ru 儒" school not "Kong 孔" school. This is quite unique among various philosophical schools of Pre-Qin Days before 221 B.C., which are named after either the founder's name, such as Mohism named after its founder Mo Tzu, or its core idea, such as Taoism named after its core idea Tao. In this case, the philosophical school of Confucius should have been named as either "Kong 孔 school" or "Ren 仁"[143] school not "Ru 儒" school. But why it is not "Kong 孔" school nor "Ren 仁" school but "Ru 儒" school?

Is Confucius the founder of Confucianism? The answer reads Yes and No! Confucianism, in Chinese, is "The 'Ru 儒' school". "Ru 儒" was a title of job for some people who had their origin in the literati responsible for holding traditional ceremonies based on traditional history, etc.. Confucius was one of those *Ru*, but he was not the first *Ru*. However, in his period, many people did not care traditions anymore. Confucius wanted to resume the tradition. Confucius did want to not only resume this Chinese (Early Zhou) tradition, but he also gave some new connotations and interpretations to this tradition. The new interpretations from him are mainly related to moral philosophy. In this sense, Confucius is the founder of Confucianism.

143 Ren or Benevolence 仁 is the core idea of Confucianism.

8.2.2 Shape: From "Xu 需" to "Ru 儒"

"Xu 需" originated from primitive worship of Thunder and Lightening. "Xu 需", written as  in bronze script and  in lesser seal script, an associative compound, indicates a human under rain， and reflects the ceremony of praying for rain when offering sacrifices to gods of Thunder and Lightening. The 而 in the regular script 需 is possibly a mistaken or wrong form of 天.

"Xu 需" originally was used as both a noun and a verb, and thus bears two meanings: one refers to female shamans who were responsible for offering sacrifices to Thunder and Lightening by burning to pray for rainfall, which had been transformed into "Ru 儒" by strengthening the meaning of "Ren 人" or human, the lower part of 需, by supplementing the signific 亻; the other has been used as a verb up till today, means "wait for, need".

8.2.3 Pronunciation: From "Xu 需" to "Ru 儒"

The pronunciation of "Xu 需" was in the line of Xin-Mu-Hou in ancient times; while that of "Ru 儒" was in the line of Ri-Mu-Hou in ancient times. The sinogram 儒 shares one meaning of 需, but their initial consonants of their syllables are different. In bronze scripts, 需, actually, kept these two pronunciations: Xin-Mu and Ni- Mu, the prototype of Ri Mu. "需 pronounced as Ni-Mu" can be inferred from its interchangeable uses, e.g. "To use fully grown good rice and glutinous (common) sorghum 用成米隹稻需粱", where 需 was used for 糯; "The King should not listen to his report if the messenger is strong, while the King should follow his advices if the messenger is weak 其健者来使，则王勿听其事；其需弱者来使，则王必听之", where 需 was used for 懦. The sinograms 糯 and 懦, the proper sinograms of 需, both were pronounced as in the line of Ni-Mu.

Why did "Xu 需" bear the two different initial consonants? This resulted from diachronic evolution in pronunciations of primitive Chinese languages, i.e., first N-, then S-, during which the position of the pronunciation of the initial consonants moved forward. The evolution process of the pronunciation of "Xu 需" went first from Ni Mu, then to Ri Mu, then gradually to Xin Mu.

It is thus clear that "Xu 需" had two pronunciations and two corresponding meanings in ancient times. In order to distinguish them from each other, "Xu 需" pronounced in the line of Ni-Mu has been written as 儒 by supplementing a human radical 亻, and thereafter has been used as a noun; while 需 pronounced in the line of Xin-Mu keeps its original writing from, and mainly used as a verb, means "wait for, need".[144]

---

144 Xu Shan. "The Origin of Ru" from www.confuchina.com.

8.2.4 Meaning: From "Xu 需" to "Ru 儒"

Generally speaking, the meanings of a certain language occur in the following order: first, an event at a certain time in a certain place, i.e. its natural, cultural meaning; then, its naming motivation for the combination of meaning and pronunciation, i.e. why this pronunciation can convey this meaning or why this meaning can bear this pronunciation; then, meanings and shapes of sinograms when writing forms came out; finally, systematizing and carding actual meanings of sinograms or words in ancient classical texts.

8.2.4.1 Natural-Cultural Meaning of "Xu 需"

"Xu 需" originated from primitive worship of Thunder and Lightening in the remote antiquity. The primitive way of offering sacrifices to Thunder and Lightening was "Liao Ji 燎祭" or Burning[145], and its direct purpose was praying for rain. The cultural background of "Xu 需" was primitive worship of Thunder and Lightening in the remote antiquity.

The shape of "Xu 需" reflects such a ceremony of praying for rain. As explained before, "Xu 需", an associative compound, shows a human under rain, and reflects the ceremony of praying for rain when offering sacrifices to gods of Thunder and Lightening.

Therefore, the natural-cultural meaning of "Xu 需" is "a ceremony of praying for rain".

8.2.4.2Naming Motivation of "Xu 需"

The prototype of 需's pronunciation was "Na", later on its vowel evolved into 'Aou'. As regards to reconstruction of 需's naming motivation, that's actually a question of why one segment of the ceremonies of offering sacrifices to Thunder and Lightening was expressed with the pronunciation "Na". You cannot find the answer through inquiring into the relationships among the elements of 需. This question can only be answered in the ancestry of Chinese language.

One of the meanings of the primitive pronunciation "Na" was "female", which in modern Chinese is written as 女, pronounced as NÜ. "女, NÜ" (Female) comes from the pronunciation line of NI MU YÜ of the remote antiquity. *The Origin of Chinese Characters* reads that "女 NÜ refers to the females". , the oracle script of 女, is an image of a human being kneeling down with one's hands before the chest.

The prototype of 需's pronunciation was "na", showing that its meaning originated from or was derived from "女 NÜ". Actually, the original meaning of

145 "Liao Ji 燎祭" or Burning: one of the ancient ceremonies for offering sacrifices to gods or ancestors, in which jades, silks, and beasts slaughtered for sacrifice were put on the rick, and were burnt to offer sacrifices.

需 was the female who offered sacrifices or held ceremonies of offering sacrifices to Thunder and Lightening.

The pronunciation of "巫 WU" also originated from "女 NÜ" , whose original meaning was witch, sorceress, or female shaman.

8.2.4.3"Xu 需" in Ancient Classical Chinese Texts

① Hexagram "Xu 需" in *The Book of Changes*

The hexagram[146] *Xu* is the No. 5 in *The Book of Changes,* which can be translated into Waiting, Nourishment, or Attendance. The image of *Xu* is composed of two trigrams: the upper *Kan*, Water or Rain ☵, and the lower *Qian*, Heaven ☰, just like the original meaning of the sinogram "praying for rain from the heaven". When you pray for rain, you have to wait; when rain comes it can provide nourishment for the beings on the earth; when a ceremony of praying for rain was holding, one should attend the ceremony. Now you can understand why "Xu 需" is translated into Waiting, Nourishment, or Attendance.

In *The Book of Changes,* the image reads that "Clouds rise up to heaven, which is the image of *Xu* or WAITING". The interpretation reads that "It is going to rain, just needs some time".

The description of the hexagram reads that

"Nine at the beginning means: waiting in the meadow. It furthers one to abide in what endures. No blame.

"Nine in the second place means: waiting on the sand. There is some gossip. The end brings good fortune.

"Nine in the third place means: waiting in the mud. Brings about the arrival of the enemy.

"Six in the fourth place means: waiting in blood. Get out of the pit.

"Nine in the fifth place means: waiting at meat and drink. Perseverance brings good fortune.

"Six at the top means: one falls into the pit. Three uninvited guests arrive. Honor them, and in the end there will be good fortune".[147]

The "Xu 需" here all refers to its original meaning "praying for the rain", of course WAITING was necessary when you prayed for the rain. The description of the hexagram shows that different places of praying for rain have different implications: waiting in the meadow and the sand indicates lucky; while waiting in the mud or blood unlucky.

146 A hexagram is a figure composed of six stacked horizontal lines (爻 yáo), where each line is either Yang (an unbroken, solid line, signified with "nine"), or Yin (broken, an open line with a gap in the center, signified with "six"). The hexagram lines are traditionally counted from the bottom up, so the lowest line is considered line 1 while the top line is line 6. Hexagrams are formed by combining the original eight trigrams in different combinations. Each hexagram is accompanied with a description, often cryptic, akin to parables. Each line in every hexagram is also given a similar description.

147 Wilhelm, Baynes. 1997: 25-27.

② "Xu 需" in *Zuo's Spring Autumn Annals*

In the chapter of *The Sixth Year of Aigong's Reign of Zuo's Spring Autumn Annals*, it reads that "I have thought it over. The best way is to kill them all. Waiting (XU, 需) is an unwise decision".[148]

③ "Xu 需" in *The Origin of Chinese Characters*

The Origin of Chinese Characters reads that "Xu 需, follows 雨 (Rain) and is pronounced as Er (而); means 'encounter rain, and then stop and wait '". According to the above discussion, the interpretation of 需's shape and meaning in *The Origin of Chinese Characters* is wrong.

8.2.4.4 The Noun Use of "Xu 需" and "Ru 儒"

"Xu 需" as a noun was written as "Ru 儒", whose original meaning is the person who offered sacrifices for the purpose of praying for rain. *The Origin of Words* (辞源) explains the earliest meaning of "Ru 儒" in classical texts as "persons who separated from witches, historians, prayers, and visionaries, also known as *Ru* scholars (Shu Shi, 术士), later on in a broad sense, refers to scholars (Xue Zhe, 学者)".

In the chapter of *Zhong Zai* of *Tian Guan* of *The Book of Rites* 周礼.天官.冢宰, it reads that "*Ru* scholars (Ru, 儒) gained people's support with their Tao ". Its Annotation reads that "Ru 儒, who educated people with six arts (rites, music, shooting, riding, books, mathematics) in the feudal princes".

In *The Analects of Confucius,* Confucius said to Zi Xia, "You should be a noble-minded 'Ru 儒', not just be a small person who takes 'Ru 儒' as his profession". "Ru 儒" referred to a profession of Zhou Dynasty, who had the knowledge of six arts (rites, music, shooting, riding, books, mathematics) and was responsible for education and rites, i.e. holding ceremonies.

When Confucius was alive, his thoughts were not popular, and there were no such names as "Ru 儒 school" or "Ru 儒 learning". Confucius was regarded as the founder of "Ru 儒 school" by the later generations for "RU 儒" was his profession he occupied himself in. Therefore it is different from other philosophical thoughts of schools, which were named after the surname of its founder like Mohism by Mo Tzu, or its core idea like Taoism of Lao Tzu and Chuang Tzu.

The Analects of Confucius talks more on "Li 礼 (ceremony or rite)" and "Ren 仁 (benevolence, love, humanity)" than others. Confucius devoted his late life to systematizing ancient Chinese classics and education, and thus studied and disseminated the spirit of Chinese culture. The highest form of the spirit of Chinese culture was "Li 礼 (ceremony or rite)", which ranked the first in the

148 The translation accords with the modern Chinese version by Yang Bojun. See Yang Bojun, Xu Ti. Zuo's Spring Autumn Annals in Modern Chinese. Changsha: Yuelu Book Company, 1993.

teaching of six arts. At the same time, Confucius devoted his major efforts to expounding and propagating “Ren 仁 (benevolence, love, humanity)”, which can make good interpersonal relationships and thus help to realize the social order with “Li 礼 (ceremony or rite)”. His professional spirit focuses on “Li 礼 (ceremony or rite)”, and so the “Ru 儒” school (Confucianism) in this sense can be traced to the origin of the ceremony of worship of thunder and lightening in the primitive society, and forms a direct line of succession with the original meaning of “Ru 儒”. The prototype of “Ru 儒” was a product of man worshiping the nature, from which a set of sacrificial rites were derived. The set of sacrificial rites influenced all the aspects of the social life of that time. The sense of gods and ghosts of Confucius’s time had been fading away, but the cultural spirit originating from offering sacrifices to gods in the primitive society was still going on with the norm of “Li 礼 (ceremony or rite)” and was passed on with the practice of “Ru 儒”. As regards to return and restoration of traditional “Li 礼 (ceremony or rite)” and deep-going understanding of “Ren 仁 (benevolence, love, humanity)” in the human nature, Confucius fully deserves the first one in the history of Chinese culture to serve as a link between past and future.

In one word, the evolution from “Xu 需” to “Ru 儒” reflects deep influences of Worship of Thunder and Lightening on Chinese Culture.

Language is an outcome of the culture.

- Claude Levi Strauss

Language is redefined as "*the means and process of man cognizing, understanding and stating the world*".

- Pan Wenguo

9 Reflections of Philosophy of Chinese Medicine in Chinese Characters

Chinese philosophy and science (including Chinese medicine) presupposes Chinese Culture. Classical Chinese philosophy focuses on the study of "Tao", probing into the "Tao of the Universe" and the "Tao of Man" from various perspectives. Philosophy of Chinese medicine is an important component part of Classical Chinese philosophy, and also an original philosophy of science originated from Chinese culture, which produces Classical Chinese science. In this chapter I would like to reflect philosophy of Chinese medicine in Chinese characters from its ontology, methodology, and ultimate aim, and concludes that Chinese medicine can be correctly and fully understood in the network of intercultural philosophy.

Introduction

The word "philosophy" is of Greek origin "φιλοσοφία, *philosophía*", composed of "philien (love)" and "sophia (wisdom)", and so originally means "to love wisdom". Philosophy is defined as "the rational investigation of the truths and principles of being, knowledge, or conduct". [149] Chinese translation of "philosophy" is 哲学 (zhe xue), and came into Chinese vocabulary about 100 years ago via translation. But Chinese philosophy evolved from the remote antiquity - the late period of patrilineal clan commune, and formed in the Shang-Zhou dynasties (ca.1600-221B.C.), so has at least over 3,000 years of history. Classical Chinese philosophy, in brief, focuses on the study of "Tao", probing into the "Tao of the Universe" and the "Tao of Man" from various angles.

Philosophy is in principle a product of a specific culture, including a specific cultural need and cultural convictions based on philosophy, and this statement is valid for all forms of philosophy, including European philosophy and Chinese philosophy. Pointedly speaking, European philosophy and science (science emerges from philosophy, historically seen) presupposes necessarily European culture; while Chinese philosophy and science presupposes Chinese Culture.[150]

149 Webster's Encyclopaedic Unabridged Dictionary of the English Language (New Revised Edition) [Z]. 1994: 1082.

150 Wallner, Friedrich G. Intercultural Philosophy: The Viennese Program. In Wallner F.G., Schmidsberger F. & Wimmer W.F. (eds). 2010: 13-20.

I support the viewpoint that the philosophy, science, and medicine are pluralistic just like the cultures are diverse. China has her own unique culture, philosophy, science, and medicine, which are very different from that of the West. Chinese medicine, the only live form and also the representative of classical Chinese sciences, no doubt presupposes Chinese philosophy and Chinese culture.

9.1 Cultural Connotations of Philosophy of Chinese Medicine

Philosophy of Chinese medicine is an important component part of Chinese philosophy, and also an original philosophy of science from Chinese culture.

9.1.1 Philosophy of Chinese Medicine: An Important Component Part of Chinese Philosophy

Chinese medicine emerges and develops in the soil of Chinese classical culture, of which Chinese philosophy is the core, and so in essence Chinese medicine presupposes Chinese philosophy. It can be easily seen from that *Qi*, Yin-Yang, and five phases, the major concepts of the philosophical structure of Chinese medicine, all underwent the evolution from philosophy to medicine through metaphorizing.[151]

Actually, philosophy of Chinese medicine is in essence the same as Chinese philosophy, in specific, is mainly the application of the philosophy of *The Book of Changes*, of Taoist School in the field of Chinese medicine, which demonstrates the great significance of cultural and philosophical dependency of Chinese medicine. Philosophically speaking, *The Book of Changes*, *Lao Tzu*, and *Huang Di's Inner Classic* present with the systematic intimate relationship with Tao as the focus: *The Book of Changes* lays the philosophical foundation for Tao of all kinds; *Lao Tzu* proposes that Tao abides by the nature; and *Huang Di's Inner Classic* advocates that medicine abides by Tao, i.e. the nature.

9.1.1.1 *Tian Ren He Yi:* the Philosophical Foundation for Tao of All Kinds

The theme of Chinese philosophy is to probe into the relationship between the "universe and man", or the relationship between "the Way of Universe and the Way of Man", regarding the Universe as Man's Universe and Man as Universe's Man.[152]

The Book of Changes establishes *Tian Ren He Yi* 天人合一 or the Universe and Man uniting and resembling each other by making a farfetched comparison between them. It states that "In the remote antiquity when Fu Xi 伏羲 ruled the

151 Note: Metaphorizing: *Qu Xiang Bi Lei* is the methodology to form metaphors in Chinese medicine, therefore I propose that *Qu Xiang Bi Lei* is the metaphorizing process and the way to form metaphors in Chinese medicine. See Part 3 The Importance of Metaphors in Chinese Medicine for details.

152 Note: *Tian* in *Tian* Dao and *Ren* Dao or *Tian Ren He Yi* is usually translated into Heaven, but actually not the same as in the West, the better translation is Universe.

country, he raised his head to observe images on the heaven, bowed his head to observe phenomena on the earth, observed images of birds and beasts and those of the earth, took near images from man and far images of other things from the universe, on the basis of which he then started to make the Eight Trigrams to illustrate the phenomena.", which lays the philosophical foundation for Tao of all kinds in Chinese culture and medicine, which formed through metaphorizing.

Here the formation of the Tao of Chinese medicine is the case in point. So, how the Tao of Chinese medicine formed? Or what is the relationship between *The Book of Changes* and Chinese medicine – one deals with *Xiang Shu* (images and numbers, 象数) and their implicit meanings in the universe, while the other talks about health and illnesses of man? Actually they are talking about the same thing in essence by applying metaphors or metaphorizing: life – one on the life of the cosmos and the other on the life of man. Both are open systems, both are communicated with and related to each other, and both should be in a state of harmony in itself and with the other, otherwise problems or illnesses will ensue, which is radically different from the strict divisions between the life and the inanimate, the subject and the object, the man and the nature etc. in the Western culture. Maybe it is fantastic for the Westerners that *The Book of Changes* and Chinese medicine do not reduce life or being to something material like cells, proteins, genes, etc., instead they understand life or being by establishing and interpreting something symbolic like *gua* 卦 and *yao* 爻, Qi, yin and yang, the eight trigrams, the five phases, the images and numbers, the visceral image, and so on.

It's worth to note that most of the thinking ways of Chinese medicine originate from *The Book of Changes* and are established through metaphorizing:

① The Thinking Way of *Xiang Shu* (images and numbers, 象数): The *Zang Xiang* (Visceral Image, 藏象) theory is established on the basis of elementary understanding of the organs to explain physiological functions of man through *Qu Xiang Bi Lei* (taking image and analogizing, 取象比类); and "pattern identification and treatment" is set up by summarizing and generalizing various symptoms and signs into a certain "pattern image" also through *Qu Xiang Bi Lei.*

② The Thinking Way of *Bian Yi* (changing, 变易): Chinese medicine regards life, health and illnesses as constantly changing processes, and stresses not only the transmission and transformation of illnesses, but also institutes corresponding treatments to meet the changes.

③ The Thinking Way of Holistic Approach: *The Book of Changes* establishes *Tian Ren He Yi* 天人合一 or the Universe and Man Uniting and Resembling each other, on the basis of which the theoretical system of Chinese medicine has formed. Chinese medicine regards man as an organic whole, and also studies the physiology and pathology of man in the unity and mutual relations of man, nature and society, thereby administers corresponding healthcare methods.

To sum up, *Tian Ren He Yi* is the philosophical foundation for Tao of all kinds in Chinese culture and science. Here medicine is the case in point. Metaphorizing is the way to bridge the thinking ways and metaphors of *The Book of Changes* and Chinese medicine such as "—" and "- -" and yin-yang, the eight trigrams and the five phases, the five phases and the visceral image, etc.[153], and the way to establish the Tao of Chinese medicine.

9.1.1.2 Tao 道: The Way of the Nature and Medicine

"*Huang Di's Inner Classic* is the highest authority on philosophy of Chinese medicine, and also one of the most important classics on Taoism of Chinese philosophy".[154] Taoist school focuses on the study of "Tao", and *Lao Tzu* and *Chuang Tzu* are the most important classics of Taoist philosophy.

Tao 道 was originally written as "", following the part of "辵", which actually shows an image of a man walking on a way with his eyes big open, metaphorizing "the only way you must follow or take in order to go ahead" . Its original meaning is explained in *The Origin of Chinese Characters* as "the way to walk", which indicates the direction for the walker, is the route to a certain destination, and then is metapharized to mean law, rule, or principle. Besides, Tao 道 in the ancient times had several other extended meanings: "thinking system or theory" such as in *The Analects of Confucius • Living in brotherliness* that "My **thinking system** is run through by a central idea"; "to govern or manage" explained in *Guang Ya • Shi Gu* 广雅 • 释诂; "way or method" such as in *Shang Jun Shu* or *The Book of Shang Yang's Ideas* that "There is not just one **way** to govern the society". Also, the sinogram 道 resembles the shape of 首 head, thereby bearing the meaning of start or beginning. You see that Tao 道 bears so many meanings, therefore, as a fundamental philosophical concept; its connotations are deep, subtle and complicated.

It is *Lao Tzu* that discusses Tao as an abstract concept and endows it with a philosophical meaning of "embracing all". *Lao Tzu· Chapter 25* states that "Therefore, Tao is great. Heaven is great. Earth is great. Man is great. In the universe, there are four great things, and man is one of them. Man abides by the earth. Earth abides by the heaven. Heaven abides by Tao. Tao abides by the nature"; The Chapter 42 states that "Tao begets One (*Qi*). One begets Two (Yin-Yang). Two begets Three (the integration of Yin and Yang). Three begets all things. All things carry Yin and embrace Yang, where the central and harmonious *Qi* makes them in harmony", which shows the generation of all things in the universe from Tao (*Wu* 无 or Non-Being) to all things (*You* 有 or Being). That

153 Lan Fengli. Metaphorizing: the Way to Bridge *The Book of Changes* and Chinese Medicine. In Wallner F.G., Schmidsberger F. & Wimmer W.F. (eds). 2010: 177-192.

154 Ni, Maoshing. 1995: Back-Cover. I think here Taoism refers to Taoist School not Taoist Religion. See "Part 2 Fundamental Concepts of Classical Chinese Philosophy" for their differences.

is to say, Tao is the origin of all things in the universe and the Way which must be observed by all.

In Chinese medicine, *Huang Di's Inner Classic* states that "Yin and yang are the Tao or Way of the heaven and earth, the fundamental principles of the myriad things, the origin of all changes and transformations, the root of generating and killing, the palace of man's spirit" in *Basic Questions• Comprehensive Discourse on Images Corresponding to Yin-Yang.*[155] It also states that "Of all things in between the heaven and earth, nothing is more precious than man. Man lives on the *Qi* in between the heaven and earth, and grows in accordance with the law of the seasons" in *Basic Questions• Discourse on Protecting Life and Preserving Physical Appearance*. *The Origin of Chinese Characters·Man Part* also states that "Man is the most valuable being in between the heaven and earth".

Thereby, it can be seen from the above quotations that "Heaven", "Earth", and "Man" are independent from and closely related to each other, and they compose a whole system, in which man plays the leading role; and that the thinking way of the "heaven-earth-man" in *Lao Tzu* embodies the thinking way of the universe, which is specified in the *Inner Classic* as the thinking way of the Chinese medicine, which shows that the great progress of natural philosophy in the aspect of the nature replacing the God. In *Lao Tzu*, Tao abides by the nature; In the *Inner Classic*, medicine abides by the Tao; In essence, medicine abides by the nature. Holistic approach and individualized treatment based on pattern identification with the aim for the central and harmonious state in health care and disease treatment are all embodied in *Lao Tzu* and *the Inner Classic.*

Chuang Tzu carries on *Lao Tzu*'s Tao of the nature, and advocates that man was born in between the heaven and the earth, and so should follow the way of the nature, i.e. the way of Yin-Yang and the seasons, in health care. It also states the way of cultivating the spirit - "to do nothing that is left undone" and "to be indifferent to any fame or gain". These ideas are all embodied in the *Inner Classic.*[156] Therefore, Tao abides by the nature, and medicine abides by Tao, and so medicine abides by the nature, which is the Tao of Chinese medicine.

9.1.2 Philosophy of Chinese Medicine: An Original Philosophy of Science Originated from Chinese Culture

There is a major misunderstanding that Chinese philosophy mainly discusses society, politics, and ethics, but neglects the nature. Actually, agriculture, astronomy, geography, mathematics, and medicine of the ancient China were very

---

155 Note: The translations of the quotations from *Huang Di Nei Jing Su Wen* all accord with Guo Aichun's interpretation in his book *Textual Criticisms, Annotations, Modern Language Interpretation of Huang Di Nei Jing Su Wen* (2nd Ed.), published by Tianjin Science and Technology Press (Tianjin, China) in 1999.

156 See the chapters of *Tian Shi* 天适 and *Ke Yi* 刻意 of *Chuang Tzu* 庄子, and the chapter *Discourse on the Prenatal True Qi of the Remote Antiquity* of *Basic Questions* 素问 • 上古天真论 for more details.

advanced, and even more advanced than that of the West esp. before 15th century. That is to say, Chinese philosophy of the nature and life in probing into the relationship between the Universe and Man produced all of the classical Chinese natural sciences, which worked very well before or even have worked quite well until today. For example, Du Jiang Yan 都江堰, the water control and irrigation dam, which has been listed in the World Inheritance Name List and was designed and built in accordance with the classical scientific ideas, has been working so well in preventing serious flooding for over 2,000 years, and even survives the Sichuan Earthquake in 2008; While cracks appeared in a modern big dam made of concrete mixer after the earthquake in 2008, which was designed and built nowadays according to the modern science. So, it's clear that classical Chinese sciences have their own unique values.

Today, only Chinese medicine survives ever after facing the serious challenges from Western medicine, and almost all of the other Chinese classical natural sciences like agriculture, astronomy, geography, and mathematics etc. have declined and are totally replaced by the corresponding Western natural sciences. It is a great pity. But the fact also indicates philosophy of Chinese science fits much better with the living system than with the other systems, and the living system is the only one which is always in a state of constant changing and transforming.

There is a common Chinese misinterpretation of philosophy of Chinese medicine, which is extensively written into the textbooks of Chinese medicine for higher education of China. That is, Chinese medicine is established on the rudimentary materialism and dialects, which actually results from understanding Chinese medicine with the framework of Western philosophy. Thereby, some scholars believe that Chinese medicine still lingers in the stage of pre-science or infancy of modern science, and advance that Chinese medicine must get rid of its philosophical concepts like *Qi*, yin-yang, five phases if it needs to be modernized in the so-called scientific way. Actually, it's totally wrong. Chinese medicine will definitely lose its strong points if it is modernized and studied in this way.

Chinese medicine must be rationale or scientific for it has worked so well in prevention and treatment of so many illnesses for thousands of years. The point is that Chinese medicine goes closer to humanities rather than science in the common Western sense, and it's based on an original philosophy of science originated from Chinese culture.

Then, how to define philosophy of Chinese medicine? It is a kind of original philosophy of science originated from Chinese culture with the focus on *Xiang* 象 (phenomena and images) and relationships. It stresses phenomena, images, and functions more than morphological structures, stresses relationships among the beings esp. among the live man, the nature and the society more than causality (whys), stresses integration more than separation, stresses the constant changes and transformations more than unchanged features, and stresses perceptual understanding more than quantified measurement, etc. So philosophy of Chinese medicine is not at all rudimentary materialism for materialism will definitely lead to reductionism; and yin-yang theory emphasizes phenomena and images (such as the images corresponding to yin-yang) and dynamic harmony in a whole system, while dichotomy stresses separation and opposition, and so philosophy of Chinese medicine is not at all rudimentary dialectics.

What philosophy of Chinese medicine mainly deals with is the Tao, *Qi*-Yin-Yang-Five Phases, thinking way, methodology, perspectives on life, disease, and treatment of Chinese medicine, which are applied to construct the theoretical system of Chinese medicine, to expound the physiology (normal state, "ping 平") and pathology (diseased states, "bing 病") of man, and to guide diagnosis and treatment of illnesses. Thereby, philosophy and medical knowledge, i.e. the basic correct understanding of the being (composed of body and mind), health and illnesses are integrated into an organic whole, i.e. Chinese medicine, a unique medical system originated from Chinese culture. So, we can say that Chinese medicine is the product of the integration of science (medical knowledge) and culture (its philosophical foundation), bearing both cultural and scientific connotations.

Why do the majors of Chinese medicine always go back to the Four Great Classics of 2,000 years ago? That is to say, why is there no breakthrough but only development and enrichment since the establishment of the knowledge system? Why has Chinese medicine not been developed along the similar procedure to Western medicine? The answer is that the philosophy of Chinese medicine makes the system of Chinese medicine into a self-contained and fruitful paradigm, which can be enriched and developed in the same framework – *Qu Xiang Bi Lei* guided by *Tian Ren He Yi* established at that time, and survive up till today. You can get clearer idea from the following Table.

Heart	*Hippocratic Corpus*[157]	*Huang Di Nei Jing*[158]
General Understanding	Two atriums and two ventricles;	The organ as a Monarch, from which spirit originates; the root of life, the seat of the spirit; the greater yang within yang;
Main Functions	The right atrium provides lungs with blood, accepts air from lungs, exchanges air;	Rules the body's blood and vessels; opens into the tongue; it's brilliance manifests in the face;
Relations to Others	There is only air, no blood in the left atrium; the left atrium is the location of intrinsic heat.	South, summer, hot & fire, bitter, red, *zheng*, elation, laughing, and the Heart, etc. are all attributed to fire in the five elemental phases; the heart (fire) engenders the spleen (earth).
Outcome	A Morphological Heart Organ: Focuses on the morphological structure of the heart, thus providing direction, possibilities and leaving space for the further study on its anatomical structure and corresponding physiological functions	A Heart Complex System: Separates "Heart" from the organ "Heart" in anatomical sense, integrates "Heart" with the theories of Yin-Yang and Five Phases, social phenomena (Monarch), natural phenomena (season, direction, climate, flavor, color), and other aspects of man (spirit, joy, tongue, face, spleen) into "A Heart Complex System
Analysis	Guides Western medicine to develop on the philosophical foundation of reductionism, mechanism and dichotomy, thus embodying the analytical thinking	Establishes the Visceral Image theory, embodying the holistic approach "Four Seasons - Five *Zang* Organs – Yin-Yang" guided by "Universe and Man Uniting and Resembling Each Other"
Conclusion	Western Medicine continuously refreshes itself because of the application of advanced scientific technology and instruments (tools)	Chinese Medicine has formed a self-contained fruitful paradigm, so can be enriched and developed in the same framework - *Qu Xiang Bi Lei* guided by *Tian Ren He Yi* established about 2,000 years ago, survive up till today.

Table 5 *Different Views of Heart in Hippocratic Corpus and Huang Di Nei Jing*[159]

157 Note: Here the contents from *Hippocratic Corpus* are translated into English from the Chinese translation.

158 *Huang Di Nei Jing* came out at about the same time as *Hippocratic Corpus* about 2,000 years ago. As Unschuld said in "Prefatory Remarks" of "HUANG Di NEI JING SU WEN: Nature, Knowledge, Imagery in an Ancient Chinese Medical Text" (University of California Press, 2003: IX) that it "plays a role in Chinese medical history comparable to that of the Hippocratic writings in ancient Europe. Progress and significant paradigm changes have reduced Hippocrates to the honored originators of a tradition that has become obsolete. In contrast, many practitioners of Chinese medicine still consider the *Su Wen* a valuable source of theoretical inspiration and practical knowledge in modern clinical settings. "

159 Lan Fengli. Intercultural Philosophy and Chinese Medicine: Reflections of Philosophy of Chinese Medicine in Chinese Language. In Wallner F. G., Lan Fengli, Jandl M.J (eds.). 2011: 14-34.

Now I would like to take *Qi* 气, *Xiang* 象, and *He* 和 to illustrate the ontology, the methodology, and the ultimate aim of philosophy of Chinese medicine.

9.2 *Qi* 气 Explains Ontology of Philosophy of Chinese Medicine

Chinese philosophy applies the concept of *Qi* to explain the nature of existence. *The Origin of Chinese Characters • Qi Part* states that "*Qi* refers to thin, floating clouds. The sinogram 气 [160] is a pictograph." The sinogram 气 in *Jia Gu Wen* 甲骨文, the oracle inscription of the Shang Dynasty (ca. 16th-11th century B.C.), was written as "", which resembles air current, evaporating and rising, whose image is just like cloud, will disappear very soon and become invisible. Therefore, *Qi* is invisible and formless, exists everywhere, can be gathered into a form, for instance, *Qi* can be condensed into water.

Soon afterwards, the *Qi* which surrounds and congests the Man's space was abstracted into the *Qi* which bears a philosophical sense. Philosophers of the Spring Autumn and Warring States Periods (770-221B.C.) believed that *Qi* is the basic ingredient constituting the world, and also the basic ingredient constituting the Man and that everything in the universe comes into being by the movement and mutation of *Qi*, as stated in *The Book of Changes* "everything is transformed and generated by the enshrouding [*Qi*] of the heaven and earth".

The Book of Changes establishes *Tian Ren He Yi* 天人合一 or the Universe and Man Uniting and Resembling Each Other by making a farfetched comparison between them. *Tian Ren He Yi* actually indicates that the Universe and the Man constitute in the same way, i.e. being composed of the same ingredient – *Qi* in the same order. Therefore, *Qi* becomes the foundation of *Tian Ren He Yi*.

Later on, ancient Chinese medical experts introduced "*Qi*" into the medical field at the right moment. In the time of *Huang Di's Inner Classic*, "*Qi*" is regarded not only as the basic ingredient constituting the world, but also as the basic ingredient constituting the Man which can be transformed into blood, essence, and body fluid, etc., and the normal functional activities of the life which is governed by "*Qi*" is known as *Shen* or spirit.

According to *A Concise Dictionary of Chinese Medicine*, *Qi* in Chinese medicine bears the following meanings: ① nutritious, essential substance flowing inside the body, such as food *qi*, breathed air; ② functional activities of the *zang fu* organs in a general sense, such as visceral *Qi*, i.e, the functional activities of the *zang fu* organs; *Qi* can also be classified into original *Qi*, nutritive *Qi*, defensive

160 The sinogram **氣** is not the original form of 气 but a mistake during the evolution of Chinese characters, which means "feed and grain for the guests" according to *The Origin of Chinese Characters • Rice Part.*

Qi, pectoral *Qi*, etc. according to its source, distribution, and function; ③ the location or stage of pattern identification of warm diseases.[161]

That is to say, *Qi* in philosophy of Chinese medicine is to make man become man, and the logic function implied in the *Wei* (Defense) – *Qi* – *Ying* (Nutrient) – Blood Pattern Identification for treatment of warm diseases is the condition of processes and activities of life, i.e. *Qi* is the condition for what it is conditioned, which is similar to Plato's ideas. Plato's ideas are the conditions of the understanding of things and of the beings of the things. Some conceptual aspects of *Qi* have the same argumentative function as Plato's theory of ideas.[162]

Be aware, ancient Chinese philosophy regards *Qi* as the ontology of the universe, and stresses *Qi*'s material characteristics - the basic ingredient constituting the universe; while in philosophy of Chinese medicine, *Qi* is the unification of material aspect and functional activities – *Qi* is not only the basic ingredient constituting the Man, but is also used to expound the dynamic processes and functional activities of the life.

Here is worth to note that the concept of *Qi* in Chinese culture is radically different from the concept of material in Western culture, a Chinese misinterpretation. *Guan Tzu* states that "*Qi* can be limitedlessly small and limitedlessly big". Therefore, *Qi*, the origin of the universe and life, is formless without any boundaries or any separation of two opposites (dichotomy). So man can feel *Qi* for man is a being of the integration of the body and the mind, of the subject and the object, of the material and function. The concept of material in the Western culture must be something with a form even with the rapid development of understanding the structure of materials. Materialism is a philosophical foundation of Western natural science, which stresses the separation and opposition of the body and the mind, of the subject and the object, and greatly promotes the development of modern Western science.

It's necessary to know that Yin-Yang, the five phases, and the eight trigrams are all the subdivisions of *Qi* of different levels from the viewpoint of *Qi*, which indicates a gradual generating and evolving process from *Qi* to Yin-Yang then to the Five Phases then to the Eight Trigrams. *The Book of Changes* states that "The changes have *Tai Ji* (the Supreme Ultimate, the Absolute in ancient Chinese cosmology, presented as the primary source of all created things, i.e. *Qi*), *Tai Ji* generates yin and yang, yin and yang generate the four images, i.e. the greater yang, the greater yin, the lesser yang, and the lesser yin, and the four images generate the eight trigrams". That is to say, *Qi* can be transformed into yin and yang, yin and yang can generate and be transformed into the five phases which are composed of two pairs of yin and yang (water and fire, wood and metal) plus one

161 Li Jingwei, Ou Yongxin, Yu Ying'ao, et al. 2001: 173.
162 Note: The ideas here are enlightened by personal talks with Prof. Dr. Friedrich G. Wallner.

middle soil. Actually, the four images and the eight trigrams indicate the five phases although the term "five phases" does not appear in this quotation: The four images can be regarded as four phases, i.e. water, fire, wood, and metal; the eight trigrams can be regarded as water (yin), fire (yang), wood (yin wood and yang wood), metal (yin metal and yang metal), and soil (yin soil and yang soil).

Therefore, the formless *Qi* explains the ontology of philosophy of Chinese medicine, i.e., in the structure of Chinese philosophy, *Qi* has the corresponding place of the Western ontology, and is also the foundation of the model of *Qi*, Yin-Yang, and the Five Phases.

9.3 *Xiang* 象 Implies Methodology of Philosophy of Chinese Medicine[163]

Xiang 象, one of the most important metaphors of Chinese culture, runs through almost every aspect of Chinese culture like philosophy, medicine, logographic writing, arts and other sciences. Then, what is meant by *xiang*? The original meaning of "*xiang*" as stated in *The Origin of Chinese Characters* "*xiang*, with long nose and teeth, is a big mammal in the Southern *Yue* area", refers to elephant. In remote antiquity, the elephant had lived in the Central Plains of China. Later on, the elephant had to migrate south because of the changes in climate, so the people in the Central Plains had few opportunities to see elephant again. Han Fei, a famous philosopher and the representative of the Legalist School of the late Warring States Period (475-221B.C.), said in his *Jie Lao Pian* 解老篇 that "people seldom see the live elephant, but has gained the skeleton of a dead one, so they can imagine what it is like after investigating the picture or image of its skeleton. Therefore, all in people's imagination is known as '*xiang*'". This quotation also reveals the mystery of the origin of the Chinese compound "xiang xiang" (想象，literally "thinking or imagining elephant", means imagination), setting off "xiang 象"'s "imagining" cultural connotations.

In the meanwhile, we can see that "*xiang*" originally evolved from "seeking similarities" between things from the angle of genetics, which is also stated in *The Book of Changes*: "*xiang* refers to something being alike or resembling this thing". Transforming *xiang* into a cultural symbol is related to divining activities - *Bu* 卜 with tortoise shell and *shi* 筮 with stalk of *shi* grass – the two main ways to hunt for information of the cosmos in the Yin-Zhou dynasties (ca.1600-256B.C.). *Zuo's Spring and Autumn Annals ·the Fifteenth Year of Xi Gong's Reign* states that "tortoise is *xiang*"; *The Book of Changes* states that "change is *xiang*". That is to say, the omens on the tortoise shell and the trigrams were called *xiang* for they were regarded as being capable of communicating the *Tian* 天 with the Man and

163 Lan Fengli. Metaphor, *Qu Xiang Bi Lei* and Chinese Medicine. In Wallner F.G., Lan F.L. & Jandl M.J. (eds.). 2010: 63-88.

ruling all of the cultural information. Thereafter, *xiang* has become a symbol which carries all the cultural information. In classical Chinese culture, all of the sceneries, the sun, the moon, the stars, even Man's pulses, tongues and viscera are termed together with *xiang* like "jing (scenery) *xiang*", "ri (sun) *xiang*", "yue (moon) *xiang*", "xing (star) *xiang*", "mai (pulse) *xiang*", "she (tongue) *xiang*" and "zang (visceral) *xiang*"; Tao, the primitive motive force of the origin of everything in the universe, is also known as *xiang,* the big *xiang*.

Xiang implies a vital methodology of philosophy of Chinese medicine: *Qu Xiang Bi Lei* 取象比类 or taking image and analogizing, which can be summarized into four steps as stated in *The Book of Changes*:

① Observing object or phenomenon (*guan wu* 观物): directly observing an object or phenomenon;

② Taking image (*qu xiang* 取象): summarizing and refining the *image* of the object or phenomenon after repeatedly observing and feeling it;

③ Comparing and analogizing (*bi lei* 比类): comparing the things which need to know with the "*image* (*xiang* 象)";

④ Understanding the Way or Rule (*ti dao* 体道): finding the rules.

Qu Xiang Bi Lei results in the formation of metaphors, and such metaphors show the process of *Qu Xiang Bi Lei* and the relationship of the involved things or objects or phenomena or images. In other words, *Qu Xiang Bi Lei* is the metaphorizing process and the way to form metaphors in Chinese medicine.

Qu Xiang Bi Lei is the core methodology of philosophy of Chinese medicine to know the cosmos and man, to construct and develop the theoretical system and clinical explorations of Chinese medicine. We can say that Chinese culture is *Xiang* culture, and Chinese science is *Xiang* Science, and Chinese medicine is a *Xiang* medicine, which stresses relationships among beings in the universe.

9.4 *He* 和 Shows Ultimate Aim of Philosophy of Chinese Medicine

"*He* 和" is usually translated into "harmony" in the Western world, which shows a simplified and reduced understanding of this concept by the Westerners. This concept as shown by its original form bears two aspects of meaning: the first is different, the second is harmonious. That is to say, being both different and harmonious can be termed "*He* 和".

It is really indeed the case that the simplified Chinese characters (the popular style of writing now in China) have also reduced the cultural connotations implied in their original forms. "He 和" is the simplified form of the sinogram 龢. As stated in *The Origin of Chinese Characters*, its original form is composed of two parts: the left part is a pictographic part symbolizing a musical instrument made of bamboo with three holes used to harmonize different tones, and the right part 禾 is phonetic part, indicating its pronunciation "He"; Its original meaning refers to harmony of different music tones.

The development of Chinese characters shows that harmony of different foods is known as 𤯍 [164], that harmony of different medicinal herbs is known as 藥 (medicine), and that harmony of different tones is known as 樂 (music). One of the variant forms of the sinogram 療 (treat) also has the 樂 part, which shows that restoring harmony is the goal of all the Chinese medical treatments.

It is well known that Chinese medicine uses mixtures of different medicinal substances formulated according to a certain strategy in a holistic approach to disease, i.e. *Yao* or Medicine 藥, which is different from *Ben Cao* or Materia Medica 本草. *Ben Cao*, the materia medica, refers to all of the individual medicinal substances with healing properties, i.e. the medicinal substances or the medicinals, including herbs, minerals and animal parts. While *Yao,* 藥, its original Chinese character, is explained to be "harmony of different medicinal substances", and is used to "treat illnesses" (the sinogram is 疒 with 樂 inside it, a variant form of 療, the simplified sinogram is 疗), i.e. restoring the harmonious state to the individual. Thus, it is clear that *Yao* 藥 refers to the medicine ready to be taken for treating illnesses, which is composed of more than one medicinal substances formulated according to the strategies of *Jun Chen Zuo Shi* or Chief, Associate, Assistant and Guide medicinals, i.e. formula.

Therefore, "*he* 和", the ultimate aim of philosophy of Chinese medicine, is in direct line with Chinese culture, which implies the man in a harmonious state or can be achieved to such a harmonious state by applying *Yao* 藥 or non-medication therapies such as acupuncture, moxibustion, and Chinese massage.

Conclusion

Chinese medicine is an integration of Chinese philosophy and plain understanding of the human life, body and diseases. That is to say, Chinese medicine takes the basic correct understanding of the being – composed of body and mind, health and illnesses as its prerequisite, *Qi* as its ontological foundation, *Xiang* as its methodological approach, and *He* as its ultimate aim, thereby the Tao of Chinese medicine has formed by following the Tao of the nature under the guidance of *Tian Ren He Yi* or Universe and Man Uniting and Resembling Each Other.

Therefore, it's clear that Chinese medicine presupposes Chinese culture and philosophy; and that philosophy of Chinese medicine cannot be correctly interpreted by Western philosophy, and Chinese medicine cannot be correctly interpreted or proved by Western medicine; and the network of intercultural philosophy provides a correct way to make Chinese medicine fully understandable, can work as a bridge for better mutual understanding of different cultures and different sciences.

164 The upper part means to harmonize; the lower part 甘, means sweet, which is applied to harmonize the other tastes i.e. sour, bitter, pungent and salty. See *The Origin of Chinese Characters*·甘 *part,* 说文解字•甘部.

Chief References

1 Britannica Concise Encyclopedia (Chinese Version), 2010.

2 Dictionary of Commonly Used Sinograms in Archaic Chinese [Z]. Beijing: Commercial Press, 1998.

3 Kaptchuk, Ted J. Chinese Medicine: The Web That Has No Weaver [M]. Revised ed. London, Sydney, Aukland, Johannesburg: Rider, 2000.

4 Guo Aichun. *Huang Di Nei Jing Su Wen* with Annotations and Modern Interpretations [M]. Tianjin: Tianjin Science and Technology Press, 1999.

5 He Jiuying, Hu Shuangbao, Zhang Meng. A Grand Exposition of Culture of Chinese Characters [M]. Peking University Press, 1995: 195-196.

6 He Yumin. Differences, Perplexity and Choice: A Comparative Study of Chinese Medicine and Western Medicine [M]. Shenyang: Shenyang Press, 1990.

7 Lan Fengli. Influence of *Huang Di's Inner Classic* on *The Origin of Chinese Characters* [J]. Chinese Journal of Medical History. 2006, 36(4): 201-205.

8 Lan Fengli, Wallner Friedrich G., Wobovnik Claudia (eds.). Shen, Psychotherapy and Acupuncture: Theory, Methodology and Structure of Chinese Medicine [C]. Frankfurt am Main: Peter Lang, 2011.

9 Li Jingwei, Ou Yongxin, Yu Ying'ao, et al. A Concise Dictionary of Chinese Medicine [Z]. Beijing: China Press of Traditional Chinese Medicine, 2001.

10 Liang Donghan. Sinograms [M]. Shanghai: Shanghai Education Press, 1984.

11 Liang Fanrong. Acupuncture and Moxibustion. Beijing: China Press of Traditional Chinese Medicine, 2005.

12 Ling Shu Jing. Taiyuan: Shanxi Science and Technology Press, 1992.

13 Ma Boying. A History of Medical Culture in China [M]. Shanghai: Shanghai People's Publishing House, 1994.

14 Originally by Matteo, Ricci. Translated by He Gaoji, Wang Zunzhong, Li Shen. Matteo Ricci's Reading Notes on China [M]. Beijing: Zhonghua Book Company, 1983.

15 Ni, Maoshing. The Yellow Emperor's Classic of Medicine [M]. Boston, Massachusetts: Shambhala, 1995.

16 Nida, Eugene A. Language, Culture and Translating [M]. Shanghai: Shanghai Foreign Language Education Press, 1993.

17 Ong Bendick. M.A. Thesis: A Study of Pre-Qin "Daoist" Thoughts: From Guodian to Jixia [D]. National University of Singapore, 2004.

18 Pan Wenguo. Sinogram as the Basic Unit and Chinese Language Study [M]. Shanghai: East China Normal University Press, 2002.

19 Ren Jiyu. History of Buddhism in China (Volume1) [M]. Beijing: China Social Sciences Press, 1985.

20 Sun Baozhi. Introduction to Clinical Medicine [M]. 2nd Ed. Beijing: Higher Education Press, 2003.

21 Wallner Friedrich, Schmidsberger Florian, Wimmer Franz Martin (eds.). Intercultural Philosophy: New Aspects and Methods [C]. Frankfurt am Main: Peter Lang, 2010.

22 Wallner Friedrich G., Lan Fengli, Jandl Martin J. (eds.). The Way of Thinking: Theory, Methodology and Structure of Chinese Medicine [C]. Frankfurt Am Main: Peter Lang, 2010.
23 Wallner Friedrich G., Lan Fengli, Jandl Martin J. (eds.). Chinese Medicine and Intercultural Philosophy: Theory, Methodology and Structure of Chinese Medicine [C]. Frankfurt Am Main: Peter Lang, 2011.
24 Webster's Encyclopedic Unabridged Dictionary of the English Language (New Revised Edition) [Z]. New York: Gramercy Books, 1994.
25 Wei Zhengtong. A History of Chinese Thoughts [M]. Shanghai: Shanghai Bookstore Publishing House, 2003.
26 Wilhelm, Baynes. Bollingen Series. The I Ching. Princeton: Princeton University Press, 3rd ed., 1967; 27th printing in 1997.
27 Wiseman Nigel, Zhang Yuhuan. Chinese Medical Characters Volume One: Basic Vocabulary [M]. Brookline, Massachusetts and Taos, Mexico, 2003.
28 www.zdic.net
29 Xiao Jiansheng. Chinese History Revisited [M]. Hong Kong: New Century Press, 2009.
30 Xu Shan. The Origin of *Ru*. www.confuchina.com.
31 Xu Shan. Worship of Thunder God: Exploration into the Origin of Chinese Culture [M]. Shanghai: Shanghai Joint Publishing House, 1992.
32 Composed by Xu Shen (Han Dynasty), Annotated by Duan Yucai (Qing Dynasty). The Origin of Chinese Characters [Z]. Shanghai: Shanghai Ancient Books Press, 1987.
33 Xu Youyu. "Copernican" Revolution: Linguistic Transfer in Philosophy [M]. Shanghai: Joint Publishing House, 1994.
34 Yang Bojun, Xu Ti. Dictionary of Zuo's Spring Autumn Annals [Z]. Beijing: Zhonghua Book Company. 1985: 559.
35 Yang Bojun, Xu Ti. Zuo's Spring Autumn Annals in Modern Chinese [M]. Changsha: Yuelu Book Company, 1993.
36 Ye Shuxian, Tian Daxian. The Mysterious Numbers in Ancient China [M]. Beijing: Social Sciences Academic Press, 1998.
37 Yin Huihe. The Fundamental Theories of Chinese Medicine[M]. Shanghai: Shanghai Scientific & Technical Publishers, 1984.
38 Zuo Min'an. Detailed Interpretation of Chinese Characters: Origin and Evolution of 1,000 Sinograms [M]. Beijing: Jiuzhou Press, 2005.

II Fundamental Concepts of Classical Chinese Philosophy (180367)

Our present-day historical consciousness, as well as our consciousness of our present situation, is determined … by the conception of the Axial Period.

- Karl Theodor Jaspers[165]

Introduction

The years from 800 B.C. to 200 B.C., esp. from 600 B.C. to 300 B.C. are the period of emergence of great philosophers of different cultures, which are named as the Axial Age in *The Origin and Goal of History* (1953) by Karl Theodor Jaspers. The Axial Age is a turning point in human history. In the years centering around 500 B.C., great advances in religion, philosophy, science, democracy, and many forms of art occurred independently and almost simultaneously in China, India, the Middle East, and Greece.

India experienced a dramatic socio-political and intellectual transformation, and produced the teachings of the Buddha (563-483 B.C.?) and Mahavira (599-527 B.C.). Like China, new teachings ran the whole gamut of philosophical thoughts of school, including even skepticism, materialism, sophism, and nihilism.

In Palestine, the prophets Elijah (9th century B.C.), Isaiah (8th century B.C.), Jeremiah (645-585 B.C.?), and *Book of Isaiah*[166] made their appearance. The law and moral code of the Israelites dates back to before this age.

In ancient Mesopotamia, cultural developments were relatively close to those in ancient Israel. However, concepts including the belief in a transcendent creator God, and full subservience of the political rulers to a God did not materialize.

In Greece, developments were more philosophical than spiritual. Greece witnessed the appearance of Thales (624-545 B.C.?), Xenophanes (431-355 B.C.?), and Heraclitus (540-470 B.C.?) who regarded all existence to be in a state of flux - one cannot step in the same river twice; Parmenides (515-450 B.C.), who discoursed on the nature of permanent being as opposed to becoming; and Democritus (470-370 B.C.), who devised the first atomic theory of the nature. These were philosophers whose teachings subsequently influenced Socrates (469-399 B.C.), Plato (427?-347 B.C.) and Aristotle (384-322 B.C.). What all

165 Karl Theodor Jaspers (1883-1969) was a German psychiatrist and philosopher who had a strong influence on modern theology, psychiatry and philosophy. See Jaspers, Karl. 1977: 21. The first print of the work: *The Origin and Goal of History*. translated by Michael Bullock. New Haven, CT: Yale University Press, 1953.

166 *Book of Isaiah*, also spelled Isaias, one of the major prophetical writings of the *Old Testament*. The superscription identifies Isaiah as the son of Amoz and his book as "the vision of Isaiah . . . concerning Judah and Jerusalem in the days of Uzziah, Jotham, Ahaz, and Hezekiah, kings of Judah." According to 6:1, Isaiah received his call "in the year that King Uzziah died" (742B.C.), and his latest recorded activity is dated in 701B.C.. Only the chapters 1–39, however, can be assigned to this period. The chapters 40–66 are much later in origin and therefore known as Deutero-Isaiah (Second Isaiah). Sometimes a further distinction is made between Deutero-Isaiah (chapters 40–55) and Trito-Isaiah (chapters 56–66).

these thinkers had in common was a thirst for discovering the fundamental principles of existence and the implications they had on human life and behavior. A major break-through from pre-axial beliefs involved their recognition of the great chasm between the transcendental/cosmic order, and ordinary human existence.

In China, this was the classical period during which various thoughts of schools contended for attention and classical Chinese philosophy came into being. These schools were born under the backdrop of tumultuous social chaos in the Spring-Autumn and Warring States Periods (770-221 B.C.) when the Chinese social structure experienced major changes. Many individual thinkers, such as Confucius (551-479B.C.), Lao Tzu (580?-500B.C.), Mo Tzu (470?-391?B.C.), Mencius (372?-289?B.C.), Chuang Tzu (369?-286? B.C.), Xun Tzu (300?-230? B.C.), and Han Fei Tzu (281?-233 B.C.), et al.[167] began to reflect on the ethical and metaphysical implications of human existence as well as how to restore order to the chaotic society. From their teachings arose Confucianism, Taoist School, Mohism, and the Legalist School.

According to the importance, influence, relevance to the theme of all the visiting lectures as well as the limit of class hours, this course mainly deals with the following topics: 1 Intellectual Flowering in Early China: The "Hundred Schools of Thought"; 2 Backgrounds of Classical Chinese Philosophy; 3 Confucianism and Its Influences on Chinese Medicine; 4 Taoist School and Its Influences on Chinese Medicine; 5 The Yin-Yang Theory; 6 The Five Phases Theory.

167 Tzu or Zi means Master.

The time of Master Philosophers and Hundred Schools is a time of pluralistic development of classical Chinese thinking.

- The Author

1 Intellectual Flowering in Early China: "The Hundred Schools of Thought"

Many nations have their own unique wisdoms, and have splendid times in their histories. In China, the Spring Autumn and Warring States periods (770-221 B.C.), also known as Pre-Qin Days, are the golden times of Chinese history, during which different thoughts of schools came out for the purpose of building a better surviving environment for human beings. They have left so much precious cultural heritage on thinking, many ideal proposals for building a harmonious society with diversity, thinking resources of dealing with reforms, a value system of cohering the common aspiration of the Chinese people, and wisdom pearls of guiding life, as well as guidelines for developing its own sciences.

1.1 Sima Tan Identified Six Schools of Thought

The so-called "the Master Philosophers and the Hundred Schools 諸子百家", which are known and remembered together today, actually result from the rise of private schools. Different schools were, in real fact, education organizations with different thoughts. There were originally six schools identified by Sima Tan 司马谈[168] (?-110 B.C.), father of Sima Qian 司马迁 (145 or 135 ? - ca. 86 B.C., the author of *Shi Ji* or *The Historical Records* 史记, China's first dynastic history, completed ca. 86 B.C.). He was the first scholar to classify the "Hundred Schools" into the following six: "The Schools of Yin-Yang 阴阳, Literati (Confucianism) 儒, Mohism 墨, Names 名, Legalists 法, and Tao Te 道德 (i.e. Taoist School) to strive on government's behalf, i.e. to take governing as their task".

1.2 Liu Xin Identified Ten Schools of Thought

Liu Xin 刘歆（50 B.C.?- A.D.23）added four in his *Qi Lue* 七略[169], which is preserved now in the *Han Shu Yi Wen Zhi* or *Treatise on Literature* of *History of*

168 Here, Sima is the family name.

169 Liu Xiang 劉向 (78-8 B.C.) and his son Liu Xin 劉歆 (50 B.C.? - 23 A.D.) are the first two persons in the history of China to systematize the available books, which were presented to the Han Imperial Court from the whole country after the event of burning books (of poetics, master philosophers and their school thoughts) 焚诗书 in 213 B.C. and burying practitioners of occult arts alive 坑术士 in 212 B.C. in Qin Shi Huang's reign. They were put in charge of writing a catalogue of the books that were stored in the imperial library in the late first century B.C. Their survey began in 26 B.C. Their catalogue, called the *Qi Lue* 七略, was later lost, but not before it was used by Ban Gu 班固 (A.D. 32-92) to compile the bibliographical monograph -"*Yi Wen Zhi*" or *Treatise on Literature* 藝文志, a part of *The History of the Former Han Dynasty* (Han Shu, 漢書). This is where the passage cited now appears, in a section called the "master philosophers" (*Zhu Zi* 諸子).

the Former Han Dynasty 汉书．艺文志: the School of Political Strategists 縱横家, the Eclectics 雜家 (literally "the School of Miscellaneous Teachings"), the School of Agriculturalists 農家, and the School of Story Tellers 小說家. These are the "Ten Schools" which later came to be called the "Hundred Schools" or "the Master Philosophers and the Hundred Schools 諸子百家". The order of the "Ten Schools" in the *Han Shu Yi Wen Zhi* or *Treatise on Literature* of *History of the Former Han Dynasty* 汉书．艺文志 is as follows: the Schools of Literati (Confucianism) 儒家, Taoists 道家, Yin-Yang 阴阳家, Legalists 法家, Names 名家, Mohists 墨家, Political Strategists 纵横家, the Eclectics 杂家, Agriculturalists 农家, and Story Tellers.小说家. But Liu Xin concluded that "The various master philosophers make up ten schools, but only nine are worth to be noticed", which excludes the School of Story Tellers. That is to say, the School of Story Tellers is much less important than the other nine schools. Later on the Nine Schools were given a name as *Jiu Liu* 九流 or Nine School of Thoughts.

1.3 Lǚ Simian Identified Twelve Schools of Thought

Lǚ Simian 吕思勉 (1884-1957), a former Professor of East China Normal University in Shanghai, added "the School of Militarists" 兵家 and "the School of Medical Practitioners" 医家 to make up altogether "Twelve Schools". His monograph entitled *Xian Qin Xue Shu Gai Lun* or *Introduction to Learnings of Pre-Qin Days* 先秦学术概论 reads that "Therefore, as regards to the learnings of the Pre-Qin Days, in real fact, it can be classified into the Schools of Yin-Yang, Literati (Confucianism), Mohists, Names, Legalists, Taoists, Political Strategists (Zong Heng, literally "Vertical and Horizontal"), Eclectics, Agriculturalists, Story Tellers, Militarists, and Medical Practitioners, which are collectively known as the 'Twelve Schools'". I think that "Twelve Schools of Thought" are also true to the real history of that time.

Actually, 191 works on Chinese medicine, amounting to 2,529 volumes, are put under the division of philosophy of the *Si Ku Quan Shu* or *The Complete Library of the Four Branches of Literature* 四库全书 completed by 4,000 Confucian officials by Emperor Qianlong's order 乾隆 (1711-1799) in 1782 and comprising the four traditional divisions of Chinese learning - classics, history, philosophy, and belle-letters.

1.4 Brief Introduction to Twelve Schools of Thought

Hereafter is a brief introduction to the "Twelve Schools". The order of the first ten schools accords with the order in the *Han Shu Yi Wen Zhi* or *Treatise on Literature* of *The History of the Former Han Dynasty* 汉书.艺文志, and then is followed by "the School of Militarists" 兵家 and "the School of Medical Practitioners" 医家 .

The School of Literati or Confucianism 儒家: Actually *Ru Jia* 儒家 should be the School of Literati, but it is well known in the West as Confucianism.

Confucius 孔子 (551-479 B.C.) was the first teacher, and he proposed "Don't do unto others what you don't want others do unto you", which has been written in the Hall of the United Nation's Building since 1993. If all observe this proposal, then there would be no war at all in the world. Mencius 孟子 (372?-289?B.C.) represented the idealistic wing of Confucianism and advocated "The human nature is good"; Xun Tzu 荀子 (300?-230?B.C.) stood for the realistic wing of Confucianism, and held that "The human nature is evil; his goodness is acquired through training and education". Actually, Confucianism 儒家 carries forward and focuses on traditional culture, promoting *Ren Ai* (仁爱, Benevolence and Love or Charity), *Zheng Yi* (正义, Justice), and *Zi Qiang Bu Xi* (自强不息, Making Unceasing Efforts to Improve Oneself), thus establishing the core value for the Chinese people. Briefly, the School of Literati or Confucianism, also known as the Way of Confucius and Mencius, advocates "Benevolent Government" and "The people are more important than the ruler", and thus representing Literati's Philosophy.

The School of Taoists, or The Taoist School 道家: Yang Zhu's ideas are the first phase of the Taoist School. The principle of Yang Zhu 杨朱(?-? B.C.) is that "Each one for himself". "Though he might have profited the whole world by plucking out a single hair, he would not have done it". We can get Yang Zhu's two fundamental ideas, one is "Each one for himself", and the other is "the despising of things and valuing of life". *Lao Tzu,* also known as *Tao Te Ching* is the second phase of the Taoist School. Actually, it is *Chuang Tzu* that synthesized and brought the Taoist School to its highest development. *Chuang Tzu* is the third phase of the Taoist School. Taoists cared little about social improvement and believed that the path to human happiness lay in the individualistic pursuit of harmony with nature. Taoist School focuses on life, pursuing living a real, free and lenient life, thus seeking the existing value of life. In short words, the Taoist School, also known as Learning about Lao (Tzu) and Chuang (Tzu), advocates "According with the nature" and "Governing with effortless action", and thus being Recluses' Philosophy.

The Yin-Yang School 阴阳家: In Sima Tan's essay *Lun Liu Jia Yao Zhi* or *On the Essentials of Six Schools* 论六家要旨, the Yin-Yang School was mentioned at the first place before the other five schools - the Schools of Literati (Confucianism), Mohists, Names, Legalists, and Taoists, which is reasonable no matter from the time or logical order for Yin-Yang is the beginning of everything in the universe and interaction of Yin-Yang results in all the phenomena in the universe. The Yin-Yang School advocated explaining all the natural and social phenomena as well as human relations with Yin-Yang and the Five Phases. Zou Yan 邹衍 (305?-240 B.C.) "deeply observed the waning and waxing of Yin-Yang" (*Shi Ji* or *The Historical Records*), remoulded the Five Phases into Five *Te* or Five Virtues 五德, and collaborated Yin-Yang with Five Phases, which were applied to explain the rise and decline of the past dynasties in the history and to provide theoretical foundation for a new reunification government of the country, i.e. Qin reunified China by annexing the other six states. The Yin-Yang and the Five Phases have certain rationality for classical Chinese natural sciences such as astronomy, calendar, meteorology, geography, and medicine for it is originally based on and contains such knowledge of the above mentioned subjects.

The School of Legalists, or The Legalist School 法家: Han Fei Tzu 韩非子 (281?-233 B.C.) is the synthesizer of the Legalist School. The Legalists represent the economic and political philosophy of the Qin Dynasty – "Abolish the field dividing system, value farming and belittle trading, encourage and reward farming and fighting in wars" and "Rule by law, and thus strengthen centralization of the state power," and advocate "stern rule of law and harsh punishments". The Legalist School believed that human nature was naturally selfish, intellectualism and literacy was discouraged by forbidding all the other thoughts of schools and advocating the teachings of the Legalist school and officials as the only teachings and only teachers respectively, law was the superior authority and replaces morality, the ruler must rule with a strong and punishing hand, and war was the means of strengthening a ruler's power. In one word, the Legalist School focuses on the way of governing and strengthening a country, and then seeking to govern a country by laws, and thus pursuing an open and fair justice – "No matter the dear or the estrangement in relations, no matter the high or the low in positions, all will be judged according to the law" (*Shi Ji* or *The Historical Records*). The Legalist School made a huge contribution to strengthen the state of Qin and help it reunify the whole country by wars. The Legalist School stood for Advisors' Philosophy.

The School of Names (or The School of Logicians) **名家:** There are two sources in this origin of the thought, Confucianism and Mohism. In addition, the Legalist School and Taoist School also influenced this school in their own ways. The Logicians dealt with the relation of names to realities. They were thought to have emerged from officers concerned with rank and position in the court and with the ceremonies to which such rank and position entitled an officer.

Gongsun Long Tzu 公孙龙子 (320?-250? B.C.), a noted member of the School of Names in Chinese philosophy, lived during the Warring States Period. The most famous argument from him is called *Bai Ma Fei Ma* 白马非马, literally, "A white horse is not a horse". The book named after his name - *Gongsun Long Tzu* is structured as a conversation between two parties, with one party proclaiming truth in the statement and the other questioning it. The argument plays upon the dual semantic meanings of informal language, in particular the dual interpretations of 'is', being either: "Is a member of the class entitled (x)", or "Is identical to concept (x)". Thus, a white horse is not a horse, because the concept of a white horse is not the same as the concept of a horse. Hence, The School of Names represented Debaters' Philosophy.

It is said that the philosophy of the School of Names has parallels with that of the Ancient Greek sophists or dialecticians. However, the school does not enjoy a very high position in classical Chinese studies, and its influence is very limited.

Mohism 墨家: Mo Tzu 墨子 (470?-391? B.C.) and his followers - the Mohists advocate "Universal Love or All-Embracing Love", even towards enemies, and seeking equality and mutual benefit in the society; "Esteeming virtuous and able persons as well as the sameness", "Denouncing aggressive warfare" in the political affairs; and "Strengthening the root and encouraging frugality" in the economy. The Mohist School focuses on society, and most of its followers were from a lower social grade. Mohism stood for Knights' Philosophy.

The School of Political Strategists 纵横家: "Zong Heng 纵横" means vertical and horizontal. Those of this school originally were politicians, diplomats, or advisors of feudal rulers of the Warring States Period (475-221 B.C.). They went to different states to lobby rulers to take the opposite theories of vertical (north-south) and horizontal (east-west) alliance of states with the state of Qin as pivot to resist Qin. Their activities exerted very important influences on the political and military setup of that time. As Liu Xin 刘歆（50 B.C.?- A.D.23）said in his *Qi Lue* 七略 that "Those of the School of Political Strategists may have their origin in the Ministry of Embassies …. They taught the art of following general orders in political strategies (such as diplomacy) instead of following literal instructions. That is where their strength lies".

The Eclectics 杂家: Liu Xin said that "Those of the Eclectics may have had their origin in the councilors. They adopted strong points of the Schools of Literati, Mohists, Legalists and Names for they knew that the nation needed all of these and saw that kingly government should not fail to unite all. That is where their strength lies". Lǔ Buwei 吕不韦 (292?-235 B.C.), a prime minister of the state of Qin, gathered his *Men Ke* 门客 (hangers-on of an aristocrat) from various fields of study to compile a book entitled *Lǔ Shi Chun Qiu* or *Lǔ's Spring and Autumn Annals*[170] 吕氏春秋, which is actually a typical representative work of the Eclectics.

The School of Agriculturalists 农家: Liu Xin said that "Those of the School of Agriculturalists may have their origin in the Ministry of Soil and Grain. They taught the art of sowing various kinds of grain and urged people to plow and cultivate the mulberry to ensure the people to have sufficient supply of clothing and food …That is where their strength lies". This school embodies the idea of valuing farming in a social and political sense, and its teachings are kinds of records and summarizations of farming skills and experiences. Several chapters in *Lǔ Shi Chun Qiu* or *Lǔ's Spring and Autumn Annals* such as *Shang Nong* or

---

170 *Lü Shi Chun Qiu* or *Lu's Spring Autumn Annals*, is an encyclopedic classical Chinese text compiled around 239 B.C. under the patronage of the Chancellor of Qin Dynasty Lu Buwei 吕不韦.

Valuing Farming, *Bian Tu* or *Differentiating Soils*, *Shen Shi* or *Observing Seasons*, etc. are regarded as important materials to study the thought of the school.

The School of Story Tellers 小说家: Liu Xin said that "Those of the School of Story Tellers may have their origin in the Petty Offices. This School was created by those who picked up street gossips and hearsays". Confucius commented that "it is a trivial art hardly worth mentioning although there must be something worth to take a look. … Men with honor would not like to do it". Liu Xin also concluded that "The various master philosophers make up ten schools, but only nine are worth to be noticed", which excludes the School of Story Tellers. That is to say, the School of Story Tellers is much less important than the other nine schools. Later on the Nine Schools were given a name as *Jiu Liu* 九流 or Nine School of Thoughts.

The School of Militarists 兵家: This school is supposed to direct battles and apply military force to achieve a proper purpose. Sun Wu 孙武 (535? B.C.-?) is regarded as the founder of the school. He authored the world famous work *Sun Zi Bing Fa* or *The Art of War* 孙子兵法, the earliest military monograph of China and the globe as well, which has been highly esteemed as "Holy Classic of Military Strategies" by military commanders of the later generations. Now it has been translated into various foreign languages such as English, French, German, Japanese, etc., and thus becoming the most famous international paradigm of military strategies.

The School of Medical Practitioners 医家: The formation of the Medical School takes nearly seven hundred years from the 5th century B.C. to the 3rd century A.D.. This art of healing actually arose from its specific cultural, geographical, and philosophy backgrounds such as the introduction of *Qi*, Yin-Yang, and Five Phases into the medical field. For example, *Yi Fa Fang Yi Lun* or *Methods of Treatment Differing in Different Regions,* the whole chapter 12 of *Huang Di Nei Jing Su Wen*, elaborates different methods of treatment – stone needles, herbal remedies, moxibustion, nine types of needles (esp. very fine needles), and Chinese massage therapy (*Dao-Yin* or guiding-pulling and *An-Qiao* or pressing-lifting) originated in the East, West, North, South, and Center respectively to meet the needs of patients due to the differences or variables in geography, weather, lifestyle, and diet, which also accords with the ideas of the Yin-Yang and the Five Phases theories (See the appendix reading of this chapter).

1.5 The Master Philosophers and the Hundred Schools

The Master Philosophers and the Hundred Schools 諸子百家 are a collective name for all the schools of teachings and thoughts in the Spring and Autumn and Warring States Periods (770-221 B.C.). During the Spring and Autumn Period (770-476 B.C) the Zhou's reign was declining and all the states were competing to be the strongest and most powerful one, and therefore scholars travelled to all the states to provide suggestions, strategies and methods on how to make them stronger and more powerful, thus forming the situation of "Contention of a hundred schools of thought" until the Warring States Period (770-221 B.C.).

Generally speaking, the Master Philosophers and the Hundred Schools were supposed to propose political strategies for the rulers of the states. The School of Literati or Confucianism advocated educating people with *Te* (De, Virtue). Taoist School advocated governing with effortless actions. Legalist School advocated drawing a clear cut between reward and punishment. The School of Names opposed to reunify the country with wars. Since the Han Dynasty (206 B.C.-A.D.220), the Schools of Mohism and Names had perished, the School of Agriculturists has transformed into a separate practical art of farming, and the Yin-Yang school had transformed into occult arts and has been introduced into medicine. Therefore, the Schools of Literati (or Confucianism), Taoists and Legalists have remained the most influential ones on the politics, culture, and society of a unified country of the later times.

Be aware the above thoughts of schools came out around 2,500 years ago. They focus on different aspects of the society, life, and well-being from different angles with the same purpose: to build a harmonious society which is composed of healthy beings with diversity, which accords well with the trends of the 21st century world civilization.

Appendix Reading: The Chapter 12 of *Huang Di Nei Jing Su Wen*
Methods of Treatment[171]

Huang Di asked, "When doctors treat conditions, even though they may be illnesses of the same nature, they use different methods and techniques. But they all succeed. Why is this?"

Qi Bo replied, "This is because of differences or variables in geography, weather, lifestyle, and diet. For example, the east is the direction of the birth of the heaven and the earth. The weather there is mild, and it is close to the water. Many varieties of fish and salts can be found, so the local people eat many kinds of fish and like the salty flavor. But because they eat so much fish, which is considered a hot food, heat accumulates and stagnates in the body. They also eat too much salt, which dries, exhausts, and drains the blood. This is why people of the east often have dark skin. The commonly suffered illnesses are boils and carbuncles. The treatment of this disease often utilizes needles made of stone, which are thicker, and bleeding, which releases the heat. Thus, the method of stone needles comes from the east.

"In the west, many mountains and plateaus and thousands of miles of desert produce a wide variety of metals or ores. This natural environment is similar to the season of autumn. It has an astringent, or conserving, nature. The natives here live

171 Translated by Ni, Maoshing. See Ni, Maoshing. 1995: 48-49.

naturally and simply by the mountains. They are not concerned about their clothing; they wear wool and sleep on straw mats. They eat food that is often heavy, such as meats and fatty milk and cheese products. Thus they are usually obese people. Externally they are not easily invaded, because they are strong. That is why their illnesses tend to be internal. So the treatment for them is herbal. It can be said, therefore, that herbal treatment comes from the west.

"In the north we have high mountains. The majestic energy of solemn solitude is similar to the season of winter, where the atmosphere is one of calm and reserve. The weather is cold and snowy. Native people here are often nomadic and live amidst nature, exposed to the weather. Their diet also consists of meat and milk products. In this environment, their internal organs are often invaded by cold, and their conditions are excess and distended. The proper method of treating these conditions is moxibustion. It is therefore said that the method of moxibustion comes from the north.

"In the southern regions the weather is hot, and the yang qi is at its utmost. The geography consists of low mountains and valleys. Fog and mist often converge here. The local people like to eat sour and overly ripe foods, such as fruit. Their skin often shows redness. Conditions common in these areas are spasms, numbness, paralysis, bi/arthralgia syndrome, and wei/flaccidity syndrome. The correct treatment employs very fine needles. Thus, the art of the nine types of needles comes from the south. These are metal needles.

"In the center are flatlands, which are often damp. Many varieties of foods abound, and living is peaceful. Conditions that manifest most are colds, influenza, cold and heat conditions, wei/flaccidity syndromes, and atrophy. One should utilize Dao-in exercise, manipulation, adjustment, tuina, and massage. It is said therefore that Dao-in exercise and manipulation come from the center of China.

"A superior doctor is able to gather all techniques and use them either together or separately, to flexibly adapt to a changing environment, lifestyle, and geography, and to consider many variables in the treatment of a condition. Thus, it is understood that even though treatment methods are different, all can succeed in healing a condition. This is dependent on the ability of the doctor to consider all variables and select the proper principle of treatment."

The wise delight in water; the good delight in mountains. The wise move; the good stay still. The wise are happy; the good endure.

- *The Analects of Confucius*

2 Backgrounds of Classical Chinese Philosophy

Philosophy is a kind of systematic reflective thinking on life and the nature. In thinking, the thinker is usually conditioned by the surroundings in which he lives. Being in certain surroundings, he feels life and the nature in a certain way, and there are therefore in his philosophy certain emphases or omissions, which constitute the characteristics of that philosophy. This is true of an individual, and it is also true of a people.[172]

Here I would like to discuss first the cultural, economic, geographical, and social background of Chinese culture in general and Chinese philosophy in particular.

2.1 Cultural Background: Rise of "Literati"

"The Son of Heaven (King) lost his power, and the schools were distributed over the country". Before and during the Western Zhou Dynasty (ca. 11th century – 771 B.C.), the government had the full control of the schools – Different knowledge could be learned only from feudal officials of different duties. Moreover, the common people were not allowed to learn knowledge, only children of kings, princes and aristocrats were qualified for the school, as stated in *The Book of Rites* "All the schools are controlled by the government". Since the King Ping of Zhou (Zhou Ping Wang) moved the capital from Gaojing (the west of Xi'an today) to Luoyang, the king gradually lost his power, then rites and music were in ruins, and the society were in total disarray. Some officials of the central government went into different feudal princes or dukes, and some were stranded among the people. The situation that "All the schools are controlled by the government" was broken, and private schools rose up luxuriantly. Take Confucius as an example. He set up a private school, where anyone no matter noble or common people could come to be his disciple provided that he brought him a piece of bacon as tuition fee. As a consequence knowledgeable people had become much more than before, they were collectively known as "Literati", which were actually from different social classes.

During the Spring Autumn and Warring States Periods (770-221 B.C.), the princes vied for supremacy, and therefore they all needed "Literati" to provide new ideas to make their countries richer and their military forces more efficient. Thus, "keeping Literati" and free academic atmosphere became a very popular social mode at that time. Under such conditions, thoughts of different schools

172 Fung Yu-Lan. 1948; 2010: 26.

flourished by writing and propounding ideas, which composed the foundation and the essence of Chinese culture.

2.2 Economic Background: Agriculture as Foundation of the Country

China is a continental country. The Chinese people have to make their living by agriculture. The ancient China had a large population. For example, 12,230,000 families and 59,590,000 persons were recorded in the 2 A.D. of the Western Han Dynasty (206 B.C.-A.D. 24), which marked the first peak in the population history of China.

In an agrarian country, land is the primary basis of wealth. A large population and limited area under cultivation forced farmers make a living by intensive and meticulous farming in a piece of narrow and small land, which resulted in the development of national character of the Chinese people: being attached to one's native land and unwilling to leave it, resting satisfied with one's life, and remaining in one's proper sphere. Hence social, economic thinking and policies have centered on the utilization and distribution of land as well as the proportion of population and land through the whole Chinese history,. The portion of the rural population has still been the majority of the whole even up till today in China.

As regards to the economic thinking of ancient Chinese philosophers, there was a distinction between the Root and the Branch: Agriculture the Root while Commerce the branch. The reason lies in that agriculture results in production, while commerce deals with exchange. If without production there would be no exchange. In an agrarian country, agriculture is the major form of production. Thus the position of farmers was much higher than that of merchants in ancient China.

Guan Tzu states that "Literati, farmers, craftsmen, traders are the pillars of the country", which also reveals characteristics and the ranking of the social classes in the Spring Autumn and Warring States Periods (770-221B.C.). That is to say, Literati came to the first, farmers secondary, craftsmen third, and traders last. It is thus clear that traders had no place in the society at that time. Hereafter are several Chinese idioms on traders: "No trader is not fraudulent"; "Traders seek nothing but profits"; "Traders value profits but despise parting from his love (the affections)".

The Literati did not actually cultivate the land themselves, but since they were usually landlords, their fortunes were tied up with agriculture. Therefore their reaction to the universe and their outlook on life and values were essentially those of farmers.[173] The fact is that most of the Chinese were farmers, which also partly explains why China failed to have an industrial revolution. The lifestyle of

173 Fung Yu-Lan. 1948; 2010: 28-31.

farmers is to follow the nature. They admire the nature and condemn the artificial, and are easily made content. Farmers desire no change, nor can they conceive of any change.

2.3 Geographical Environment: Relative Isolation

2.3.1 Geographical Environment of China vs. Independent, Continuous, and Plural Chinese Culture

The geographical location of a nation exerts direct and important influences on the initial formation of its culture. China is a huge country with vast expanse in length and breadth of land, and it is bounded and isolated by the Pacific in the east, Himalayas in the south-west, and deserts in the north-west. Geographical environment is the first factor and the basis of forming Chinese culture. Actually, Chinese culture formed and developed independently in its specific geographical conditions, its influences were mainly limited in the South-East Asia and influences of other cultures on it were likewise limited in ancient times due to its geographical relative isolation from the outside world.

There are four ancient civilizations in the world, which all originated from reaches of big rivers, i.e. the ancient China originating from the Yellow River Valley, the ancient Egypt from the Nile River Valley, the ancient Babylon from Euphrates and Tigris (known as Mesopotamia Civilization), and the ancient India from the Indian River Valley. But among them the Chinese civilization might be the only one which has never broken off but survived and continued up till today. What's the reason? This has to be attributed to the vast territory and long-term unified culture and administration of China. The territories of the other three ancient civilizations were very narrow and small or big but varied too much like India, so there was no room for maneuver when they were invaded by other nationalities. And thus the three civilizations discontinued. While China is very different for Chinese culture flourishes in its vast land, which can be well preserved and carried on in at least a part of it. Even when it was fully occupied and governed by some foreign nationalities or minority ethnic groups, such as Yuan Dynasty by Mongolians (1206-1368) and Qing Dynasty by Manchu nationality (1644-1911), Chinese culture was well preserved and spread over the rulers. That is to say, the rulers were forced to accept and learn Chinese culture for a better administration of the country.

Chinese culture has been plural since its formation due to the complicatedness of its geographical conditions. A varied topography, configurations of the ground and climatic conditions make the whole territory fall into many lands of different sizes, as a Chinese idiom says that "Hundred miles make folkways different, thousand miles make customs different, and ten thousand miles make foods different", which actually means that "The customs and habits of people differ in each locality". This is indeed the case with China. As early as the Pre-Qin Days, cultures of different regions bore different characteristics based on some common features, such as culture of Central Plains (comprising the middle and lower reaches of the Yellow River) being a gathering place of talents and being broad and profound; culture of Yan-Zhao 燕赵 (mainly Hebei province, still including Beijing, Tianjin, the north of Henan and Shanxi provinces, and the south of Inner Mongolia) being like chant in a heroic but mournful tone; culture of Jing-Chu 荆楚 (Hubei province) being light, clever, excellent and wonderful; etc. Different geographical environments make lifestyles, thinking ways and customs as well as food, clothing, shelter and means of traveling all different. But the same writing language bridges the gap among all the different local cultures.

2.3.2 Continental Culture vs. Maritime Culture

The human beings can be roughly classified into continental people and maritime people according to general geographical environments. In a typical maritime country such as the ancient Greece, the living space was relatively narrow and small, and then the people had to seek how to survive and develop by going out of sea and expanding to the outside, as a consequence its commerce was usually very well developed and the people there were easy to meet the people of different cultures by so doing.

China is a continental country. To the ancient Chinese their land was the whole world. They live on the land, agriculture has always been the foundation of the country and farmers have always been the majority of the population. There are two expressions in Chinese language to express the world. One is “all beneath the sky” or “the land under the heaven” and the other is “all within the four seas” or “the land within the four seas”. To the people of a maritime country such as the ancient Greece or the Britain, it would be inconceivable that such expressions like these could be synonymous. See Illus. 17. The farmers are always in contact with nature, so they observe and follow the way of the nature, which is the central idea of the Taoist School, as stated in the Chapter 25 of *Lao Tzu* that "Man abides by the earth. Earth abides by the heaven. Heaven abides by Tao. Tao abides by the nature”.

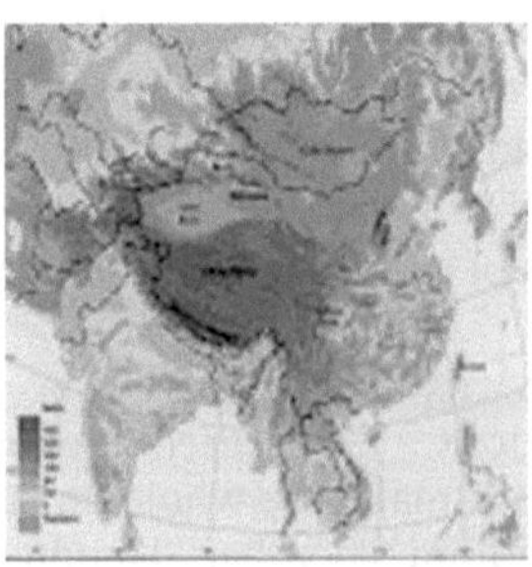

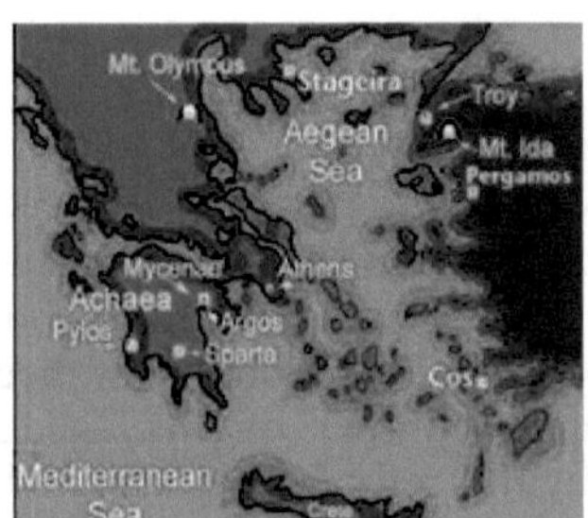

[174]

Illus. 17 Maps of China and Ancient Greece

174 The Ancient Greek world included parts of modern-day Greece, Turkey, Egypt, and Italy.

China has also a very long coastline of 32,000 km, in which the continental coastline is 18,000 km and the island coastline is 14,000 km. Why the ancient Chinese did not go out of the ocean and make business with people of different cultures etc.? The map of China clearly shows that what China faces in the east is the Pacific Ocean. And then how far could the ancient Chinese travel in a time without machinery power and engineering? Navigation in the Pacific Ocean was an impossible task until the Ming Dynasty (1368-1644), which also reflects in an idiom from the chapter of *Autumn Water* of *Chuang Tzu* "to lament one's littleness before the vast ocean - bemoan one's inadequacy in the face of a great task".

Why was the thinking of ancient Chinese so different from that of ancient Greeks? From the time of Confucius until the end of the 19th century, no Chinese thinkers had the experience of venturing upon the high seas. Confucius and Mencius lived not far from the sea, but in *The Analects of Confucius*, he mentions the sea only once.

Confucius is recorded as saying: "If my way is not to prevail, I shall get upon a raft and float out to the sea. He who will go with me will be [Zhong] You[175]." When Zhong You heard this statement, he was much pleased. Confucius, however, was not so pleased by Zhong You's over-enthusiasm, and remarked: "[Zhong] You is braver than me. I do not know what to do with him."

Even in this case, where Confucius was going to go was not any part of the world across the Pacific but the Korean Peninsula just across the Yellow Sea. Confucius implied that he would like to spread his way in Korean Peninsula if his way had failed in disseminating in the mainland China for it was the only possible place he could reach at that time by boat.[176]

Mencius's reference to the Sea is likewise brief. He lamented his littleness before the vast sea. He said, "He who has seen the sea, finds it difficult to think anything about other waters; and he who has wandered to the gate of the sage, finds it difficult to think anything about the words of others." Mencius is no better than Confucius, who thought only of "floating out to the sea".

How different were Socrates, Plato, and Aristotle, who lived in a maritime country and wandered from island to island! Yes, they could easily reach other parts or islands by boats or ships even without machinery power, and had much more and greater opportunities to see different people with different customs and different languages!

The ancient Greek people lived in a maritime country and maintained their prosperity through commerce. They were primarily merchants. As merchants they

---

175 Zhong You 仲由 (542-480B.C.), also known as Zi Lu 子路, one of Confucius 72 favorite disciples of virtue. He was straightforward, brave, faithful, ambitious, and always handled affairs in a decisive manner.

176 Ge Jianxiong. Influences of Geographical Environment on History and Culture of China. Lecture at Tsinghua University (Beijing), Nov. 1st, 2009. Ge Jianxiong 葛剑雄 (1945-), a famous professor of historical geography of Fudan University, Shanghai.

have to deal with first are the abstract numbers used in their commercial accounts, and only then with concrete things that may be immediately apprehended through these numbers. Such numbers are what Northrop [177] called concepts by postulation. Hence Greek philosophers likewise took the concept by postulation as their starting point. So, they developed mathematics and mathematical reasoning. That's why they had epistemological problems and why their language was so articulate.

As merchants, in order to have a good sale for their goods, they have to encourage novelty in the manufacture of what they are going to sell. Therefore, they are accustomed to change and are not afraid of novelty. It's no accident that in the West, the industrial revolution was first started in England, which is also a maritime country maintaining her prosperity through commerce.

Besides, China was a state composed of families, while Greece was a state composed of cities. The family system was the social system of China. In ancient China, the whole country was composed by big and small families. Out of the five traditional social relationships, which are those between sovereign and subject, father and son, elder and younger brother, husband and wife, and friend and friend. Among them three are family relationships, and the remaining two can be conceived in terms of the family - the relationship between sovereign and subject can be conceived in terms of that between father and son, and the relationship between friend and friend in terms of that between elder and younger brother. In a family, the authority of the father, elder brother, and husband is always naturally superior to or more important than that of the son, the younger brother, and the wife for they are of different hierarchical levels. Ancestor worship, loyal to the throne, filial obedience to parents, observation of masters and authorities etc. all developed for this reason. The ancient Greek people lived on commerce, and they were merchants living in cities. All the people were of the same class without hierarchic distance, so no one was more superior to or more important than, or had

177 Filmer Stuart Cuckow Northrop (1893 – 1992) was an American philosopher, was appointed Sterling Professor of Philosophy and Law at Yale University in 1947. Northrop's major contribution to philosophy is in the area of epistemology, specifically his theory of concepts. He divided all concepts into two kinds: intuition and postulation. A concept by intuition is one which denotes, and the complete meaning of which is given by, something which is immediately apprehended. Northrop gave blue in "the sense of the sensed color" as an example of a concept by intuition. The other kind is concepts by postulation. A concept by postulation is one the meaning of which in whole or in part is designated by the postulates of the deductive theory in which it occurs. Blue in the sense of the frequency or wavelength in electromagnetic theory is a concept by postulation. According to Northrop, these two types of concepts exhaust the available concepts (i.e., providing terms with meanings) from which any scientific or philosophical theory can be constructed and therefore provides a means to do comparative philosophy, analyze and solve the problem of world peace, tame nations, provide a philosophical anthropology, explain why economists from Smith to Marx were incapable of providing a dynamics to supplement their statics, and to ground art and religion as well as legal and ethical theory. See *The Logic of the Sciences and the Humanities*. One early claim by Northrop in "The Meeting of East and West" was that Concepts are in the west "by postulation," while in the East "by intuition."

more say than the others. Therefore they had to form a country based on their common interests. This can also partly explain why Western science (usually based on the common features of objects and seeking for universal) and democracy developed in the West, while Chinese science (e.g. Chinese medicine as a master-oriented medicine) and autocracy developed in China.

The Analects of Confucius reads that "The wise delight in water; the good delight in mountains. The wise move; the good stay still. The wise are happy; the good endure." We can paraphrase this quotation by saying that "the people of maritime countries are the wise, while those of continental countries are the good".[178]

2.3.3 Climactic Extremes and the Five Phases

The land of China is vast and with clear definition of the five directions – East, West, South, North, and Center. And it is located in the North Temperate Zone, where there are four distinctive seasons such as hot summers and freezing winters. These features are preconditions for the formation of the Five Phases theory. Obviously the five phases can not be conceived in the Equator where it is extremely hot all the year round or in the North and South Poles where it is terribly freezing cold through the whole year. See detailed analysis in the Chapter 6 "The Five Phases Theory".

2.4 Social Background: The Crisis in the Zhou (ca. 771-221 B.C.) Order

After 771 B.C., Zhou rule was weakened by foreign invasions and internal divisions. The years of 770-476B. C. was known as the Spring and Autumn Period, which was a period of unstable feudal coalition; the years of 475-221B.C. was known as the Warring States period, which was a period of constant civil war among feudal lords competing to impose rule and restore unity of Zhou territory. Intense pressure arose for social harmony.

The Hundred Teachings or School of Thoughts arose in response to cultural crisis and "free market" for political, philosophical, and ritual expertise, and thus making the Spring Autumn & Warring States Periods (Pre-Qin Days, 770-221 B.C.) become the Golden Times of Chinese Philosophy in the History.

2.5 Logographic Writing Language and Image thinking

Chinese characters (or sinograms) are the only logographic writing (as opposed to phonetic writing) which has been preserved for over 6,000 years. The shape of a Chinese character is directly related to its meaning, and both integrate into a unity. The formation of a Chinese character, an organic whole of the shape and the meaning, is one-step made following the rule of nature, reflecting the direct

178 Fung Yu-Lan. 1948; 2010: 42-44.

communication between and integration of the subject and the object. The formation also implies an important thinking way, i.e. the imaging thinking. Integration of the subject and the object is a thread running through the classical Chinese culture and science, on the basis of which Universe and Man Uniting and Resembling Each Other (*Tian Ren He Yi*, 天人合一) constitutes the foundation of the classical Chinese culture and sciences. The imaging thinking is a specific thinking way of classical China, whose process, methods, and rules make up the methodology of Taking Image and Analogizing (*Qu Xiang Bi Lei*, 取象比類), the core methodology of classical Chinese culture and science. Developed on the basis of the pictographic writing, Chinese characters and their meanings are quite stable and conservative, which greatly promotes the development of the imaging thinking in classical China in different fields of study.

For example, in medicine, such a thinking way was set up in the *Huang Di's Inner Classic* and has greatly influenced experts of Chinese medicine of the later generations. The logographic writings of yin-yang 陰陽, *wu xing* or *five phases* 五行, *qi* 气 and blood 血, the extensive analogizing and abundant imaging thinking examples in the *Huang Di's Inner Classic*, and criticism, proofreading, annotations for sinograms from the aspects of the "shape", "pronunciation", and "meaning" in the ancient medical classics made esp. in the Ming (1368-1644 A.D.) and Qing (1644-1911 A.D.) Dynasties, all demonstrate the far-reaching influences of the logographic imaging thinking way on the development of Chinese medicine.

Don't do unto others what you don't want others do unto you.

- *The Analects of Confucius*

Medicine is an art of practicing Benevolence.

- Yu Chang[179]

3 Confucianism and Its Influences on Chinese Medicine

Confucius is the first and the most influential philosopher in China. "Contention of all schools of thought" started because of him and ended with him. He took what "the ancients" - the forebears had left him but as a departure for new inventions by systematizing and re-interpreting the old classics, or in other words, he inherited the past and forged ahead into the future, and served as a link between past and future.

Socrates, Buddha, Confucius, Jesus: From The Great Philosophers[180] is a part of Jaspers's planned universal history of philosophy, focusing on the four paradigmatic individuals who have exerted a historical influence of incomparable scope and depth. The four "paradigmatic individuals" by being what they were, did more than other men to determine the history of man; Their influence extends through two millennia down to our own day; They became the foundations of powerful philosophical movements; they were not philosophers themselves, but they have had extraordinary impact for all philosophies.

The 100: A Ranking of the Most Influential Persons in History[181] by Michael H. Hart gives a list of the one hundred most influential people in history, and features descriptions of the careers, contributions, and accomplishments of the political and religious leaders, inventors, writers, artists, and others who changed the course of history. Confucius comes the fifth after Muhammad (570-632), a secular and religious leader, prophet, the founder of Islam, and the author of the Koran; Isaac Newton (1642-1727), a scientist who made many scientific and mathematical inventions and theories; Jesus Christ (ca.6 B.C.-ca.30), a prophet, spiritual leader, and the founder of Christianity; and Buddha (563-483 B.C.), a spiritual leader and the founder of Buddhism.

What was Confucius? "Confucius did not create 'a religion' in the sense that the Buddha, Jesus, or Mohammed did a movement for the masses… His doctrines

179 Yu Chang 喻昌 (1585-1664), also known as Yu Jiayan 喻嘉言, a famous medical expert of the late Ming and early Qing Dynasties. The quotation is taken from his work entitled *Yi Men Fa Lu* 医门法律 or *Laws of Medicine*.

180 Jaspers, Karl Theodor. *Socrates, Buddha, Confucius, Jesus: From The Great Philosophers* [M]. Volume I. Mariner Books, 1966.

181 Actually this ranking is quite controversial, for example, why Muhammad comes the first? But as regards to Confucius there is a common viewpoint in the international intellectual circle. See Hart, Michael H. *The 100: A Ranking of the Most Influential Persons in History* [M]. Citadel, 2000.

assume the framework of traditional Chinese religion... Chinese religion was a function of government, the governing class was the nearest thing to priesthood, and so the philosophy of the governing class was an integral part of the religion. Confucius created a philosophy and a set of values which in its broad outlines was adopted by the Chinese scholarly and administrative class for some 2,000 years."[182]

What was he? Was he a politician - a conservative or a reformer or a revolutionary? A philosopher who created Confucianism? Or a teacher?

Hereafter is a self-description from *The Analects of Confucius*: "At fifteen I set my heart upon learning. At thirty I had planted my feet upon the ground. At forty I had no more doubts. At fifty I knew the Will of the Heaven. At sixty my ears were attuned to it. At seventy I could follow the desires of my own heart for what I desired would not overstep the line". That is to say: At fifteen, Confucius wholeheartedly devoted himself to learning; At thirty, he accomplished a solid foundation in the learning, and then had good manners and full confidence in his words and deeds; At forty, he grasped all kinds of knowledge, and thus had no more doubts and no longer suffered from perplexities; At fifty he knew the Will of the Heaven for he studied *The Classic of Changes* at this age[183]; At sixty the function of his ears could understand his own and others minds, telling true from false, distinguishing clearly between right and wrong, and understanding the intention by words; At seventy he could follow the desires of his own heart, and do what is natural and rightful.

3.1 Confucius and His Historical Contexts

Confucius lived at the end of the Spring and Autumn Period (770-476 B.C.). The central government was in a state of collapse and the society was in a state of social anarchy; The kingdom broke up into many independent states, among which constant wars occurred; That was a time of various calamities, such as wars, fires, and floods. In *Shi Jing* or *The Classic of Poetry* it reads that "Compassionate Heaven rages in fury, sending down death and afflicting with famine. The people wander about and perish. Everywhere destruction reigns."

Confucius was a descendent of a noble family. The ancient state of Lu (the south-east part of Shandong Province today) was where he was born and spent most of his time.

---

182 T. Patrick Burke. *The Major Religions: An Introduction with Texts* [M]. Blackwells, 1996: 107.

183 The story of Confucius studying *The Classic of Changes* is cited in the *Shi Ji* or *The Historical Records* by Sima Qian that Confucius read *The Classic of Changes* in his old age so frequently that the leather ropes fixing the pages (actually the bamboo slips) were fractured three (Here "three" means many) times (韦编三绝), which indicated that he studied the book very diligently.

3.1.1 A Brief Account of Confucius's Life

When Confucius was born in 551 B.C., his father Shuliang He 叔梁纥[184] was 70 years old while his mother Yan Zhengzai 颜征在 was just 18 years old. His father died when he was three. Since then he lived a poor life with his mother. His mother died when he was 22. He had made a living by doing various kinds of jobs such as a shepherd, a tally man and a librarian.

Actually there is little historical information on Confucius in his time but much legend. It is well known about his failure as a politician, but great success as a philosopher, teacher, and transmitter of tradition. The most detailed account of Confucius's life is the biography which comprises the 47th chapter of *Shi Ji* or *The Historical Records*. From this we learn that Confucius was poor in his youth, but entered the government of Lu and by the time he was fifty had reached a high official rank. Then he was soon forced to resign from his post and go into exile. For the next 13 years he traveled from one state to another, tried to persuade rulers of different states to accept his thoughts, always hoping to find an opportunity to realize his ideal of political and social reform. Nowhere, however, did he succeed, and finally as an old man he returned to Lu, where he died three years later in 479 B.C..

3.1.2 Confucius as a "Homeless Dog" Politician

Undoubtedly, Confucius's lifetime experiences show that his life dream was to be an official to realize his political blueprint, his moral ideals and his scholar proposals as well as his life value. He traveled from one state to another, and tried to persuade rulers of different states to accept his proposals. But unfortunately nowhere did he succeed in so doing.

The 47th chapter of *Shi Ji* or *The Historical Records* records a story about Confucius, where an allusion "homeless dog" comes from, which means “miserable and distressed”. The story reads that "Confucius arrived in Zheng Kingdom (the middle part of the north of Henan Province today), but was separated from and lost touch with his disciples, and so he stood alone at the east gate of the outer city. A citizen of Zheng kingdom saw him and told Zi Gong, one of his disciples, that ‘There is a person standing at the east gate, whose forehead looks like Tang Yao[185], neck like Gao Yao[186], and shoulder like Zichan[187]. But his

---

184 “He” was his first name and “Shuliang” the styled name given usually at 20.

185 Tang Yao, also known as Yao 尧, a legendary king in the remote antiquity. According to legends, he set up officials for government administration, season control and calendar formulation. He abdicated and handed over the crown to Shun 舜 as long as he died.

186 Gao Yao 皋陶, a legendary figure of the remote antiquity. The legend reads that he was the first judge of the Yu Shun's Reign (Shun living in between ca. 2179-2079 B.C.), and later his name was often taken as a substitution for prison official or god.

187 Zheng Zichan 郑子产 (?-522 B.C.), a famous politician and a grandson of Duke Mu of Zheng State (Zheng Mu Gong).

part below the waist was 3 cun shorter than Yu[188], and he seemed to be extremely awkward, dispirited and discouraged just like a homeless dog'". Zi Gong told Confucius what this citizen said about him. Confucius happily agreed that "What he said about my appearance may be not right, but it is really indeed the case that he metaphorized me as a homeless dog".

He failed as a politician but succeeded in becoming a happy teacher. Notice that not many people could be educated at that time. So Confucius was actually a pioneer in education because he was willing to teach every person, not only Nobles. Although he did not achieve success in politics, he was good in education. Or in other words, he cultivated his disciples to practice his political proposals.

3.1.3 Confucius as a Successful Teacher

Lun Yu or *The Analects of Confucius* 論語 is the book with the collection of conversations mainly between Confucius and his disciples. As the single most important Confucian work, *Lun Yu,* in Chinese, means "Conversation", and focuses on practicalities of interpersonal relationships and the relationship of the role of rulers and ministers of the government.

What we can see from *The Analects of Confucius* is that Confucius was a teacher, who wished to educate and enlighten his disciples to be "rounded men" who could be pillars of the state and society, and therefore he taught them various branches of knowledge based on different classics.

He said "I am a transmitter, not an innovator; I believe in antiquity and love the ancients". (Arthur Waley's translation) D.C. Lau's translation of the same passage reads that "I transmit but do not innovate; I am truthful in what I say and devoted to antiquity."

It is said that Confucius set up the first private School in history. It is thus clear that he was the supreme and the first teacher.

The Master said, "He who by reanimating the Old can gain knowledge of the new is fit to be a teacher…"

The Master said, "As to a Divine Sage or even a Good Man, far be it from me to make any such claim. As for unvarying effort to learn and unflagging patience in teaching others, those are merits I do not hesitate to claim."

According to *Biography of Confucius* by Qian Mu[189], he started to recruit disciples when he was 30 (522 B.C.). As a teacher what and how did he teach?

188 Yu 禹 was a legendary leader of an ancient tribe union. His father Gun 鲧 was killed by Shun 舜 at Yushan mountain for he failed in preventing floods by water control. He carried on his father's duty in taming rivers, but took a different method - dredging instead of blocking rivers (his father's way), and finally succeeded in water control. He was then chosen by Shun 舜 as his successor. His son Zi Qi 子启 succeeded to the throne and set up the first slaver-owners' state in ancient China, the Xia Dynasty (ca. 2070-1600 B.C.).

189 Qian Mu 钱穆 (1895-1990), a historian, educator, Confucianism scholar, and a master in studies of Chinese ancient civilization.

According to *The Analects of Confucius,* what he taught was the four teachings and the four subjects. The four teachings refer to historical documents, social practice, moral training, and behavioral principles, the so-called *Wen* 文, *Xing* 行, *Zhong* 忠, and *Xin* 信 in the chapter of *Shu'Er* 述而; The four subjects refer to ethics, language, politics, and literature as stated in the chapter of *Xian Jin* 先进. All in all what he taught was ethics and politics, i.e. he aimed at educating his disciples how to become "rounded men" and "qualified officials". The teaching

methods he used were mainly two, one was questions and answers and the other was group discussion.

He advocated "education for all without discrimination", and as a consequence he had 72 of outstanding worth in 3,000 disciples. His disciples again had disciples, who carried on and developed Confucius's thoughts and teachings.

3.1.4 Confucius as a Transmitter of Chinese Culture and the Founder of the School of Literati (Confucianism)

Confucius claimed to derive his teachings from "the Ancients," whose wisdom is embodied in "The Five Classics". Confucius did not write any book himself. But he "edited or compiled" several books, what is the so-called "the spirit of originating through transmitting 以述為作". He was not the author but was believed to be the editor and compiler of "The Six Classics" by systematizing the documents he collected at that time, which are known as "The Five Classics" by later generations for *The Classic of Music* (*Yue Jing*, 乐经） had been lost long time ago.

The Classic of Poetry (*Shī Jīng,* 詩經), translated variously as *The Book of Songs* and *The Book of Odes*, is the earliest existing collection of Chinese poems and songs. It comprises 305 poems and songs, with the earliest range from the 10th to the 7th centuries B.C.. The collection is classified into three parts according to their genre, namely *feng* 风, *ya* 雅 and *song* 颂, with the ya genre further divided into "small" and "large": Feng 风, 160 folk songs of different localities on political darkness, weal and woe of the masses, and love; Xiao Ya 小雅, 74 minor festal songs or odes traditionally sung at court festivities; Da Ya 大雅, 31 major festal songs, sung at more solemn court ceremonies; and Song 颂, 40 hymns and eulogies, sung at sacrifices to gods and ancestral spirits of the royal house. Most of poems of ya 雅 and song 颂 parts are epics and thus bear very high historical values. Confucius commented that "In The Classic of Poetry there are [around] 300 poems. But the essence of them can be covered in one sentence: 'Have no depraved thoughts'." (The Analects of Confucius)

The Classic of Documents (Shū Jīng, 書經), also commonly known as the Shàng Shū 尚書, literally "Esteemed Documents", is the earliest compilation of documentary records related to events from the Yu Shun through Xia, Shang to

Zhou Dynasties until the reign of Duke Mu of Qin (Qin Mu Gong) in ancient history of China. The title has various translations in Western texts such as *"The Classic of History"*, *"The Classic of Documents"*, *"The Book of History"*, *"The Book of Documents"*. This book has four parts, i.e. *Document of Yu, Document of Xia, Document of Shang, and Document of Zhou*. It contains some of the earliest examples of Chinese prose. Many citations of *The Document of Shang [Dynasty]* can be found in the texts on the bamboo slips from the tombs of Guodian, in Hubei, dated to 300 B.C.. The language is archaic and differs in grammar and vocabulary from that typical of prose from the classical age of Chinese literature e.g., *The Analects of Confucius* or *The Mencius*.

The Classic of Rites (*Lǐ Jì,* 禮記), also known as *The Book of Rites, The Book of Customs, The Record of Rites*, describes the social forms, governmental system, and ancient ceremonial rites of the Zhou Dynasty (ca.1050–256 B.C.). The original text is believed to have been compiled by Confucius himself, whilst the edition usually referred to today was edited and re-worked by various scholars during the Han Dynasty (202 B.C.–A.D.220). The work should not to be confused with two other classical texts on rites: *Zhou Li* or *The Rites of Zhou* 周禮, a collection of bureaucratic establishment with characteristics of archives; and *Yi Li* or *The Book of Etiquette and Ceremonies* 儀禮, records of complicated ceremonial procedures of Zhou rulers, something like a schedule of a professional master of ceremonies.

The Classic of Changes, or *The I Ching* (Yì Jīng, 易经), also commonly known as *The Book of Changes* and *Zhou Yi*, is one of the oldest classical Chinese texts, which "was completed by three sages (namely Fu Xi 伏羲, Wen Wang 文王 and Confucius) through three eras". Fu Xi made the Eight Trigrams by observing the Heaven and the Earth; Wen Wang of Zhou Dynasty (Zhou Wen Wang) doubled the Eight Trigrams into Sixty-Four Hexagrams and gave text comments on them; Confucius composed *Shi Yi* or *Ten Wings* 十翼 to interpret the sixty-four hexagrams, and thus transforming *The I Ching* from a divination book to a philosophical masterpiece, and finally to a classic of Confucianism. The story of Confucius studying *The Classic of Changes* is cited in the *Shi Ji* or *The Historical Records* by Sima Qian that Confucius read *The Classic of Changes* in his old age so frequently that the leather ropes fixing the pages (actually the bamboo slips) were fractured three[190] times (韦编三绝), which indicated he studied the book very diligently.

The book contains a divination system comparable to Western geomancy or the West African Ifá system; in Western cultures and modern East Asia, it is still widely used for this purpose. During the Warring States Period, the text was

190 Three implies many. See Chapter “6.2.5 Three: San, 三” of the Part 1 “Overview of Chinese Culture with Chinese Characters”.

re-interpreted as a system of cosmology and philosophy that subsequently became intrinsic to Chinese culture. It centered on the ideas of the dynamic balance of opposites, the evolution of events as a process, and acceptance of the inevitability of change.

The Spring and Autumn Annals (Chun Qiu, 春秋) is the official chronicle of the State of Lu covering the period from 722 B.C. to 481 B.C.. It is the earliest surviving Chinese historical text to be arranged on annalistic principles. Its contents involve various aspects such as politics, military affairs, economics, culture, astronomy, meteorological phenomena, material production, and social life, which are original records with correct time, place and figure of that time. The text is extremely concise and, if all the commentaries are excluded, about 16,000 words long. Because of this its meaning can only be appreciated with the aid of ancient commentaries, especially the traditional *Commentary of Zuo*.

In his period, many people did not care traditions anymore. Confucius wanted to resume this tradition. Confucius did not only want to resume this Chinese (Early Chou) tradition, but he also gave some new meanings and interpretations to this tradition. The new interpretations from him are mainly reflected in *The Analects of Confucius* and interpretations of "The Five Classics", which all relate to moral philosophy and politics. In this sense, Confucius is the founder of the School of Literati (Confucianism).

The further expression of the School of Literati (Confucianism) is known collectively as "The Four Books", i.e. *Lun Yu* or *The Analects of Confucius, Zhong Yong* or *The Doctrine of the Mean,* whose authorship was attributed to Zi Si 子思, the only grandson of Confucius, *Da Xue* or *The Great Learning,* and *Mencius* or *The Book of Mencius*. Later on, the School of Literati (Confucianism), also known as the Way of Confucius and Mencius, has become the most important thought in China for more than 2,000 years.

3.2 Timeline of Confucianism

As regards to the function of Confucianism in ancient China, Li Hongqi, a professor of The City University of New York, commented that the social structure of China had been that of a closed pyramid, of which the emperor, the aristocrats, officials constituted the bricks of the different levels, and Confucianism was the adhesive power among the bricks; and that this system would be relatively harmonious and stable if without the external invasions.[191]

Hereafter is a brief timeline of Confucianism.

Confucius (551-479 B.C.) tried to resume the Chinese (Early Zhou) tradition, and Confucianism was born on the basis of his ideas during the Warring States Period in Chinese history, and thus he is the founder of Confucianism.

191 Translated into English from Chinese.

Mencius (372?-289?B.C.) spread Confucianism throughout China and developed it as the idealistic wing of Confucianism. Mencius advocates "the Goodness of Human Nature". In *The Book of Mencius* it reads that "The people are the most important element in a state; the spirits of the land and the grain are secondary; and the sovereign is the least".

Xun Tzu (300?-230?B.C.) also spread Confucianism throughout China and developed it as the realistic wing of Confucianism. Xun Tzu is best known because of his theory that "human nature is originally evil". Superficially it may seem that Xun Tzu had a very low opinion about man, yet the truth is quite the contrary. His general idea is that everything good and valuable is the product of human effort. Value comes from culture and culture is the achievement of man. It is in this that man has the same importance in the universe as Heaven and Earth. Heaven, Earth and man are the three powers of the universe, each of which has its own particular vocation. In the chapter *On Heaven* of *The Book of Xun Tzu* it reads that "Heaven has its seasons, Earth has its resources, and man has his culture. This is what is meant [when it is said that man] is able to form a trinity [with Heaven and Earth]"; and that "The stars make their rounds; the sun and moon alternately shine; the four seasons succeed one another; Yin and yang go through their great mutations; wind and rain are widely distributed; and all things acquire their harmony and have their lives". Such is the vocation of Heaven and Earth. But the vocation of man is to utilize what is offered by Heaven and Earth and thus create his own culture. Human nature should also be cultured, for, from Xun Tzu's point of view, the very fact that it is uncultured means that it cannot be good.[192] Therefore, in this sense, Xun Tzu is a pioneer of cultural philosophy for his philosophy is a kind of cultural philosophy or a philosophy of culture.

In 134 B.C., Dong Zhongshu 董仲舒 (179-104 B.C.) put forward a proposal of "To proscribe all non-Confucian schools of thoughts and to espouse Confucianism as the orthodox state ideology", which was taken by Han Wu Di, Emperor Wu of Han Dynasty. And thereafter Confucianism was established as an official religion of China and the leading philosophical thought in China until 1905.

In 300 A.D., Confucianism spread into Korea, Japan, and Vietnam.

In between 200-599 A.D., interest in Confucianism declined for the metaphysics, a philosophical sect in the Wei and Jin Dynasties and Buddhism were prosperous and popular.

Interest of Confucianism started to revive since 600. The rulers of Tang Dynasty (618-907) adopted the culture policy of making Confucianism, Buddhism, and Taoism go side by side. Achievements in systematizing, annotating, and spreading Confucian classics surpassed well beyond what had done in the former

192 Fung Yu-Lan. 1948; 2010: 234.

dynasties. Confucian civil examinations, which had started and taken Confucianism as the fundamental standard since Sui Dynasty (581-618), were enforced during the Tang Dynasty.

In between 716-916?, Japan followed China and introduced Confucian civil examinations to its nation.

Korea followed China, and held Confucian civil examinations in the years from 958 to 1894.

In 1075, Vietnam followed China and introduced Confucian civil examinations to Vietnam, which was continued until 1919.

Zhu Xi 朱熹 (1130-1200) was regarded the founder of Neo-Confucianism. In 1368 Neo-Confucianism was introduced as the state philosophy of Yuan (1271-1368), Ming (1368-1644), and Qing Dynasties (1644-1911), which marked that the feudal ideology was coming to the complete and perfect. In 1313, *The Collected Annotations of The Four Books* by Zhu Xi was determined by an imperial decree as the standard of Confucian civil examinations; In 1369, Confucian civil examinations took Zhu Xi's annotations as the principal.

In the years between 1582 and 1610, Italian Jesuit Matteo Ricci 利玛窦 (1552-1610) translated Confucian Classics into Latin, attempting to convert Chinese to Christianity by making it appear like Confucianism. In 1704 Pope Clement XI. decided against Jesuit suggestion of treating Confucianism as a form of Christianity, forbade practicing Catholic mass in Chinese language.

In 1905, the Empress Dowager Ci Xi abolished the Confucian civil examination system in China.

The May 4th Movement in 1919 proposed to "Down with Confucianism".

On Jan. 18th 1974, the Central Committee of the Communist Party of China (CCCPC) transmitted a document with the title of "*Lin Biao* 林彪 (1907-1971) *and The Way of Confucius and Mencius*" selected and compiled by Jiang Qin 江青 (1914-1991), who married Mao Zedong 毛泽东 (1893-1976) in 1938, which officially launched the "Criticizing Lin and Confucius Movement" in Communist China. Confucianism was in decline.

On Jan 11th 2011, a Confucius statue of 9.5 meters high located at the east of Tian'anmen Square was completed, and then he became the third after Mao Zedong and Sun Yat-Sen [193] who marched into the square and stationed there. The Nine-Five originates from comments on QIAN or the Creative Hexagram (䷀) of *The Book of Changes* - "Nine in the fifth place means: Flying dragon in Heaven. It furthers one to see the great man". The height of the statue of Confucius (9.5 meters) indicates the royal prerogative, the imperial throne, or the position of an emperor. But as we know Confucius was far away from taking the

---

193 Sun Yat-sen or Sun Zhongshan 孙中山 (1866 - 1925) was a Chinese doctor, revolutionary and political leader. As the foremost pioneer of Nationalist China, Sun is frequently referred to as the Founding Father of Republican China.

position of an emperor and was actually expelled by various states like "a homeless dog" during his lifetime. Moreover, he also has nothing to do with revolution. How could Confucius be compared with the other two figures that are vital for China today?

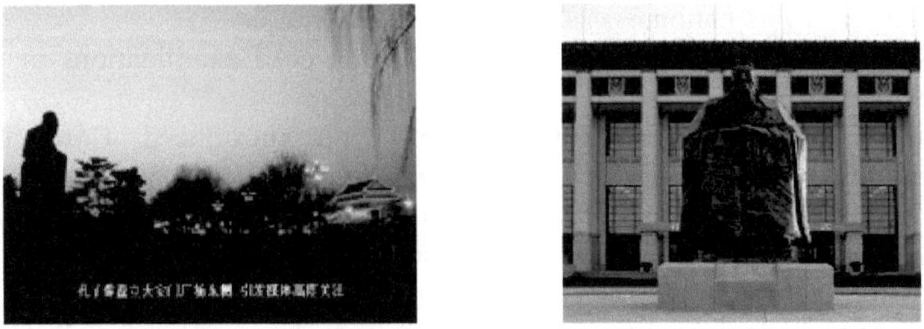

Illus. 18 The Statue of Confucius Standing in Tian'anmen Square

In fact the “Movement of Criticizing Lin and Confucius” in Communist China started with a poem to Guo Moruo 郭沫若 (1892-1978) by Chairman Mao Zedong (1893-1976) composed in the summer of 1973.

Reading *On System of Enfeoffment*. To Master Guo[194]

Advise you against condemning Qin Shi Huang[195] so much,

Events of “Burning books and burying Confucian scholars alive”[196] need to be re-discussed.

Qin[197] remained although Ancestor Dragon[198] died,

Ten Criticisms[199] is not a good article.

All dynasties followed the King of Qin[200]’s way of ruling the country,

Confucius’s teachings bear high reputation but are actually worthless like chaff.

Read carefully over and over again *On System of Enfeoffment* by Tang people,

---

194 The original title is *Du Feng Jian Lun. To Master Guo* 读《封建论》呈郭老.

195 Qin Shi Huang 秦始皇 (259?-210 B.C.) is the founding emperor of Qin Dynasty who united China and ended the Warring States period.

196 Actually, what were buried alive were not Confucian scholars but practitioners of occult arts; what were burned were not books of all kinds but books of poetics, master philosophers and their school thoughts. The original names of the events “焚书坑儒” were actually “焚诗书坑术士”, i.e. “Burning books (of poetics, master philosophers and their school thoughts)” in 213 B.C. and “burying practitioners of occult arts alive” in 212 B.C., the two important political events in Qin Shi Huang’s reign. The translation here in the poem accords with Guo Moruo’s understanding of the events.

197 Qin refers to Qin Shi Huang’s way of governing a country.

198 Ancestor Dragon refers to Qin Shi Huang.

199 *Shi Pi Pan Shu* or *Ten Criticisms* 十批判书 is a book by Guo Moruo, in which he criticizes Qin Shi Huang for he “burned books and buried Confucian scholars alive”, which reflects his viewpoint of upholding Confucianism and opposing Legalist School.

200 The King of Qin refers to Qin Shi Huang.

Don't follow Zihou to go back to Wen King [of Zhou Dynasty][201].

During the Warring States Period (475-221B.C.), Confucius's disciples were permitted to give lectures in six of the seven powerful states of that time, i.e. Qi, Chu, Yan, Han, Zhao and Wei states, with the Qin state as the only exception. But the fact is that the six states who believed in Confucius were all destroyed and annexed by Qin state, the only state which didn't follow Confucius's teachings. Did Confucius's teachings terminate the life of the other six states? In Mao Zedong's eyes, Confucianism is just like "The Emperor's New Clothes"[202], which the rulers upheld in the surface to control the common people but practiced deep into their hearts the same as Qin Shi Huang did. Mao Zedong gave a penetrating analysis of the rise and decline of the past dynasties in China - The history of the dynasties since Qin Shi Huang died from Han (206 B.C.- A.D. 220), Three Kingdoms (220-265), Jin (265-420), the Northern and Southern Dynasties (420-589), Sui (581-618), Tang (618-907), Song (960-1279), Yuan (1271-1368), Ming (1368-1644) to Qing (1644-1911) Dynasties moved in cycles. Before founding fathers of the dynasties took the throne, they were surely against Confucianism for a subject should just follow but not rebel the current emperors according to Confucianism; but they respected and advocated Confucianism as long as they took the throne in order to rule the people and to avoid their subjects rebelling them during their reign.

Actually this is a total misinterpretation of the quotation "let the ruler be ruler, the minister minister, the father father, and the son son"(*The Analects of Confucius*. *Zi Lu*) , which actually implies that things in actual fact should be made to accord with the implication attached to them by names, that every name in the social relationships implies certain responsibilities and duties, and that the ruler, minister, father, and son are all names of such social relationships, and the individuals bearing certain names must fulfill their responsibilities and duties accordingly.[203]

In *The Analects of Confucius,* besides of the quotation "The man who uses his brain will govern; while the man who uses his strength will be governed", there are much more other quotations, such as "Don't do unto others what you don't want others do unto you"; and "A man with benevolence (*ren zhe)* is one who, wishing to establish one self, establishes others, and wishing to develop one self, develops others"; etc.

---

201 *Feng Jian Lun* or *On System of Enfeoffment* is an article by Liu Zongyuan 柳宗元 (773-819) with a style name Zihou of Tang Dynasty (618-907), which upholds the system of prefectures and counties, a system of local administration which took shape during the Spring and Autumn Period and the Qin Dynasty, and opposes the system of enfeoffment.

202 The author is Hans Christian Andersen (1805-1875).

203 Fung Yu-Lan. 1948; 2010: 68.

What kind of philosophy can Confucianism be? Is it a philosophy like "The Emperor's New Clothes" or an advanced philosophy?

Actually Confucianism, originally an advanced philosophy of culture, moved towards the opposite at Zhu Xi's time, which results from the high praise and practice of Neo-Confucianism by the rulers of that time. "To Keep Principles of Heaven and Destroy Desires of Man", which originally appeared in *The Book of Rites* and later was advocated by New-Confucianism, became a traditional slogan of Chinese dictatorial system. What the May 4th Movement in 1919, an anti-imperialist, anti-feudal, political and cultural movement, criticized under the signboard of "Down With Confucianism" was actually "Down with the "Neo-Confucianism", such as "Three Cardinal Guides (ruler guides subject, father guides son and husband guides wife) and Five Constant Virtues (benevolence, righteousness, propriety, knowledge and sincerity - principle of feudal moral conduct)" as specified in the feudal ethical code, "Males were supposed to be worth more than females", "arranged marriage", and "feudal dictatorial system" etc., but advocated individuality liberation and combated personality attachment. The guiding thinking of the May 4th Movement is "science and democracy" introduced into China from the West, which actually coincides with Confucius's idea of "benevolence, i.e. loving people".

A fact worth to be mentioned here is that top philosophers, thinkers, and scholars of that time such as Fung Yu-Lan or Feng Youlan 冯友兰 (1895-1990), Guo Moruo 郭沫若 (1892-1978), Hu Shi 胡适 (1891-1962), et al., who supported the May 4th Movement, and the Kuomintang government of that time, all respected Confucius and valued him and Confucianism in a high and positive way.

In September 2004, some cultural celebrities including Xu Jialu 许嘉璐 (1937-), Ji Xianlin 季羡林 (1911-2009), Ren Jiyu 任继愈 (1916-2009), Yang Zhengning 杨振宁 (1922-), and Wang Meng 王蒙 (1934-) et al. jointly launched "*Culture Announcement of 2004*" in order to carry forward China's civilization, which became an indicative event in the culture circle of that year. And then in the recent years there has arisen a craze for classical Chinese culture, esp. Confucianism in China. I just give you one example - Confucius and Confucianism have been lectured and interpreted at least 3 times at "Lecture Room", a popular national TV program daily broadcasting at the Science and Education Channel of China Central Television (CCTV 10) by 3 distinguished scholars[204] to meet such a social need. The amount of distribution of the book "*Yu*

204 The names of the three scholars here and the titles of their lectures are as follows: Prof. Yu Dan 于丹 of Communication University of China with the title "My Personal Understanding of *The Analects of Confucius*"; Prof. Yi Zhongtian 易中天 of Xiamen University with the title "The Philosophers of Pre-Qin Days, Contention of A Hundred Schools of Thoughts"; Prof. Bao Pengshan 鲍鹏山 of Shanghai TV University with the title "How Confucius Was Tempered".

Dan's Personal Understanding of The Analects of Confucius" has reached over 5 millions, and the author Yu Dan 于丹, a female professor, is analogized as "Confucius painted with lipstick".

How do we return to Confucianism? The modern return to Confucianism should take human rights as the weapon, clear away such feudal dross as personality attachment and official-rank-oriented standard, root human rights theory into Confucianism classics, and thus return to classics at a higher point. I think that's also the implications of the statue of Confucius standing together with that of Mao Zedong and Sun Yat-Sen in the Tian'anmen Square of Beijing.

3.3 The Main Ideas of Confucius

It is always not easy to understand Chinese philosophy. *The Analects of Confucius* is not a systematic work with logical arguments in the modern Western philosophical sense. Generally speaking, Confucianism can be classified into two main parts: one on the self, i.e. how to become a full rounded man or a man of noble characters by self-cultivation; the other on the society, i.e. how to construct a good government and harmonious human relations.

3.3.1 The "Self" and the "Society"

How do we deal with a society in chaos and how can we keep ourselves from being destroyed? Here are some possible answers:

The Legalists' or realists' answer would be force for people understand force and force is the only way to control people, as the saying goes "might makes right".

The Mohists' – followers of Mo Ti or idealists' answer would be love for human beings have a great capacity for love, so they believe that the universal love or all-embracing love will solve the problem.

Confucius rejected both of these answers. His solution is that we need social structures and a collective ethos; and then people can be molded by tradition and education. How do we achieve this? What did Confucius propose on how to go from self to society?

"Cultivate individual moral character, run the family unison, manage the nation in order, and finally peace will prevail throughout the universe", which has been interpreted by "inner sage and outer king" since Song Dynasty (960-1279), which originally comes from the chapter of *Beneath the Heaven* of *Chuang Tzu.*

In Confucius's ideas "inner sage" and "outer king" are united together with the former as the foundation and the latter as the goal. Only after continuous self cultivation can a man become a full rounded man of noble character, i.e. reach and achieve the "inner sage"; and only on the basis of "inner sage" can the country be peacefully and harmoniously ruled. Confucius was recorded to say that "A man with benevolence *(ren zhe)* is one who, wishing to establish one self, establishes others, and wishing to develop one self, develops others".

After achieving the "inner sage", what is the way to practice "outer king", i.e. how to bring peace to the country and have it settled on a firm basis? Zi Xia, one of Confucius's disciples, proposed that "He who excels in doing his duty to the country should devote himself to study; He who excels in study should devote himself to the service of the country". In other words, "when a man in office finds that he can more than cope with his duties, then he studies; when a student finds that he can more than cope with his studies, then he takes office".

Self is the center of all relationships and is constantly changing and growing towards maturity. Family is where each person has a clear sense of place and purpose; Good behavior and respect for elders are important in the family. Government of a country is where the leader has acquired the moral perfection needed to lead by the power of example. Heaven represents the ultimate moral force that guides and nurtures humanity.

Da Xue or *The Great Learning* reads that

"Once things are investigated, knowledge will be completed.

Once knowledge is complete, opinions will be verified.

Once opinions are verified, minds will be rectified.

Once minds are rectified, persons will be cultivated.

Once persons are cultivated, families will be harmonized.

Once families are harmonized, states will be put in order.

Once states are in order, there will be peace all under heaven.

From the emperor to the common people, all must see the cultivation of their own person as the root of all else.

If roots are in disarray, there will never be healthy branches". (Lydia Garber)

3.3.2 Officialdom: the Natural Outlet for Good Scholars

The only way to practice Confucius's teachings is to be an official. Did Confucius want to be an official? Yes, of course. How strong of his desire? Very strong. He was so eager, itching for a try, and could scarcely wait. Zi Gong was very good at doing business, and was the only successful business man among Confucius's disciples. It is said that Confucius's travel through all the states was sponsored by him. *The Analects of Confucius* records such a conversation between Zi Gong and Confucius.

Zi Gong asked: "Here it is a piece of beautiful jade. Should we store it in a box? Or should we find a businessman who can appreciate its beauty and then sell it to him?"

The master answered: "Sell it! Sell it! I am right here waiting for such a businessman who can appreciate my talent!"

This conversation actually talks about political attitudes on whether scholars should go out to take official duties or not - That a scholar waits for being appointed as an official is just like that a beautiful jade waits for being bought by a businessman who can appreciate its beauty! Confucius's answer to this question shows how eager he wanted to be an official! Why was he so eager to be an official? Because he wanted to realize his political blueprint - to make the country the same as East Zhou in order, harmony, peace, and happiness; to practice his academic viewpoints - to educate the people to gain moral characteristics to realize his moral ideals; and to realize his life value as a man with honour - being both an official and a scholar. Was Confucius an empleomania? Would Confucius be an official in any case?

Here is worth to mention preconditions for Confucius to be an official. He said,

"If the government is well ordered and well regulated, you could work as an official and get your salary; It is shameful if you are economically poor and politically lowly in this case.

"If the government is dark ruled, it is shameful if you work as an official and get your salary; you should be a recluse; it is shameful if you enjoy untold wealth and high honour."

It is thus clear that Confucius's ideal would be: The administration of the government is well regulated; then scholars should study hard in order to work as an official to serve for the society, and thus being rich and powerful, having a high social position and honour in ranking.

The Imperial Examination System (605-1905) had been the hope for the common people to be directly promoted as officials of different rankings in China. The examination questions were all from *The Four Books* and *The Five Classics*, the classics of Confucianism, and therefore Confucius and Confucianism had been in the leading position among all the scholars and feudal bureaucrats. That "Cultivate individual moral character, run the family unison, manage the nation in order, and finally peace will prevail throughout the universe" had become the thinking and cultural perception which had dominated the literati and officialdom in feudal China for nearly 1,500 years.

3.3.3 The Five Cardinal Human Relations

The Analects of Confucius discussed in details the five cardinal human relations with the self in the center for the self involves inevitably the five human relations, i.e. Monarch-Subject, Father-Son, Husband-Wife, Elder Brother (Sister)-Younger Brother (Sister), Friend-Friend. Each relation is bounded by rights and obligations. Four of the relations involve the authority of a higher person over a lower one, and each person has to give obedience and respect to "superiors", for example, the subject to his ruler, the wife to her husband, the son to his parents, and the younger brother to the elder brother. The "superior", however, owes loving responsibility to the lower person or the inferior. Loyalty (*Zhong*) – subjects to the monarch, filial piety (*Xiao*) – children to their parents, chastity (*Jie*) – wife to her husband, popriety (*Li*) in between brothers or sisters, and sincerity (*Xin*) in between friends with *Benevolence* (*Ren*) in the center for *Benevolence* (*Ren*) involves all the human relations, constitute core values in Confucianism. This demonstrates that the physical, natural order and the social, moral order are identical and actually are often spoken as one and the same.

In more details, that is the so called *Zhong*-Loyalty, *Xiao*-Filial Piety, *Ren*-Benevolence, *Yi*-Righteousness, *Li*-Propriety, *Zhi*-Knowledge, and *Xin*-Sincerity. *Zhong*-Loyalty is the foundation of a country; *Xiao*-Filial is the foundation of a family; the other five are known collectively as the Five Constant Virtues in the feudal ethnic code, which are the foundation for the self cultivation. It is still necessary to learn, inherit and carry forward those virtues.

***Zhong*-Loyalty 忠:** It originally means to keep a solemn and respectful attitude when people were holding ceremonial activities of offering sacrifices to gods or ancestors, later on was extended to mean loyalty to the monarch and the country. In modern times *Zhong*-Loyalty advocates to be patriotic and to love one's country. Therefore *Zhong*-Loyalty is the foundation underlying all our efforts to build the country.

***Xiao*-Filial Piety 孝:** The sinogram 孝, an associative compound, is composed of two parts, the upper is the abbreviated form of 老 (pronounced as Lao, and means old) and the lower is 子 (pronounced as Zi, and means son), which indicates that son carries on his parents' career. It originally means "good at serving one's parents". This concept implies complete devotion, honor, respect, and obedience to one's parents, no matter living or deceased. China has preserved such a tradition, i.e. respect for age, which means experiences and wisdoms. *Xiao*-Filial Piety is the foundation underlying all our efforts to build the family.

In Chinese, "Guo Jia 国家", some times "Jia Guo 家国", implies that a country is composed of families, and that a country and a family are isomorphic, i.e. similar in form and relations. The institution of the family is the foundation of a well-ordered and civilized society, which is grounded mainly on respect of children for their parents.

***Ren*-Benevolence 仁:** The original meaning of "Ren 仁" is the love between people, which is shown from the sinogram, an associative compound (*The Origin of Chinese Characters*). Confucius believed that the man who really loves others is one able to perform his duties in the society. You see that the five cardinal human relationships do not indicate the hierarchical structure in the soicety, which has been misinterpreted since the Han Dynasty (202 B.C.- A.D. 220).

Benevolence (Ren 仁) is the most important ethical concept in Confucianism. The concept of *Ren* is similar to something like "love", "humanity", "benevolence", "human-heartedness", etc. What on earth is "Ren-Benevolence"? Confucius answered that "Benevolence is to love others"; that "Don't do unto others what you don't want others do unto you"; and that "A man with benevolence (*ren zhe)* is one who, wishing to establish one self, establishes others, and wishing to develop one self, develops others. To be able from one's own self to make an analogy for the treatment of others, which may be called the way to practice *Ren*". The way of putting *Ren* into effect is actually the doctrine of loyalty and consideration for others. Immanuel Kant's[205] morality and duty is similar to this. The conception of "universal conformity to law" is Kant's central notion of duty. Kant defined it as a generalized version of the Golden Rule: "Do unto others as you would have them do unto you", which is so similar to "Don't do unto others what you don't want others do unto you" advocated by Confucius.

Ancient emperors sought to practice policies of benevolence, and diligently strove to be benevolent governments. The core of *Ren*-Benevolence is people oriented, people foremost, which means to do all for caring, loving and developing people in order to make the country in the perfect harmonious state. Besides, *Ren*-Benevolence is still embodied in the equality of all the living creatures just as Confucius advanced to "make no social distinctions in teaching".

***Yi*-Righteousness 義:** The sinogram 義 is an associative compound, following 我 and 羊. "我 Wo", an associate compound, following 戈 (ge or dagger-axe, an ancient weapon), originally means weapons; and then was extended to mean insignia carried before the emperor; or flags, weapons, etc carried by a guard of honour; and basically means "to call oneself". "羊 Yang", a pictograph reflecting the image of a goat with two horns on its head, feet and tail, is a mammal usually used in animal sacrifice, implying being good and beautiful. And thus the original meaning of "義 Yi" is "righteousness; appropriate morality, behaviour, or principle", and was the ancient writing form of "儀 Yi".

It is a universal and "holistic" expression of all the general virtues in the Confucian system. Any failure to actualize a potential virtue and any infraction against or non-fulfillment of loyalty, filial piety, chastity, or even the principle of faithfulness among friends disqualifies a person from being considered "righteous." The attainment of it represents a moral completion.

Yi-Righteousness refers to the moral disposition to do good. *Yi* connotes a moral sense, i.e. the ability to recognize what is right and good; the ability to feel under the circumstances what is the right thing to do. Some actions ought to be performed for the sole reason that they are right - regardless of what they produce; not for the sake of something else.

Yi-Righteousness and *Li*-Profit are in Confucianism diametrically opposed terms: "The man with honor comprehends *Yi*-Righteousness; the small man comprehends *Li*-Profit".

---

205 Immanuel Kant (1724–1804) was a German philosopher, researching, lecturing and writing on philosophy and anthropology at the end of the 18th Century Enlightenment. His ideas influenced many thinkers in Germany during his lifetime. He settled and moved philosophy beyond the debate between the rationalists and empiricists. The philosophers Johann Gottlieb Fichte (1762-1814), Friedrich Wilhelm Joseph von Schelling (1775-1854), Georg Wilhelm Friedrich Hegel (1770-1831) and Authur Schopenhauer (1788-1860) amended and developed the Kantian system, thus bringing about various forms of German idealism. He is seen as a major figure in the history and development of philosophy. German and European thinking progressed after his time, and his influence still inspires philosophical work today.

***Li*-Propriety 禮:** "*Li* 禮" means holding ceremony or offering sacrifices to gods or ancestors to pray for good fortunes. *Li* then was used to refer to the (rules governing the) religious rites associated with the worship of deities or ancestor veneration that characterized traditional Chinese religion, particularly with regards to those rites performed by the emperor. Later on, *Li* came to denote all of the emperor's duties as well as a wide range of other rituals, such as marriage, and military and government festivals.

Confucius included in his discussions of *li* such diverse topics as learning, tea drinking, titles, mourning, and governance. *Li* can also be used to refer to common moral prescriptions and "customary law", or anything which orders human conduct. *Li* is what the sage uses to find that which is appropriate; it is both the means which sets the example for others, and the end which maximizes understanding, pleasure, and the greater good. The core of *Li* is respect - respect the self and respect others.

***Zhi*-Knowledge 知-智:** The sinogram 知 is the ancient writing form of 智, means knowledge, wisdom, ability. So one should cultivate the self to become a person with knowledge, wisdom, and ability in order to serve the society.

***Xin*-Sincerity 信:** The sinogram 信 is an associative compound, following 人 (Ren, human) and 言 (Yan, words, speech). Its original meaning is "sincerity" for none of the human words were not sincere in ancient China. Confucius took *Xin*-Sincerity as a vital embodiment of *Ren*-Benevolence. Moreover, he promoted it up to the level of national government - the most important one among the three essentials of administering a country, i.e. "adequate food, powerful military army, and the sincerity of the people in the government". The full story reads that:

Zi Gong asked about how to run a country.

The Master answered, "Adequate food, powerful military army, and the sincerity of the people in the government".

Zi Gong said, "If one of these must be dispensed with, which of the three should be foregone first?"

The Master answered, "The military army".

Zi Gong asked again, "If one of the remaining two must be dispensed with, which of them should be foregone?"

The Master answered, "The food. Since death is unavoidable to everyone throughout the history. But if the people have no sincerity (faith) in their rulers, there is no standing for the state."

All in all, discussion on the five cardinal human relations in Confucianism is a system of intense moralism and humanism, which is people oriented, advocates humanism, stresses self cultivation, identifies politics with ethics, and attempts to restore the social order. As regards to the social order, Confucius thought "rectification of names" is of the first importance for a society to be on the right track and in good order.

3.3.4 Rectification of Names

Once Zi Lu, a disciple of Confucius, asked him, "The Duke of Wei State expects you to administer his state, and then what are you going to do first"? Confucius replied: "The first thing needed is the rectification of names"(*The Analects of Confucius. Zi Lu*). In order to have a well ordered society, the most important thing is to carry out the rectification of names.

How to rectify names? On another occasion the Duke of Qi State (Qi Jing Gong) of that time asked Confucius the right principle of government, to which he answered: "let the ruler be ruler, the minister minister, the father father, and the son son"(*The Analects of Confucius. Zi Lu*). Things in actual fact should be made to accord with the implication attached to them by names. Every name contains certain implications which constitute the essence of that class of things to which this name applies. That is to say, there is an agreement between name and actuality. Every name in the social relationships implies certain responsibilities and duties. Ruler, minister, father, and son are all names of such social relationships, and the individuals bearing certain names must fulfill their responsibilities and duties accordingly.[206]

3.4 Dispute between Confucius and Mo Tzu: Literati and Knights

Since Confucius founded Confucianism, the Mohist, Taoist, and Legalist Schools arose to criticize Confucius's points of view, while Confucian scholars defend, carry on, modify and develop them. The dispute between Confucianism and Mohism focused on that between *Ren Ai* 仁爱 or Benevolence and *Jian Ai* 兼爱 or All-Embracing Love; The dispute between Confucianism and Taoist School focused on that between *You Wei* 有为 or Having Action and *Wu Wei* 无为 or Having Effortless Action; The dispute between Confucianism and the Legalist School focused on that between *De Zhi* 德治 or Rule with Virtue and *Fa Zhi* 法治 or Rule with Law.

The contention of a hundred schools of thought started with the dispute between Confucianism and Mohism. Mo Tzu 墨子 (470?-391 B.C.?) is the first who criticized Confucius and Confucianism in public for Chuang Tzu 庄子 (369?-286?B.C.) and Han Fei 韩非 (281?-233 B.C.) were surely later than Mo Tzu, while *Lao Tzu* (also known as *Tao Te Ching*) does not criticize Confucius nor have any conflict with Confucianism.

In real fact, Mo Tzu's reputation and influences were equally matched with Confucius's reputation in China of that time. But the destiny of Mohism cannot even be compared with Confucianism in the later over 2,000 years. What is the reason? Let's take a look at some differences between Confucius (551-479 B.C.) and Mo Tzu (470?-391 B.C.?).

---

206 Fung Yu-Lan. 1948; 2010: 68.

3.4.1 Living in Different Times: Spring and Autumn Period vs Warring States Period

First they lived in different times, i.e. Confucius lived in the Spring and Autumn Period (770-476 B.C.), while Mo Tzu lived in the Warring States Period (475-221 B.C.). During the former period, the states still respected the Zhou Dynasty, but until the latter period - the Warring States Period, most of states ignored the existence of the Zhou Dynasty, and such a respect to the Zhou dynasty was gone, and wars frequently broke out, that's way this period was so named "Warring States" Period (475-221 B.C.). That is to say, the conditions were much worse in many aspects in the latter period than in the former period - the political administration was much darker, the society was much more turbulent and upheaval, wars broke up much more frequently in between different states, and the people had much more sufferings.

In the Spring and Autumn Period (770-476 B.C.), Confucius still had a hope to restore the Zhou order by reform and education, and thus always tried to persuade rulers to apply policies of benevolence, to improve and reform the way of administration by giving advices and criticisms in a mild tone.

But Mo Tzu lived in this turbulent Warring States Period, he was deeply affected by people's sufferings and experienced some himself, so he never concealed his attitudes and always took a clear-cut stand when criticizing, which can be seen from titles of some chapters of *Mo Tzu*[207]: *Anti-Attack* (against all unjust wars), *Anti-Music* (against indulgence in music), *Anti-Destiny*, *Anti-Confucianism*, etc. which are just like to say "I Oppose!"

As regards to "Anti-Attack", *Mo Tzu* records a story known as "Mo Tzu Relieved *Song* State from Being Attacked by *Chu* State". Gongshu Ban, a noted mechanical inventor and the earliest master carpenter also known as Lu Ban, employed by the state of *Chu* 楚, invented and completed a new weapon - scaling ladder for attacking city walls. The state of *Chu* was going to attack the state of

207 *Mo Tzu*, the book bearing his name and the main source for the study of Mohism, is a collection of writings by himself and his followers. It is rich in content and well-knit in structure in general, and some topics are closely elaborated with an incisive, penetrating analysis and sound argument. It not only deals with humanities such as epistemology, logics, economics, sociology, and social history etc., but also contains knowledge of natural sciences such as time and space, material structure, mechanics, optics, and geometry, thus having important scientific values. James Legge 理雅各 (1815-1897) was the first Western scholar to pay close attention to it by discussing its philosophy and presenting his translation of its three chapters on "All-Embracing Love" (1-3) in his work "*The Chinese Classics*". Hereafter are its 4 main English translations: ① Mei Yipao, Trans. *The Ethical and Political Works of Motse*. London: Probsthain, 1929; ② Watson, B., Trans. *Basic Writings of Mo Tzu*. New York: Columbia University Press, 1963; ③ Wang Rongpei, Wang Hong, Trans. *Mozi*. Changsha: Hunan People's Press, 2006; ④ Wang Rongpei, Wang Hong. Trans. *The Mohist Canons*. Shanghai: Shanghai Foreign Language Education Press, 2011. Up till 2009, Alfred Forke (1867-1944), a German sinologist, remained to be the only one who gave the full translation of *Mo Tzu* in a Western language (German) in the 1920s (See Wang Rongpei, Wang Hong. *English Translation of Chinese Classics*. Shanghai: Shanghai Foreign Language Education Press, 2009: 48).

Song 宋 with this new weapon. Mo Tzu heard of this information, and came to *Chu* from a very far place *Lu*, which took him ten days and ten nights on the way, to meet Gongshu Ban. He persuaded him to stop attacking *Song* by arguing that such an attack would be not wise for war killed people, nor benevolent for *Song* did nothing wrong, nor loyal for he did not make his king understand the truth, nor strong if he did not achieve this goal.

Then Gongshu Ban introduced him to his king. He tried to persuade the king to desist from attacking, and said to the king that *Chu*'s attack on *Song* was just like that a man abandoned his magnificent cart, splendid clothes, grain and meat to steal a broken cart, crash clothes, and poor men's foodstuffs for *Chu* was ten times of bigger in the size of territory and much richer in natural resources than *Song*, etc. But the king answered that "I have to attack *Song* for Gongshu Ban has created this scaling ladder for me although that is the case and you are right".

And then there he and Gongshu Ban made a demonstration of their weapons of attack and defense before the king. Mo Tzu first united his belt and laid out a city with it, and used a small stick as a weapon. Gongshu Ban applied nine different miniature machines to attack, but Mo Tzu nine times repulsed him. Finally, Gongshu Ban had used up all his machines of attack, while Mo Tzu was far from being exhausted in the defense. But Gongshu Ban still did not want to admit defeat, and then said, "I know how to defeat you, but I will not say it". While Mo Tzu replied, "I know what you mean, but I will not say it either". The king then asked them what was meant by that. Mo Tzu answered, "Gongshu Ban is thinking of murdering me. But my disciples - Qingu Li 禽滑厘[208] and others, numbering three hundred men, are already armed with my implements of defense, waiting on the city wall of *Song* state for the invaders from *Chu*. Even if I were murdered, you cannot exterminate them". Finally the king exclaimed, "Well, let us give up attacking *Song*.

This story shows us several points: 1) How Mo Tzu spared no efforts to successfully realize his proposal of "Anti-Attack" by convincing arguments and meticulous arrangement; 2) Mo Tzu himself was a much greater engineer than Gongshu Ban, and the Mohists were originally a group of Knights;[209] 3) This story enlightens us a brilliant way to settle disputes between two countries in the present world - turning a war into a competition between scientists and engineers of the two countries by demonstrating their laboratory weapons and techniques of attacking and defense!

---

208 Qingu is the family name, and Li is the first name.

209 It is said that Mo Tzu had worked as a carpenter with superb craftsmanship when he was young, and also an inventor and a scientist for his inventions and achievements in optics, mathematics, and mechanics. See his teachings *Mo Tzu* for detailed information.

3.4.2 Standing for Different Social Groups: Literati vs. Knights

Now comes the second difference, i.e. what they stood for were different. Confucius stood for literati, scholars; while Mo Tzu stood for knights. Literati participated in political affairs; while knights participated in military affairs. They may live on a powerful aristocrat as advisers, secretaries, or generals, body guards, assassins, or just hangers; or exist as free lance scholars or knights. What Confucius actually stood for were free lance scholars, and he found a way out for them - Officialdom is the natural outlet for scholars; While what Mo Tzu actually stood for were also free lance knights, and he also found an outlet for them - earning their own living in normal times and being chivalrous and fond of doing good deeds in emergent cases.

The history demonstrates that Confucius's way is workable, while Mo Tzu's way failed to work for earning one's own living could not distinguish oneself and being chivalrous and fond of doing good deeds was forbidden by the government. That's why Mohism declined afterwards.

During the feudal age of the Zhou dynasty (1066 B.C.?-256 B.C.), kings, princes, and feudal lords all had their military specialists. These were the hereditary knights who continued the backbone of the armies of that time. And they got regular salaries. With the disintegration of feudalism that took place in the latter part of the Zhou dynasty, however, those warrior specialists lost their positions and titles, scattered throughout the country, and made a living by offering their services to anyone who could afford to employ them. This class of people was known as *Xia* 侠 or *You-Xia* 游侠, terms which can both be translated as "knights-errant", i.e. war-waiting knights, knights waiting for employment for fight.

Concerning such "knights-errant", *Shi Ji* or *The Historical Records* says, "Their words were always sincere and trustworthy, and their actions were always quick and decisive. They were always true to what they promised, and without regard to their own persons, they would rush into dangers threatening others." Such was their professional ethics. A large part of Mo Tzu's teaching was an extension of this ethics.[210] The following table shows the major differences of Mo Tzu and his followers from the ordinary Knights-errant.

210 Fung Yu-Lan. 1948; 2010: 85.

Points	Ordinary Knights-Errant	Mo Tzu and His Followers
War	Were ready to engage in any fighting whatever, only provided that they were paid for their efforts or favored by the feudal lords;	Were strongly opposed to aggressive wars; hence they agreed to fight only in wars that were strictly for self-defense;
Professional Ethnics	Confined themselves wholly to their code of professional ethics.	Elaborated this professional ethics, gave it a rationalistic justification, and therefore, founded a new philosophical school of thought: Mohism.

Table 6 Differences of Mo Tzu and his followers from Ordinary Knights-Errant

In Chinese history both *Ru* or literati and *Xia* or knights-errant originated as specialists attached to the houses of the aristocrats, and were themselves members of the upper classes. In later times, *Ru* continued to come mainly from the upper or middle classes, but *Xia*, on the contrary, more frequently were recruited from the lower classes.

3.4.3 Taking Different Stands: Ruling Class vs. Labourers

Now comes the third difference - They took different stands. Confucius mainly took the stand of aristocrats, the ruling class; while Mo Tzu took the stand of common people, labourers. Therefore, Confucius tried to find a solution for the ruling class on how to achieve the long lasting political stability, and thus he advocated that "let the ruler be ruler, the minister minister, the father father, and the son son".

In ancient times, social amenities as rituals and music were all exclusively for the aristocrats; but from the point of view of the common people, they were luxuries that had no practical utility. It was from this point of view that Mo Tzu and the Mohists criticized the traditional institutions and their rationalizers, Confucius and the Confucianists. Mo Tzu's viewpoints on economics such as frugality in use, in funeral arrangements, and anti-music fully embodied his stand of common people. The chapter of "*Anti-Confucianism*" of *Mo Tzu* reads that "Even those with long life cannot exhaust the learning required for their [Confucianists] studies. Even people with the vigor of youth cannot perform all the ceremonial duties. And even those who have amassed wealth cannot afford music. They [Confucianists] enhance the beauty of wicked arts and lead their sovereign astray. Their doctrine cannot meet the needs of the age, nor can their learning educate the people".

It is interesting to note that Mo Tzu's criticism on Confucius and Confucianism is very fierce and sharp, and argues one point to death. *Mo Tzu* records arguments between the two schools and each ended with Confucianists at a disadvantage. This might be the reason: If Mo Tzu or his followers lost in a debate, they would not write it down nor include it into the book. *The Analects of Confucius* is different in this point, others ridicule, disciples' discontent, Confucius in a dilemma etc. are all naturally and vividly recorded into the book.

3.4.4 Confucius and Mo Tzu: Benevolence vs. All-Embracing Love

Benevolence is a very important part of Confucianism; while all-embracing love is the central idea of the Mohism. Both Confucius and Mo Tzu advocated letting the world be filled with love. The difference lies in that Confucius's benevolence is a kind of hierarchic love based on genetic connection, centered on oneself, and starting with self cultivation; while Mo Tzu's all-embracing love is a kind of equal love by making no distinction between family and non-family, rich and poor, high and low, noble and common, me and others, etc., that is to say, everyone in the world should love everyone else equally and without any discrimination. Benevolence is thus much more logical and practical; while all-embracing love is an ideal state of the world which is impossible to be realized in the real world, just like a moon in the water or a flower in the mirror which is very beautiful but not to be reached forever.

According to Mo Tzu, "the principles of the Confucianists ruin the whole world in four ways": ① The Confucianists did not believe in the existence of God or of spirits, "with the result that God and the spirits are displeased"; ② The Confucianists insisted on elaborate funerals and the practice of three years of mourning on the death of a parent, so that the wealth and energy of the people were thereby wasted; ③ The Confucianists laid stress on the practice of music, leading to an identical result; ④ The Confucianists believed in a predetermined fate, causing the people to be lazy and to resign themselves to this fate.

The first point reflects that belief in Gods & Ghosts had been given up by some well-educated people, and that common people of the lower class was generally behind the new thoughts in the society; The second and third points confirmed again their differences in social background and what stands they took; But the fourth point was really irrelevant - *Ming* (Fate, Destiny, Decree) of the Confucianists did not refer to "the predetermined fate", but signified something that is beyond human control for there are other things that remain within man's power to control if he will exert himself; Only after man has done everything he can himself, therefore should he accept with calm and resignation what comes thereafter as inevitable; Such is what the Confucianists meant when they spoke of "knowing *Ming*".[211]

---

211 Fung Yu-Lan. 1948; 2010: 85-86.

To sum up, Confucius and Mo Tzu advanced different remedies for this chaotic society - the former took the rulers' stand, advocated monarchical power, benevolence, and reform; while the latter took the labourers' stand, advocated democratic rights, all-embracing love and revolution. What was the proper remedy? What did the Taoist School propose? We will discuss in the next topic, which would be "The Taoist School and Its Influences on Chinese Medicine".

3.5 English Translation and Dissemination of *Lun Yu* in the West

Confucius and his teachings travelled to the Europe first through missionaries. Matteo Ricci 利玛窦 (1552 -1610), a celebrated Italian missionary, arrived in Macau in 1582, and then opened the prologue to the first large scaled cultural exchange between China and Europe in the world's history. He authored a book with the aim of introducing the Four Books - *Lun Yu* or *The Analects of Confucius*, *Da Xue* or *The Great Learning*, *Zhong Yong* or *The Doctrine of Mean*, and *The Mencius* to Europe. But this book is actually far beyond a translation, more like an intercultural monograph on classical Chinese philosophy.

According to a scholar's statistics, as regards to the number of the western languages being translated into, *Lun Yu* is only secondary to *Tao Te Ching* among the Chinese classics.[212] The first translation of *Lun Yu* in Western language was published in Paris in 1687, which was in Latin and entitled *Confucius Sinarum Philosophus, sive Scientia Sinensis Latine Exposita*. Latin translations of *Lun Yu* or *The Analects of Confucius*, *Da Xue* or *The Great Learning*, and *Zhong Yong* or *The Doctrine of Mean* are included in this book. Philippe Couplet 柏应理 (1623-1693), a Belgium missionary of the Jesuits, translated and compiled the book with the other three missionaries in China. This book was translated into English and published in 1691 in London with the title of *The Morals of Confucius, A Chinese Philosopher*, which should be the first English translation of *Lun Yu*.[213]

Since then, over 40 English translations of *Lun Yu* have got published until today.[214]

An English missionary named Joshua Marshman 马士曼 (1768-1837) translated the first nine chapters of *Lun Yu,* and published it with the title of *The*

---

212 Stephen W. Durrant. On Translating *Lun Yu*. *Chinese Literature: Essays, Articles, Reviews* 3:1(1981): 109.

213 It was reprinted in 1818, but the title was changed as *The Life and Morals of Confucius, A Chinese Philosopher*. See David Mungello. *Curious land, Jesuit Accommodation and the Origins of Sinology*. Wiesbaden: Franz Steiner, 1985, 247-299.

214 According to Cui Yujun's paper "English Translation of *Lun Yu* by British Sinologists: History and Problems", there were 41 English versions of *Lun Yu*. [See Research Center of Unearthed Documents and Ancient Writings of Fudan University (editor). Interpretation of Unearthed Documents and Classics That Will Be Handed on from Age to Age[C]. Shanghai: Shanghai Ancient Books Publishing House, 2010.] But there are some new ones coming after the time, for example, Lin Wusun's translation published by Foreign Languages Press (Beijing) came out in March 2010.

Works of Confucius in 1809 in India.[215] Rev. David Collie 高大卫 (?-1828), again an English missionary, translated and published *The Chinese Classical Work, Commonly Called The Four Books* (1828), which may be the first English translation of *The Four Books.*[216] Academically judged, translations of this time misinterpret or distort the original maybe because of lack of Chinese language knowledge, or are confused or mixed with their religious purpose. For example, Walter Henry Medhurst 麦都思 (1796-1857), an English missionary and scholar, inserted paragraphs from *The Old Testament* and *The New Testament* into his translation of *Lun Yu.* But because of lack of good translations in this period, their translations still arose interests in some scholars of the English-speaking world. For example, Ralph Waldo Emerson (1803-1882)[217] became interested in Confucius's thoughts when he read *The Works of Confucius* by Joshua Marshman, and then selected and published 21 quotations from Confucius on the journal he was editing - *Dial*; Samuel Wells Williams 卫三畏(1812—1884), a missionary, diplomat-translator, famous American sinologist and the first professor of Chinese language and literature at Yale University and of the America as well, referred to *The Four Books* by David Collie in his famous work *The Middle Kingdom.*[218]

James Legge 理雅各 (1815-1897), a widely known Scottish missionary, sinologist and the first professor of Chinese at Oxford University (1876-1897), started to translate Confucian classics in 1848 with the assistance of Wang Tao 王韬（1828-1897）[219]and Hong Rengan 洪仁玕 (1822-1864)[220] among some other Chinese scholars. Many volumes of Chinese classics gradually got published, the first of which includes translations of *Lun Yu*, *Da Xue*, and *Zhong Yong* published in 1861 in Hong Kong.[221] By so doing he became the first person ever who translated *the Four Books* and *the Five Classics* into a western language.[222] His translation purpose was to make Europeans and missionaries in China understand better the Chinese moral, social, political thoughts, and thus helping missionaries

215 Joshua Marshman. *The Works of Confucius, Containing the Original Text with a Translation* (Vol.1). Serampore: the Mission Press, 1809.

216 David Collie, trans. *The Chinese Classical Work, Commonly Called the Four Books.* Malacca, 1828.

217 Ralph Waldo Emerson (1803–1882) was an American essayist, lecturer, thinker, and poet, who led the Transcendentalist movement of the middle 19th century. He disseminated his thoughts through dozens of published essays and more than 1,500 public lectures across the United States.

218 See Samuel Wells Williams. *The Middle Kingdom.* New York and London: Wiley and Putnan, 1848: 654.

219 Wang Tao 王韬 (1828-1897) was a Chinese translator, a reformer, a political columnist, a newspaper publisher and a writer in the late Qing Dynasty.

220 Hong Rengan 洪仁玕 (1822-1864) was an important leader of the Taiping Heavenly Kingdom (1851-1864). He was the cousin of the movement's founder and spiritual leader Hong Xiuquan 洪秀全 (1814-1864). His position as the Prince Gan 干王 resembled the role of a Prime Minister. He is a noted figure in history because of the sweeping reforms attempted under his rule, and because of his popularity in the West.

221 James Legge, trans. *The Chinese Classics* (Vol. I). Hong Kong: Hong Kong University Press, 1960.

222 Besides, he still translated other classics such as *Zhou Yi* or *The Book of Changes*, *Tao Te Ching*, *Chuang Tzu*, and so on.

fulfill their duties. Without any doubt his translations have exerted important and extensive influences on the studies on Confucianism in the West, and his translation of *Lun Yu – Confucian Analects* has become the foundation and basis of all the scholarly translations of *Lun Yu* afterwards.

Later on, Some British scholars such as Lionel Giles 翟林奈 (1875-1958), William Edward Soothill 苏慧廉 (1861-1935), Leonard Arthur Lyall 赖发洛 (1867-?), and William Jennings 詹宁斯 (?-?) had translated *Lun Yu* into English, too.[223] But few have shown interest in their translations for they were just occasionally or even seldom listed in the reference parts or bibliographies.

And then Arthur Waley (1889-1966)'s translation of *Lun Yu* came out in 1938, which has remained one of the most popular very few ones even until today among English readers in the world since its publication.[224] Arthur Waley was regarded as the greatest British sinologist after James Legge.[225] His understanding of classical Chinese thinking is far beyond the others of his time although he had never come to China in his life time.

Hereafter is a list of some other translations of *Lun Yu* (in chronological order):

KU Hung-Ming, trans. *The Discourse and Saying of Confucius*. Shanghai: Kelly and Walsh, 1898.

Ezra Pound, trans. *Analects*. New York: Kasper & Horton, 1951; published as *The Confucian Analects*. P. Owen, 1956; in Square Series, 1957.

Raymond Dawson, trans. *Confucius: The Analects*. New York: Hill and Wang, 1982.

Raymond Dawson, trans. *The Analects*. Oxford and New York: Oxford University Press, 1993.

HUANG Chichung, trans. *The Analects of Confucius: A Literal Translation with an Introduction and Notes*. Oxford and New York: Oxford University Press, 1997.

Simon Leys, trans. *The Analects of Confucius*. New York: Norton， 1997.

Roger T. Ames, Henry Rosemont, trans. *The Analects of Confucius: A Philosophical Translation*. New York : Ballantine Pub. Group, 1998.

David Hinton, trans. *The Analects*. Berkeley: Counterpoint Press, 1999.

LAU, D.C., trans. *The Analects*. Hong Kong: The Chinese University Press, 2000.

---

223 William Jennings, trans. *The Confucius Analects, A Translation with Annotations and An Introduction*. London: George Routledge and Sons, 1895; Lionel Giles, trans. *The Sayings of Confucius: A New Translation of the Greater Part of the Confucian Analects*. London: John Murray, 1907; Leonard Arthur Lyall, trans. *The Saying of Confucius*. London: Longmans, Green and Co.,1909; William Edward Soothill, trans. *The Analects of Confucius*. Shansi, 1910.

224 Elva Huang. *Translation Literature Culture*. Beijing: Beijing University, 1999: 132.

225 David B.Honey, *Incense at the Alter: Pioneering Sinologists and the Development of Classical Chinese Philology*. New Heaven, Conn.: American Oriental Society, 2001: 224.

Edward Gilman Slingerland, trans. *Analects, with Selections from Traditional Commentaries*. Indianapolis: Hackett Publishing, 2003.

Burton Watson, trans. *The Analects of Confucius*. New York: Columbia University Press, 2007.

LIN Wusun, trans. *Getting to Know Confucius: A New Translation of The Analects*. Beijing: Foreign Languages Press, 2010.

Different translators of different times of different culture backgrounds result in different translations. You see, translators involve missionaries, sinologists as well as professors and scholars from both China and English speaking world. Their cultural status, intended readers, translation motives and purposes etc. all differ from each other. Influences of Christianity, Europe Centralism (or West Centralism), and Orientalism etc. on translating *Lun Yu* as well as interpretation and/or translation of the original *Lun Yu* are all worth for further studies.

3.6 The Influences of Confucianism on Chinese Medicine

Confucianism is generally considered as an important factor in hindering the birth and development of science and technology in modern China partly for Confucianism excluded and rejected science and technology in ancient China. But this viewpoint is in fact not right. Actually, Confucianism exterted significant influences on classical Chinese science and technology in both positive and negative ways. Confucius established the paradigm of unity of *Ren*-Benevolence and *Zhi*-Knowledge, i.e. unity of epistemology and ethics, and thereby making scientific and technical knowledge being ethical, which, on one hand, restricted the scope and depth of objects of scientific cognition and ignored the independent value that scientific and technological knowledge deserves, while, on the other hand, formed a tradition of stressing the subjects of medicine, agriculture, astronomy, and mathematics in ancient China for these subjects themselves embody the unity of *Ren*-Benevolence and *Zhi*-Knowledge. That is to say, Confucianism provides a philosophical support for the birth and development of these four subjects. For example, the establishment of the practical systems of astronomy and mathematics was very much influenced by "knowing the will of Heaven" of Confucianism. For the same reason, classical Chinese sciences are generally good at solving practical problems, but have not devloped into independent subjects with complicated deep-going theories.[226]

Another notable influence from Confucianism on classical Chinese sciences is that the composition of scientific works followed the way of Confucian classics, such as interpreting and annotating the former classical texts, wording, and abundant use of metaphors, which integrates inheriting the past and creating the new into one, thus forming a tradition of developing a subject in the same

226 Chen Weiping. On the Dual Role of Confucianism in the Development of Traditional Science and Technology. In: Collected Papers of Traditional Chinese Medicine International Forum[C]. Shanghai, 2010.

framework and with one principle running through it, and finally giving classical Chinese sciences a feature of humanities.

These are also true with Chinese medicine. Chinese medicine arose from the ancient Chinese culture, and the culture of Confucianism had been the mainstream of the ancient Chinese culture for over two thousands of years until the May 4th Movement in 1919. Therefore, the influences of Confucianism on Chinese medicine are a very important topic in the culture history of Chinese medicine.

3.6.1 Scholar Physicians

3.6.1.1 Preconditions and Cultural Roots of Scholar Physicians

In 134 B.C., the Emperor Wu of Han Dynasty (Han Wu Di) accepted Dong Zhongshu's proposal of "Proscribing all non-Confucian schools of thought and espousing Confucianism as the orthodox state ideology". Confucian Classics had been approved as official textbooks for imperial examinations since Sui-Tang Dynasties (581-907). Thereafter, large numbers of Confucian Scholars arose for this reason, as Confucius pointed out that officialdom is the natural outlet for scholars. In fact officialdom is the goal of studying Confucian classics.

The metaphor "Being A Physician Is only Secondary to Being A Good Prime Minister" first appeared in *Mo Tzu,* and was clearly formulated by Fan Zhongyan 范仲淹 (989-1052). It has been a motto for Confucian scholars even up till today. For example, Wu Yi 吴仪 (1938-), a former deputy prime minister of the Chinese government retired in 2008, announced that she would go to learn medicine (esp. Chinese medicine) to be a good physician since she retired from his post as a deputy prime minister.

Why do Confucian scholars claim "Being A Physician Is only Secondary to Being A Good Prime Minister" as their motto?

① They abandoned Confucianism and then were engaged in medicine for they or their parents were maltreated by quacks. For example, Huangfu Mi[227] 皇甫谧 (215-282) suffered from wind paralysis (rheumatism in modern Western medicine) when he was 30, nearly died after taking Hanshi Powder 寒食散 by mistake. Since then, he studied medicine and devoted himself to acupuncture, compiled *Zhen Jiu Jia Yi Jing* or *The Systematic Classic of Acupuncture and Moxibustion* 针灸甲乙经, the first monograph exclusively on the subject.

Another example is Li Dongyuan 李东垣 (1180-1251). He was determined to follow Zhang Yuansu 张元素 to learn medicine after his mother died of a malpractice. His masterpiece is *Pi Wei Lun* or *Treatise on the Spleen and Stomach* 脾胃论. He held that "Diseases, apart from external changes, were mainly caused by internal injury to the spleen and stomach", and advocated "Cure by regulating the spleen and stomach and nourishing the original qi", and by so doing became the founder of the School for Strengthening the Spleen and Stomach.

227 Here, Huangfu is the family name, and Mi is the first name.

② They turned to medicine for they always failed in Imperial Examinations. For example, Li Shizhen 李时珍 (1518-1593), the author of *Ben Cao Gang Mu* or *The Compendium of Materia Medica* 本草纲目, which was appraised as the "encyclopedia of China published in 1596" by Charles Robert Darwin (1809-1882). Joseph Needham (1900-1995) compared him to Galileo Galilei (1564-1642) and Andreas Vesalius (1514-1564) of the Europe, and said he was the greatest scientist outside the Europe at that time.

③ They felt frustrated as officials. For example, Wang Kentang 王肯堂 (1549-1639) had served as a court official for some years, but frequently felt frustrated as an official, and then devoted most of his time to studying medicine until he became a famous physician. He authored *Liu Ke Zheng Zhi Zhun Sheng* or *The Standards of Diagnosis and Treatment in Six Branches of Medicine* 六科证治准绳, which had the largest circulation of all medical books in the 17th century in China.

3.6.1.2 Characteristics of Scholar Physicians

Generally speaking, scholar physicians bear the following characteristics:

① They were proficient in medical classics. Generally speaking, scholar physicians were well-educated, expert in Confucian classics, history, philosophy and literature, and very good at independent studying, and thus proficient in medical classics.

② They liked to explore the rules (hows and whys) in diagnosing and treating diseases. A bell practitioner, who shook a bell to call on notice from patients or their family to provide medical service, stressed simple and convenient therapies with quick therapeutic effects, but did not care so much hows and whys; While a scholar physician valued rational thinking, liked to explore the rules or hows and whys when diagnosing and treating diseases, devoted particular care to the all complete of "*Li* or Theories, *Fa* or Methods, *Fang* or Prescriptions and *Yao* or Medicinal agents (acupoints in acupuncture treatment) 理法方药", and was capable of making rational prognosis. This is particular the case after the Song Dynasty (960-1279) because of the influences from Neo-Confucianism "studying the phenomena of the nature in order to acquire knowledge", and thus pursuing the very source of knowledge.

③ They were expert in writing, composing or compiling, then leaving works to posterity;

④ They elaborated medical theories with Confucian principles;

⑤ They practiced "benevolence", the core virtue of Confucianism, by relieving sufferings from patients.

All in all, scholar physicians projected high ambitions of "Cultivating individual moral character, running the family unison, managing the nation in order, and thus making peace prevail throughout the universe" into the practice of doing medicine.

3.6.1.3 Contributions of Scholar Physicians or Officials to Chinese Medicine

Contributions of scholar physicians to Chinese medicine can be summarized into the following three aspects:

3.6.1.3.1 Systematizing medical classics to preserve the former achievements. Large-scale systematizations of medical classics in the history were accomplished by scholar physicians or scholar officials. If without Confucian officials or Confucian physicians, the situation and development of Chinese medicine would be unimaginable.

Liu Xiang 刘向 (77?-6 B.C.), a great Confucian scholar, systematized available books of that time including medical books such as *Huang Di's Inner Classic*, and compiled *Bie Lu* 别录, the first work on bibliography of China, on the basis of which his son Liu Qin 刘歆(50? B.C.-23 A.D.) compiled *Qi Lue* 七略, the first comprehensive classified bibliography of China. The famous *Han Shu Yi Wen Zhi* or *Treatise on Literature* of *History of the Former Han Dynasty* 汉书·艺文志 by Ban Gu 班固 (32-92) took it as its chief source.

The transmission, circulation and application of ancient Chinese medical classics nowadays should be attributed to the success of Bureau of Rectifying Medical Books set up in 1057 by the government of the Northern Song Dynasty (960-1127), which aimed to systematize valuable medical books available at that time. In between the years of 1068-1077, several Confucian officials, Lin Yi 林亿 (?-?), Gao Baoheng 高保衡 (?-?), et al. rectified *Huang Di Nei Jing Su Wen* or *Huang Di's Inner Classic Basic Questions* 黄帝内经素问, *Shang Han Lun* or *On Cold-induced Diseases* 伤寒论, *Jin Gui Yao Lue* or *Synopsis of the Golden Chamber* 金匮要略, *Mai Jing* or *The Classic of Pulse Diagnosis* 脉经, *Zhe Jiu Jia Yi Jing* or *The Systematic Classic of Acupuncture and Moxibustion* 针灸甲乙经, *Zhu Bing Yuan Hou Lun* or *Treatise on Causes and Symptoms of Diseases* 诸病源候论, *Qian Jin Yao Fang* or *Invaluable Prescriptions* 千金要方, *Qian Jin Yi Fang* or *Supplement to Invaluable Prescriptions* 千金翼方, *Wai Tai Mi Yao* or *Medical Secrets of an Official* 外台秘要, which were then issued and widely spread. These Confucian officials are noted for their meticulous scholarship. Take *Su Wen* or *Basic Questions* as an example. They corrected many mistakes in the texts and Wang Bing's annotations, supplemented over 2,000 notes by referring widely to former versions, learning extensively from others' strong points, and tracing to its source: *Quan Yuanqi's Annotated Version of Su Wen*[228], thus preserving general pictures of former versions of *Su Wen*. The bureau did great contributions to preserve ancient medical literature and promote transmission of Chinese medicine.

---

228 Quan Yuanqi 全元起 (?-?), a famous medical expert living in the Northern and Southern Dynasties (420-589). *Quan Yuanqi's Annotated Version of Su Wen* is the earliest annotated version of *Su Wen* or *Basic Questions* in China. It lost in between Norther (960-1127) and Southern Song (1127-1279) Dynasty. A famous modern Chinese scholar Duan Yishan 段逸山 (1940-) tried to restore it based on his research, and published the outcome entitled "*Su Wen Quan Yuanqi Ben Yan Jiu Yu Ji Fu*" or "Research and Restoration of *Quan Yuanqi's Annotated Version of Su Wen*" 素问全元起本研究与辑复 in 2001.

In the years of 1057-1059, Zhang Yuxi 掌禹锡 (992-1068) and other Confucian officials, followed an imperial decree to compile *Jia You Ben Cao* or *Jiayou Materia Medica* 嘉佑本草, which includes 1,082 medicinals and preserves many lost materials on materia medica.

Tu Jing Ben Cao or *Illustrated Materia Medica* 图经本草 compiled by Su Song 苏颂 (1020-1101), a Confucian official, was issued and printed in 1061, which records over 1,000 single medicinal formulas with over 900 illustrations. It is the first block-printed edition of illustrations of material medica.

In 1082, Tang Shenwei 唐慎微 (1056-1093), a Confucian physician, compiled *Jing Shi Zheng Lei Bei Ji Ben Cao* or *Classic of Classified Materia Medica for Emergencies* 经史证类备急本草, which summarizes achievements on materia medica of the former ages, includes records on materia medica from Confucian classics, historical records, philosophical writings, and miscellaneous works as well as the Buddhist and Taoist Scriptures. It includes 1,746 kinds of medicinal agents with directions for use and preparation, and many new prescriptions. It laid a solid foundation for the development of Chinese materia medica. Li Shizhen, a Confucian physician, took it as one of the chief sources of his monumental work *Ben Cao Gang Mu* or *Compendium of Materia Medica* 本草纲目.

In 1116, Kou Zongshi 寇宗奭 (?-?), a Confucian official, compiled *Ben Cao Yan Yi* or *Augmented Materia Medica* 本草衍义 by supplementing what *Jing Shi Zheng Lei Bei Ji Ben Cao* or *Classic of Classified Materia Medica for Emergencies* 经史证类备急本草 lacks such as some medicinal agents' actions and methods to differentiate similar ones. It includes 472 medicinal agents, and suggests that the dosage of a medicinal should vary according to age, constitution, and emergent or chronic condition.

The above mentioned works on materia medica by Confucian officials or Confucian physicians altogether advanced Chinese materia medica to a new stage.

Later on, during the Ming Dynasty (1368-1644), Confucian officials or Confucian physicians compiled a lot of other monumental works on Chinese medicine, such as 52-volume *Ben Cao Gang Mu* or *Compendium of Materia Medica* by Li Shizhen, a Confucian physician; 120-volume *Liu Ke Zheng Zhi Zhun Sheng* or *Standards of Diagnosis and Treatment in Six Branches of Medicine* 六科证治准绳 by Wang Kentang 王肯堂 (1549-1613), a Confucian official, which epitomized the achievements on medicine before his time and was highly appraised by medical practitioners afterwards; 32-volume *Lei Jing* or *Classified Inner Classic* 类经, 64-volume *Jingyue Quan Shu* or *Jingyue's Complete Works* 景岳全书 by Zhang Jiebin 张介宾(1563-1640).[229]

During the Qing Dynasty (1644-1911), 10,000-volume *Gu Jin Tu Shu Ji Cheng* or *Integration of Books from Past to Present* 古今图书集成, the best and the most intact preserved classified book with the largest scale and richest materials ever extant in China compiled in 1706 by Cheng Menglei 陈梦雷

229 He is also known as Zhang Jingyue 张景岳.

(1650-1741), a Confucian official, was prefaced by Emperor Yongzheng 雍正 (1678-1735), the title of which was given by Emperor Kangxi 康熙 (1654-1722), among which 520 volumes are books on Chinese medicine; 90-volume *Yi Zong Jin Jian* or *Golden Mirror of Medicine* compiled by Wu Qian 吴谦 (1689-1748), an imperial physician, in 1742 by an imperial order, is the most complete and concise series of works on Chinese medicine with illustrations, expositions, and rhymes, etc., the title of which was given by Emperor Qianlong 乾隆 (1711-1799); The *Si Ku Quan Shu* or *The Complete Library of the Four Branches of Literature* 四库全书 completed by 4,000 Confucian officials by Emperor Qianlong's order in 1782 and comprising the four traditional divisions of Chinese learning - classics, history, philosophy, and belle-letters, contains 3,503 titles bound into more than 36,000 books with a total of 853,456 pages, thus having the world's longest hand-copied series of books, of which 191 are works on Chinese medicine under the division of philosophy, amounting to 2,529 volumes.

Therefore, the existence and development of Chinese medicine is difficult to imagine if without Confucian physicians or Confucian officials.

3.6.1.3.2 Summarizing experiences, developing the treating procedure of "*Li* or Theories, *Fa* or Methods, *Fang* or Prescriptions and *Yao* or Medicinal agents"

The history demonstrates that Confucian physicians were the main developers of Chinese medicine. For example, Zhang Zhongjing 张仲景 (150-219) developed six-meridian pattern identification and instituting treatment based on pattern identification as well as the treating procedure of "*Li* or Theories, *Fa* or Methods, *Fang* or Prescriptions and *Yao* or Medicinal agents" in his monumental works *Shang Han Lun* or *On Cold-induced Diseases* and *Jin Gui Yao Lue* or *Synopsis of the Golden Chamber* 金匮要略; Wang Shuhe 王叔和 (201-280) made a great contribution to pulse diagnosis, and his work *Mai Jing* or *The Classic of Pulse Diagnosis* 脉经 records 24 pulses; Qian Yi 钱乙 (1032-1113) is the founder of pediatrics of Chinese medicine, and his work *Xiao Er Yao Zheng Zhi Jue* or *Key to the Therapeutics of Children's Diseases* 小儿药证直诀 is the first monograph of this discipline; Li Shizhen 李时珍 (1518-1593) made great contributions to materia medica and pulse diagnosis; Wu Jutong 吴鞠通 (1758-1836) created *San Jiao* Pattern Identification to diagnose and treat warm diseases or epidemic febrile diseases; and so and so forth.

3.6.1.3.3 Launching competition to improve academic levels of the profession.

Confucian physicians broke the tradition of venerating the old and classics, proposed new viewpoints, established new schools, and thus launched competition to improve academic levels of the profession. Let us take "the Four Great Medical Schools in the Jin-Yuan Dynasties" as examples.

Liu Wansu 刘完素 (1110?-1200) turned to medicine from Confucianism because of the death of his mother, set up the Hejian School and the Cooling School by advocating the use of cool or cold medicinal agents in the practice.

Zhang Congzheng 张从正 (1156-1228), the representative of the Purgation School, authored the work *Ru Men Shi Qin* or *Confucian Scholars' Care of Their Parents* 儒门事亲, which advocated treatment of diseases with the three methods of diaphoresis, emesis and purgation.

Zhang Yuansu 张元素 (?-?) was determined to study medicine after he failed in imperial examinations, advocated Viscera Pattern Identification, meridian entries of medicinal agents, and care of stomach *qi*, and established the Yishui School, which is just as famous as the Hejian School established by Liu Wansu; Li Dongyuan 李东垣 (1180-1251), a disciple of Zhang Yuansu, advanced the theory of Spleen and Stomach and created the methods of invigorating the spleen *qi*, upbearing yang and dispersing fire to treat diseases, and thus founded the Soil-Invigorating School for the spleen is attributed to soil in the five phases.

Zhu Zhenheng 朱震亨(1281-1358) studied Neo-Confucianism in his early years and then turned to medicine afterwards. He learned strong points from both Hejian and Yishui schools, and on the basis of the climatic characteristics of the South China and his clinical experiences, advanced to nourish yin and lower fire to treat diseases, thus founding Yin-Nourishing School.

3.6.2 Medicine: An Art of Healing of Embodying & Practicing "Benevolence"

Treating diseases, rescuing human beings, and relieving the sufferings in the society were inseparable for Confucian scholars, just as the saying goes "A superior doctor administers a country; a common doctor cares the human being; while an inferior doctor treats the disease".

What is benevolence? "Benevolence is to love people". The *Xiao Jing* or *The Classic of Filial Piety* 孝经 states that "Man is the most valuable being in the universe". The *Huang Di Nei Jing* or *Huang Di's Inner Classic* reads that "Nothing is more precious than man in between the heaven and the earth". Confucian physicians had strong social responsibilities - to relieve the sufferings of the people for Confucianism stresses life and beings.

As regards to "Doctor's Cardinal Humane Care to Patients", also known as "medical morality", Sun Simiao 孙思邈 (581-682) advanced that "A great doctor should be expert in medical skills and sincere to the patients". *Da Yi Jing Cheng* or *A Great Doctor Should Be Expert in Medical Skills and Sincere to His Patients* 大医精诚, from the first volume of *Bei Ji Qian Jin Yao Fang* or *The Invaluable Prescriptions for Emergencies* 备急千金要方, reads that "When well-qualified doctors treat patients, they should be calm and concentrated without any desire or avarice. First of all, they should have great sympathy for the patients and then be determined to save people from their sufferings. When patients come to ask for help, they should not treat them differently by seeing whether they are rich or poor, old or young, beautiful or ugly, enemy or friend, Chinese or foreigner, foolish or wise. They should treat all the patients like their closest relatives.

"When treating patients, they should not think over and over for themselves and pay too much attention to the protection of their own lives. Being qualified doctors, they should regard the patients' sufferings as their own and have deep sympathy for them. They should not try to avoid danger if being confronted with it. No matter in day time or night, winter or summer, no matter they are hungry or thirsty, tired or exhausted, they should treat or save patients heart and soul without any delay or worrying about personal gains or losses. Only by so doing can they become great doctors for people".

In one word, medicine is an art of healing of embodying and practicing "Benevolence".

3.6.3 Confucian Doctrine of the Mean in Chinese Medicine

The core value of the golden mean of the Confucian school can be summarized into the following three aspects: ① Sticking to principles in the unbiased way; ② Seeking stable and harmonious state; ③ Advancing with the times, judging the hour and seizing up the situation. In one word, the core value is to seek the healthiest state of the development of things.[230]

The golden mean of the Confucian school actually refers to that man's words and deeds should accord with the middle, harmonious standard, opposing "going too far" and "not going far enough", which reflects in physiology, pathology, etiology, treatment and prevention of Chinese medicine. That is to say, with the rise of the "Hundred Schools of Thought", the intellectual flowering in early China, "Zhong Yi 中医" is interpreted as "medicine that accords with the doctrine of mean".

Physiologically, the healthy state is considered as the balance and harmony between yin and yang.

Pathologically, morbidity (unhealthy states) is explained in terms of yin-yang imbalance, relative predominance or decline of yin or yang - "when yin prevails there is cold, when yang prevails there is heat"; "when yang is deficient there is cold, when yin is deficient there is heat"; "If yang abounds, yin ails; if yin abounds, yang ails"; "Double yin becomes yang; double yang becomes yin"; "Extreme cold engenders heat; extreme heat engenders cold"; etc.

As regards to etiology, the causes of diseases, the diseased states result from failing to maintain the middle and harmony - "going too far" or "not going far enough" due to abnormal weather conditions, excessive emotional changes, improper diets, overstrain of the body, mind, and excess of sexual activities, etc.

Since imbalance of yin and yang accounts for the emergence and development of diseases, treatments must involve restoring the balance between yin and yang, such as "Treating cold with heat, treating heat with cold; Treating excess by reducing, treating deficiency by supplementing" in order to attain a state of equilibrium and harmony.

The properties, flavours and actions (effects) of medicinal agents may also be classified according to yin and yang. As to the properties, cool and cold are yin, while warm and hot are yang; As to the flavours, sour, bitter and salty are yin, while acrid, sweet and bland are yang; As to the actions, astringing, descending

---

230 Kang Zhen 康震. Eight Great Master Writers of Tang- Song Dynasties. Zeng Gong. Lecture Room of CCTV 10, 2010.

and sinking actions are yin, while dispersing, ascending and floating actions are yang.

Chinese medicine emphasizes health cultivation, as *Huang Di Nei Jing* or *Huang Di's Inner Classic* reads that "In the past, people practiced the Tao, the Way of Life. They understood the principle of balance of yin and yang, as represented by the transformation of the energies of the universe. Thus, they formulated practices such as Dao-in, an exercise combining stretching, massaging, and breathing to promote energy flow, and meditation to help maintain and harmonize themselves with the universe. They ate a balanced diet at regular times, arose and retired at regular hours, avoided overstressing their bodies and minds, and refrained from overindulgence of all kinds. They maintained well-being of body and mind; thus, it is not surprising that they lived over one hundred years".[231]

3.6.4 Major Negative Influences of Confucianism on Chinese Medicine

Confucianism has also some negative influences on Chinese medicine.

3.6.4.1 Belittling Anatomical Exploration

The *Xiao Jing* or *The Classic of Filial Piety* states that "The body, hair and skin should not be damaged for they are from parents, which is the start of filial piety". The only exceptional case is that doctor could take the chance of executing a criminal by cutting him to pieces to observe the inner structure of the body, which is any way not dissection with a purpose in anatomical sense. This not only affects the diagnosing and treating process, but also restricts the development of surgical operations.

Of course, there are still some other more important reasons to interpret why anatomy is not well-developed in Chinese medicine. See "5.2.2.5 Why Did Anatomy Decline in Chinese Medicine?" of the "Part 3 The Importance of Metaphors in Chinese Medicine" for a more detailed discussion.

3.6.4.2 Obstructing Development of Gynecology and Obstetrics

It is well known that "The men and women should keep distance" according to Confucianism, which not only restricted the way a male doctor diagnosed and treated female patients, e.g. to feel a thread which was connected with a lady's wrist to try to know her pulse's conditions, but also obstructed the development of gynecology and obstetrics in Chinese medicine.

231 Ni, Maoshing. 1995: 1.

Man abides by the earth. Earth abides by the heaven. Heaven abides by Tao. Tao abides by the nature.

- *Lao Tzu*

In *Lao Tzu*, Tao abides by the nature; In the *Huang Di's Inner Classic*, medicine abides by the Tao; In essence, medicine abides by the nature.

- The Author

4. Taoist School and Its Influences on Chinese Medicine

Here what we discuss is a major philosophical thought of school of Pre-Qin Days, Taoist school 道家 not Taoist religion 道教.

4.1 Differences between Taoist School and Taoist Religion

Actually there are two kinds of Taoism, i.e., *Tao Jia* or Taoist School 道家 and *Tao Jiao* or Taoist Religion 道教.

Taoist School 道家 is one of the major philosophical thoughts of school, stands for recluses' or hermits'[232] philosophy, and is named after its theoretical foundation and core concept - Tao 道, the source and the rule of the universe. It has exerted deep influences on the development of Chinese philosophy as a whole, as well as almost every aspect of Chinese culture. It was initiated by Yang Zhu 杨朱 (?-?), founded by Lao Tzu 老子(580?-500 B.C.?), further developed by Chuang Tzu 庄子(369?- 286?B.C.) and Lie Tzu 列子 (?-?). Its main works include *Lao Tzu* 老子, *Chuang Tzu* 庄子, *Lie Tzu* 列子, *Wen Tzu* 文子, *He Guan Tzu* 鹖冠子, *Huan Nan Tzu* 淮南子, and four chapters of *Guan Tzu* 管子 - *Xin Shu* 1 心术上, *Xin Shu* 2 心术下, *Bai Xin* 白心, and *Nei Ye* 内业. Taoist school believes that Tao is the source and the root of everything in the universe and that Tao creates everything in the universe in a complete natural way without any intervention, i.e. the nature of Tao is "Having Effortless Action", which is the fundamental rule of controlling everything in the universe. Taoist school observes the rule of the nature, and advocates a natural, simple, easy and free life. Some vital fundamental concepts such as *Tao* 道, *Te* 德, *You* (有, Being), *Wu* (无, Non-Being), *Li* 理, *Qi* 气, *Tai Ji* 太极, and *Wu Ji* 无极 are from Taoist school.

While Taoist Religion 道教 carried on the tradition of "Wu Dou Mi Tao 五斗米道", which was founded by Zhang Ling 张陵 (?-?). It was so named for whoever wanted to join the religion should donate five *dou*s (*dou*, a measure for grain) of rice. The religion formed on the basis of ideas of Taoist school 道家 together with ways on how to become supernatural beings, popular worship of

232 Neither recluse nor hermit can convey the original connotations of the word in Chinese, i.e. "Yin Shi 隐士", which actually refers to talented people who are very capable in administering and running a country but not willing to do this. But persons who live a very simple life alone and like to avoid others are not always talented people.

gods and ghosts, and witchcrafts. It regards Lao Tzu as the Guru, and has religious belief, worship of Gods, followers, organizations, as well as religious ceremonies and activities. It advocates being calm and "Having Effortless Action", pursuing immortality or eternal life, and finally achieving Tao and transforming into god. Zhang Lu 张鲁 (?-216), Zhang Ling's grandson, spread it through the country by the aid of his political influence.

Hereafter we are going to discuss is *Tao Jia* or Taoist School 道家 not *Tao Jiao* or Taoist Religion 道教, which is arranged into the following three aspects: Development of Taoist School; Translation and Dissemination of *Lao Tzu* and *Chuang Tzu* in the West; Taoist Philosophy: the Philosophical Foundation of Chinese Medicine.

4.2 Development of Taoist School

Taoist School of the Pre-Qin Days developed in three stages, each of which can be stood for by one representative: Yang Zhu, the first phase; Lao Tzu, the second phase; and Chuang Tzu, the third phase.

4.2.1 Yang Zhu: Refusing to Pluck One Single Hair

Yang Zhu 杨朱 (?-?), a famous thinker and philosopher, lived in between Mo Tzu (470?-391 B.C.?) and Mencius (372?-289 B.C.?), i.e. the Warring States Period (475-221 B.C.), during which the whole country was in a state of chaos and constant wars. He was equally famous to Mo Tzu at that time although he didn't leave any writings behind him, as *The Book of Mencius* says "Yang Zhu's and Mo Di's viewpoints enjoy equal popularity in the country. The available viewpoints [of that time] go along with either Yang Zhu or Mo Di". What made Yang Zhu's viewpoints so influential?

Under such a social circumstances during the Warring States Period, what should be done? Try to save the world or the self? The principle of Yang Zhu is to save the world by saving the self, i.e. "refusing to pluck one single hair". Actually what he advocated is "Each for the self" and "Despising of the things and Valuing of life", i.e. valuing personal life, opposing both damage to the self from the others and encroaching on the others from the self. Mencius commented him "Though he might have profited the whole world by plucking out one single hair, he would not have done it" (from the chapter of *Jin Xin* 尽心 of *Mencius*), where a Chinese idiom *Yi Mao Bu Ba* 一毛不拔 originally comes from. This idiom was originally neutral, but now is always used in a derogatory sense, means "unwilling to give up even a hair","too stingy to pull out a hair", "parsimonious", "as mean as a miser", or "extremely stingy".

Was Yang Zhu really so stingy and selfish? If it were really the case, it would have been surely unacceptable. But besides, how could his proposals prevail in the country? Hereafter is the story of "refusing to pluck one single hair" recorded in the chapter of *Yang Zhu* of *Lie Tzu*. Yang Zhu's idea of "Each for the self" had a sharp conflict with the "all-embracing love" of the Mohist proposal, so Qingu Li, the Chief disciple of Mo Tzu, went to argue with him.

Qingu Li 禽滑厘, the chief disciple of Mo Tzu, asked Yang Zhu, "If you can benefit the whole world by plucking out one single hair, will you do this"? Yang Zhu answered, "The problems of the world can definitely not be solved by plucking out one single hair"! Qingu Li asked again, "If it can save the whole world, will you do this"? Then Yang Zhu ignored his question and turned a deaf ear to him. Qingu Li came out and told this to Meng Sun Yang 孟孙阳, Yang Zhu's disciple. Meng Sun Yang commented, "You don't understand my master's motive! Let me clarify his points of view. I would like to ask, if some one proposes to beat you until your skin is damaged, but give you ten thousands gold later, will you do that"? Qingu Li answered, "Yes, I will"! Meng Sun Yang asked again, "If you are proposed to get a country preconditioned that your leg is broken apart by chopping from your body, will you do that"? Qingu Li was silent for a while. Then Meng Sun Yang said, "It is clear that compared to the skin, body hair is so small that is not worth noticing; compared to the limbs, the skin is insignificant. But without body hair there would be no skin; without skin there would be no limbs. Though a hair to the body is just like one to ten thousands, but how could it be set little by underestimating its function just because of its being little?"

The chapter then makes a very good summary of political philosophy of Taoist School in its early period with Yang Zhu's words that "In ancient time, people would not sacrifice one single hair to benefit the whole country; it is not right either to serve one person with the benefits of the whole country. If every one does not need to sacrifice one single hair to benefit the country, the country will be stable, peaceful and prosperous". That is to say, neither sacrificing the self to satisfy the society nor sacrificing the society to satisfying the self is right. The society and the self are equal, and they cannot harm each other. Only in this way will the society be well-ordered.

It is thus clear that what contains in Yang Zhu's "unwilling to give up one single hair" is a big pearl of wisdom in the human world, i.e. to govern by doing nothing that goes against the nature. In details, this wisdom can be interpreted in the following three aspects:

① The first lies in despising the empty talk but stressing solid work. Don't give oral empty promises nor do meaningless things like "plucking one hair", but be practical. Can one hair really benefit the entire world? If you need to pluck a hair today to benefit the entire world, you may need to tear off one piece of skin or cut off one piece of flesh or chop off one leg tomorrow for this purpose. Meng Sun Yang might continue to ask Qingu li, "Will you do that if you can get the whole world only on one condition that your head has to be cut off"? Therefore, Yang Zhu drove the point home: I will not give up even one single hair let along my life!

② The second lies in valuing the self most, choosing valuing the self compared to benefiting others. The self is one essential part to make up the society. If the self is sacrificed one by one, there would be no society any more. The self to the others (the entire world) is just like a hair to the whole human being. If some one does not care or value himself, how could he count on others to do so? And how could he be able to care others? Don't infringe upon or even deprive an individual's rights in the name of the entire whole!

③ The third lies in keeping one's obliged duties, neither give to nor take from others.

To sum up, Yang Zhu's refusing to pluck one single hair seems to be stingy and selfish, but in fact contains a big pearl of wisdom: "governing by doing nothing that goes against the nature".

4.2.2 *Lao Tzu*: Naming the Unnambale Tao

Lao Tzu 老子 (580 - 500 B.C.?) literally means “Old Master”. His real name is Li Er 李耳， also known as Li Dan 李聃. Legend says that when his mother gave birth to him, he was already eighty one years old, like a wise man with flowing white hair. That's why he was named as Lao Tzu. He lived in the same time with Confucius, but older than Confucius. Legend says Confucius had learned rites from him on several occasions, if it was true, then he could be considered as Confucius’s teacher. Legend also says that Lao Tzu was saddened by the evil ways of men, so he left his job as a court librarian, hopped on his trusty Ox, and went on a journey westward. At a mountain pass he was stopped and asked to write down his teachings. This became the first and most sacred Taoist text, i.e. *Lao Tzu* 老子, also known as the *Tao Te Ching* 道德经. After he finished writing, Lao Tzu continued west and was never heard from again. In fact it is not sure who really authored the book *Lao Tzu*. But what we are going to discuss here is the real author of *Lao Tzu* 老子 and the book itself.

4.2.2.1 *Lao Tzu* (or *Tao Te Jing*): Tao and Te

The authorship of *Lao Tzu* or *Tao Te Jing* is attributed to Lao Tzu. The book *Lao Tzu*, the most important Taoist text, has 81 short chapters, dating back to the 3rd century B.C.. It reads that “All things respect Tao and value Te (Chapter 51)". What is it meant by Tao and Te respectively?

Tao 道 was originally written as “[illegible]”, following the part of “辵”, which actually shows an image of a man walking on a way with his eyes big open, metaphorizing “the only way you must follow or take in order to go ahead”. Its original meaning is explained in *The Origin of Chinese Characters* as “the way to walk”, which indicates the direction for the walker, is the route to a certain destination, and then is metapharized to mean “law, rule, or principle”. Besides, Tao 道 in the ancient times had several other extended meanings: “thinking system or theory” such as in *The Analects• Living in brotherliness* (*Lun Yu • Li*

Ren 论语•里仁） that "My thinking system is run through by a central idea"; "to govern or manage" explained in *Guang Ya • Shi Gu* 广雅 • 释诂; "way or method" such as in *The Book of Shang Yang's Ideas* 商君书•更法 that "There is not just one way to govern the society". Also, the sinogram 道 resembles the shape of 首 head, thereby bearing the meaning of start or beginning. You see that Tao 道 bears so many meanings, therefore, as a fundamental philosophical concept, its connotations are deep, subtle and complicated. Hereafter is the word item Tao in *Webster's Encyclopedic Unabridged Dictionary of the English Language*: "Tao (*dou, tou*), n. 1. (in philosophical Taoism) that in virtue of which all things happen or exist. 2. the rational basis of human activity or conduct. 3. a universal, regarded as an ideal attained to a greater or lesser degree by those embodying it. [<Chin: the way]"[233].

In Taoist school, Tao is the source and the rule of the universe; it serves to reveal the underlying laws of the changes in the universe. Everything should observe the rule of the nature, and should be in harmony with the nature by "having effortless action". *Lao Tzu* holds that if one understands these laws and regulates one's actions in conformity with them, one can then turn everything to one's advantage.

Te 德, also known as "de", written as 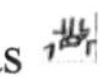 in oracle-bone script, following "彳" and "直", without the "心 heart" at the lower right part, means "To observe the hammer and take a straight line; to see whether the way is straight or not". Its original meaning is "direct and straight vision", "to look neither right nor left", "upright behavior". It was written as  in Bronze script with the heart at the lower right position, denotes "straight eye vision, upright heart"; and then is extended to mean "virtue". To sum up, Te's original meaning is the true features of objects or things, later on is metaphorized as the common behavioral principles people should observe. *Lao Tzu* 老子, also known as *Tao Te Ching* (or "*Dao De Jing*" in the current Pinyin) 道德经, where Te is regarded as the reflection, power of Tao (Way or Rule). The Te of a thing is what it naturally is.

Lao Tzu or *Tao Te Jing* is composed of two parts, *Tao Jing* and *Te Jing*. In the popular version, *Tao Jing* (1-37 chapters) is set before *Te Jing* (38-81 chapters); but in the version unearthed from Mawangdui Han Tomb, *Tao Jing* is set after *Te Jing*. The book contains altogether 5,635 sinograms, which is composed by 815 different ones. It contains many paradoxes and profound teachings on living in harmony with the nature, as the Chapter 56 reads that "Those who know do not speak; Those who speak do not know".

233 Webster's Encyclopedic Unabridged Dictionary of the English Language. 1994: 1453.

4.2.2.2 Tao, the Unnamable

It is *Lao Tzu* that discusses Tao as an abstract concept and endows it with a philosophical meaning of "embracing all" for the first time. Where does Tao actually come from? Chen Guying 陈鼓应 (1935-), a Taiwanese scholar, said in his paper *The Formation of Lao Tzu's Philosophical System* that "Lao Tzu's Tao is the principle and truth he understood and got from his own experiences in the world". I agree with this point of view.

The chapter 1 starts with

"The Tao that can be told is not the eternal Tao;
The name that can be named is not the eternal name.
The Unnamable is the beginning of the Heaven and the Earth;
The namable is the mother of all things".

The Chapter 40 states that "All things in the world come into being from Being (*You* 有); and Being comes into being from Non-being (*Wu* 无)".

It is thus clear that Tao is the first cause of the universe, and a force that flows through all the life. *The Book of Changes* makes a distinction between *Xing Er Shang* 形而上 "That which lies beyond shapes and features" and *Xing Er Xia* 形而下 "All things that lie within shapes and features". Actually the former refers to the unnamable, such as Tao and Te, while the latter refers to the namable, the concrete things in the universe. So *Lao Tzu* says "The unnamable is the beginning of the Heaven and the Earth; while the namable is the mother of all things". How do all the things come out?

The Chapter 42 states that

"Tao begets One (*Qi*).
One begets Two (Yin and Yang).
Two begets Three (the integration of Yin and Yang).
Three begets all things.
All things carry Yin and embrace Yang, where the central and harmonious *Qi* makes them in harmony".

This quotation shows the generation of all things in the universe from Tao, *Wu* 无 or Non-Being to all things *You* 有 or Beings. That is to say, Tao is the origin of all things in the universe and the Way which must be observed by all.

4.2.2.3 The Invariable Law of Nature

Among the laws that govern the changes of things, the most fundamental and the invariable is that "A thing will develop in the opposite direction when it reaches its extreme" (Chapter 55), which is the Tao, as stated in *Lao Tzu* that "Reversing (or developing in the opposite direction) is the movement of the Tao" (Chapter 40); and that "To go further and further means to revert again" (Chapter 25). I think Lao Tzu summarized and got this invariable law from his own understanding and experiences of the world.

Here I would like to tell you a famous story from *Huan Nan Tzu* 淮南子, a work mainly on Taoist School but later than *Lao Tzu*, which is known as "When the old man on the frontier lost his mare, who could have guessed it was a blessing in disguise", just like "Every cloud has its silver lining". The full story reads that

"In former times, there was a man living on the frontier, who was good at speculating good or ill luck, misfortune or happiness. One day his mare run to the Northern barbarian tribes without any reason, and then all of his neighbours came to comfort him. The father said, 'How do you know this is not a blessing in disguise'? Some months passed by, his mare came back home along with a gallant horse from the Northern barbarian tribes, [which were famous for keeping fine horses]. The neighbours then came to extend their congratulations. The father said, ' 'How do you know this is not a disaster in disguise'? The family had a fleet horse, and his son liked riding it. But on one occasion he fell off the horse and broke his thigh, [thus going lame]. The neighbours came to comfort him [once again]. The father said, 'How do you know this is not a blessing in disguise'? One year later, the Northern barbarian tribes made a massive invasion into the frontier; [as a consequence,] the able-bodied [young] men had to take bows and arrows to fight against invaders. [Consequently], nine of ten able-bodied men living near the frontier died in the war, while the father and the son of this family preserved their lives only because of being [old and] lame [respectively]".

This story actually elaborates the statement from *Lao Tzu* (Chapter 58) that "It is upon calamity that blessing leans, upon blessing that calamity rests." *Lao Tzu* believes that all things have their opposites, all things are in a state of constant moving and changing, all things have their advantages and disadvantages, good contains the seed of bad and vice versa, and there is neither pure gain nor pure loss. That's Lao Tzu's dialectics!

There are still a lot of statements from *Lao Tzu* on this law, such as

"Those with little will acquire, those with much will be led astray." (Chapter 22)

"A hurricane never lasts the whole morning, nor a rainstorm the whole day." (Chapter 23)

"The most yielding things in the world master the most unyielding." (Chapter 43)

"Diminish a thing and it will increase. Increase a thing and it will diminish." (Chapter 42)

"Nothing under the heaven is softer and weaker than water, but in attacking the hard and strong, no force can compare with it, for nothing can take its place". (Chapter 78)

...

"A thing will develop in the opposite direction when it reaches its extreme." Then, what is meant by the word "extreme"? Is there any absolute limit for the development of anything, going beyond which would mean going to the extreme? In the *Lao Tzu* no such question is asked and therefore no answer is given. But if there had been such a question, Lao Tzu would have answered that no absolute limit can be prescribed for all things under all circumstances. If a student, having just learned 3,000 sinograms, thinks that he then knows all about Chinese language, he certainly cannot make further advancement in his learning, and will as certainly "revert back".

The Chapter 9 reads that "If people of wealth and exalted position are arrogant, they abandon themselves to unavoidable ruin". Here, arrogance is the sign that one's advancement has reached its extreme limit. It is the first thing that one should avoid.

In one word, whether one reaches its or his extreme is determined by the subjective feelings and objective circumstances. That "A thing will develop in the opposite direction when it reaches its extreme" is the invariable law of the nature. You will be enlightened as long as you know this, as stated in Chapter 16 that "Knowing the invariable is named enlightenment".[234]

4.2.2.4 Understanding *Wu Wei* or Having Effortless Action

"Not to know the invariable and to act blindly is to go to disaster". (Chapter 16)
"He does not define himself, therefore he is distinct; he does not assert himself, therefore he succeeds". (Chapter 32)
"What is most perfect seems to have something missing, yet its use is unimpaired. What is most full seems empty, yet its use is inexhaustible. What is most straight seems like crookedness. The greatest skill seems like clumsiness. The great eloquence seems like shuttering." (Chapter 45)

It is thus clear that, according to Lao Tzu, Human should **have just effortless actions**. By "Having Effortless Action" it is meant that a man should restrict his activities to what is necessary and what is natural. "Necessary" means necessary to the achievement of a certain purpose, and never over-doing; "Natural" means to follow one's Te with no arbitrary effort.

Yi Zhongtian 易中天 (1947-), a professor of Xiamen University in China, summarized *Wu Wei* or Having Effortless Action into the following four points, i.e. having few desires, keeping the people in ignorance, against knowledge, and against Te 德.

Lao Tzu advocates that both the rulers and the people should have few desires. The Chapter 57 states that the people's characters will unconsciously be influenced and they will unconsciously become rich if the rulers take effortless actions and have nothing to do; and the people will go along the right track, and they will be kind-hearted, simple, and honest if the rulers have pure hearts and few desires. That is to say, if the rulers "pursue no goal as the goal, do effortless action as their activity, seek no achievement as the achievement (Chapter 63)", the people will calm down, make little turmoil, and have few desires.

234 Fung Yu-Lan. 1948; 2010: 156-158.

But if the people have too many desires they will get something which is just opposite to their intentions. In order to satisfy their desires, people will seek for happiness. In this way, they will lose their Te 德. The Chapter 12 reads that "The five colors blind the eyes. The five tones dull the ears. The five tastes fatigue the mouth. Riding and hunting madden the mind. Rare treasures hinder right conduct". "There is neither disaster worse than being greedy nor sin more serious than having desire for acquisition". That's why *Lao Tzu* advocates a pure heart and few desires.

In order to achieve "governing by having effortless actions" (or "governing by non-interference") *Lao Tzu* puts forward three principles, i.e. "Don't select and appoint talented, capable people to office" for people will learn from them, have desire to be talented and capable, and then contend; "Don't value rare treasures" for rare treasures will induce people to steal; and "Don't show off anything which could trigger or arouse avarice and lust" for people's desires are actually hidden inside (Chapter 3).

Knowledge itself is an object of desire, and is both the servant and master of desire. "When knowledge and intelligence appeared, Gross Artifice began". (Chapter 18) Thereby, *Lao Tzu* advances that "A sage governs by simplifying people's minds, feeding them to the full, weakening their ambitions, and strengthening their body; by making people lose desire for knowledge and making intellectuals lose their courage to do anything". Briefly speaking, to spend one's day in food and drink and have an empty head, and just to be an animal or return to an infant, as *Lao Tzu* states that "Not to part from the invariable Te is to return to the state of infancy"(Chapter 55).

In order to govern a country, you should keep the people in ignorance for "The difficulty of ruling people lies in that they know too much"; In order to keep the people in ignorance, you should keep the rulers in ignorance too for *Lao Tzu* is against "ruling a country with knowledge" (Chapter 65); Therefore no matter the rulers or the people should be against knowledge in order to be simple and ignorant, and just need to become natural and have no effortless actions.

As regards to "against Te", it does not mean "transgressing morality". What *Lao Tzu* is against is what Confucianism advocates for *Lao Tzu* believes Te was too fake or sham to follow. "If we abolish knowledge and wisdom, people will benefit hundredfold; If we abolish benevolence and righteousness, people will be again show filial piety to their parents; if we abolish craftsmanship and profit, thieves will no longer exist"(Chapter 19). In Lao Tzu's point of view, Being ignorant is a great virtue.

4.2.3 Chuang Tzu: Enjoying Carefree Excursions

Chuang Tzu 庄子 (369? – 286?B.C.) with his given name Zhou 周 and style name Zixiu 子休, inherited and developed Lao Tzu's thinking, and thus standing for the third phase of the Taoist school. He lived and enjoyed a poor life as a hermit for his whole life time. Be aware, almost all the master philosophers of

"Hundred Schools" were "*Shi* 士" or scholars, who lived a general good life except Mo Tzu, an ascetic, and Chuang Tzu, a hermit.

Chuang Tzu saw through the world and discarded fame and wealth. According to *Shi Ji* or *The Historical Records*, Chuang Tzu turned down the King Wei of Chu (Chu Wei Wang)'s invitation of appointing him to a position of prime minister for he preferred enjoying his own free will. Then he did not make any official after that but made a living by knitting straw sandals and propagating his thinking by telling fable stories. His main ideas are preserved in the work named after his name *Chuang Tzu*. And he was named together with Lao Tzu by later generations as "Lao Chuang".

Chuang Tzu had already been spread out during the Pre-Qin Days (before 221 B.C.). *Shi Ji* or *The Historical Records* was the earliest literature which mentioned it "with over 100,000 sinograms". As we know that *Lao Tzu* has just 5,635 sinograms, so Lin Yutang 林语堂 (1896-1976) summarized this kind of similar phenomena and commented that"Jesus was followed by St. Paul, Socrates by Plato, Confucius by Mencius, and Laotse by Chuangtse. In all four cases, the first was the real teacher and either wrote no books or wrote very little, and the second began to develop the doctrines and wrote long and profound discourses". [235]

According to *Han Shu Yi Wen Zhi* or *Treatise on Literature* of *History of the Former Han Dynasty*, it had 52 chapters, but only 33 has transmitted down until today, among which 7 are inner chapters, 15 outer chapters, and 11 miscellaneous chapters. The authorship of the inner chapters is generally attributed to Chuang Tzu himself, and the others to his followers and other Taoists afterwards. The popular version of *Chuang Tzu* with 33 chapters nowadays was compiled by Guo Xiang 郭象 (252-312) of the Western Jin Dynasty (265-316), who turned metaphors of *Chuang Tzu* into ways of reasoning and arguing.

Chuang Tzu bears very high values in both literature and philosophy. Its achievements in the literature are mainly embodied in the aspects of romantic writing, realistic description, fables in different poses and with different expressions as well as forceful, boundless, free and natural language. Prose in *Chuang Tzu* can be regarded as the beginning of the romantic writings in China. I would like to give you two short examples from the chapter *Xiao Yao You* or *Enjoying Carefree Excursions* to show how Lie Tzu and the Roc enjoy their free wills by taking carefree excursions, which reads that

"Lie Tzu can travel by flying with the aid of wind and return to the earth in fifteen days…;

"In the Northern Ocean there is a fish named KUN (leviathan). Kun is so huge that no one knows that its size covers thousands of *li* (miles); it transforms

235 See Lin Yutang's "Introduction to Chuangtse: Mystic and Humorist".

into a bird named PENG (roc), whose back, no one knows that it covers thousands of *li* (miles). When the bird rouses itself and flies, its wings are just like clouds hanging over the sky. "

The underlying truth of all the fable stories in the *Chuang Tzu* is that "All Taos conform to the nature". Guided by this principle - "All Taos conform to the nature", philosophically, *Chuang Tzu* approaches the following five couples of concept: Tao and Te; Universe and Man; Things and Me; the Others and the Self; and Mind and Body. For example, it advocates "Man and Universe Uniting Each Other". In order to achieve this purpose, "The accomplished man has no self; The spiritual has no achievement; And the true sage has no name". What are they? They are the perfect being who transcend the distinction between the self and the world, the "me" and the "non-me", and the subject and the object. That is to say, they are the ones with Tao. It further advocates "Having Effortless Action", and advances "Equalization of life with death, the identity of self with others", which means to see life and death, self and others, from a higher cosmological point of view.

4.2.3.1 Life Philosophy: Letting Nature Take Its Course

The chapter *Xiao Yao You* or *Enjoying Carefree Excursions* tells a story about a Peng (or Roc) and a Sparrow's life. The Peng (or Roc) can fly thousands of miles in the sky of 90,000 miles high, but a sparrow frequently drops down to the ground when flying from one tree to the next. But they both feel happy for they play their natural abilities to the full and enjoy so doing. That's the Chuang Tzu's life philosophy – Letting Nature Take Its Course. Things are different in their nature and their natural abilities are also not the same. But we should have a full and free exercise and development of our natural ability, and thus we all can enjoy an equally happy life when we have a full free exercise and development of our natural abilities.

If you fully understand *Chuang Tzu*, you will know the vastness of the universe and the littleness of the man and the self as well; and when you are at the end of your rope or feel helpless in your life, you may go for *Chuang Tzu* to enlighten you to find a new way. At least you can still be yourself in the natural way.

4.2.3.2 Political Philosophy: Governing by Having Effortless Action

Chuang Tzu's life philosophy presents in the administration of a country as "Governing by Having Effortless Action", which *Lao Tzu* advocates first. But what's the difference? *Chuang Tzu* emphasizes the distinction between what is of nature (natural) and what is of man (artificial). All laws, morals, institutions, and governments are artificial, which aim to establish uniformity and suppress difference. If the rulers rely on more artificial means to govern, the people will have more sufferings and miseries. *Lao Tzu* states that "Reversing is the movement of the Tao" (Chapter 40), which indicates the more the rulers do to govern, the less the rulers get their desired result.

The chapter *Zhi Le* or *Peak of Happiness* tells a story about "The Marquise of Lu Keeping a Seabird", which reads that "Of old, when a seabird alighted outside the capital of Lu, the Marquis went out to receive it, gave it wine in the temple, had the *Jiu Shao* 九韶 music[236] played to amuse it, and a bullock slaughtered to feed it. But the bird was dazed, and too timid to eat or drink anything. In three days, it was dead. This was treating the bird as one would treat oneself, not the bird as a bird … Water is life to fish but is death to man. Being differently constituted, their likes and dislikes must necessarily differ. Therefore the early sages did not make abilities and occupations uniform". In one word, one simply follows what is natural in oneself.

4.2.3.3 Enlightenments of *The Mountain Tree*: Following the Middle Course

The Chapter *Shan Mu* or *The Mountain Tree* tells such a story, which reads that

"Chuang Tzu was travelling through the mountains, when he saw a great tree well covered with foliage. A tree-cutter was standing beside of it, but he did not cut it down. Chuang Tzu asked him the reason and he replied: 'It is of no use.' Chuang Tzu then said: 'By virtue of having no exceptional qualities, this tree succeeds in completing its natural span.'

"When the Master (Chuang Tzu) left the mountains, he stopped at the home of a friend. The friend was glad and ordered the servant to kill a goose and cook it. The servant asked: 'One of the geese can cackle. The other cannot. Which shall I kill?' The host said: 'Kill the one that cannot cackle.'

"Next day, a disciple asked Chuang Tzu the question: 'Yesterday the tree in the mountain, because it had no exceptional quality, succeeded in completing its natural span. But now the goose of our host, because it had no exceptional quality, had to die. What will be your position?'

"Chuang Tzu laughed and said: 'My position will lie between having exceptional qualities and not having exceptional qualities. Yet this position only seems to be right, but really is not so. Therefore those who practice this method are not able to be completely free from troubles. If one wanders about with Tao and Te (the Way and its spiritual power), it will be otherwise.'"

Then Chuang Tzu went on to say that he who links himself Tao and Te is with the "ancestor of things, using things as things, but not being used by things as things. When that is so, what is there that can trouble him?"

236 *Jiu Shao* 九韶, the name of a music of Shun's reign, was composed of 9 chapters, that's why it was named. Confucius believed that it was perfectly good and beautiful. Shun is a name of a legendary monarch in ancient China.

This story is used to illustrate the developments of Taoism[237]:

The 1st part illustrates the theory of preserving life as practiced by Yang Zhu (Selfish);

The 2nd Part illustrates the theory of Chuang Tzu: A position between these two extremes corresponds to the middle way in the quotation; If a man cannot see things from a higher point of view, none of these methods can absolutely guarantee him from danger and harm. To see things from a higher point of view means to abolish the self. We may say that the early Taoists were selfish, but until Chuang Tzu, this selfishness became denied by abolishing the self to get a higher point of view.

Therefore, Chuang Tzu proposed to "use things as things, but not being used by things as things".

4.2.4 Major Ideas of Taoist School

It is not wrong if we say that the ideas of the Taoist school are religious and poetic, but it's at least the same strong in occult arts, science, democracy, and revolutionary in politics.[238] The major ideas of Taoist School can be summarized into the following points:

4.2.4.1 *Tao* is the first cause of the universe and a force that flows through all the beings.

4.2.4.2 A follower's goal is to unite oneself with the universe, i.e. to become one with Tao, or one with nature.

(See the chapter *Qi Wu Lun* or *On the Equality of Things* of *Chuang Tzu* for the story of "The butterfly or the man?".)

4.2.4.3 Advocate Having Effortless Action (*Wu wei)* by "Letting the nature take its course" in life, social and political activities as well as health cultivation.

4.2.4.4 Man is unhappy because he lives according to man-made laws, customs, and traditions that are contrary to the ways of the nature.

How did a man live in a world dominated by chaos, suffering, and absurdity? The School of Literati called on restoring the moral order of the former Zhou Dynasty to the society; The Legalist School advocated ruling by harsh laws and order; The Mohist School appealed for the All-Embracing Love; and The Taoist School proposed to reject formal knowledge and learning, rely on the senses and instincts, discover the nature and the rhythm of the universe, ignore political and social laws, and to conform to the Tao of the nature with the aim of uniting man with the universe by having effortless action and living a free life with a free will. That's the uniqueness of the Taoist School!

---

237 Fung Yu-Lan. 1948; 2010: 109.

238 Translated from Chinese into English. This is a comment on Taoist School from Joseph Needham. The original source is said to be: *The Tao Chia [Taoist] and Taoism*. In *Science and Civilization in China Series Volume 2: History of Scientific Thought*. pp 33-164. Cambridge: Cambridge University Press, 1956.

4.3 English Translation and Dissemination of *Lao Tzu* and *Chuang Tzu* in the West

4.3.1 English Translation and Dissemination of *Lao Tzu* in the West

Lao Tzu has long become a world-famous book for it is one of the first ancient Chinese masterpieces which were translated into foreign languages. The first foreign language version was in Sanskrit, which was translated by Xuan Zang 玄奘 (600-664), a famous monk, translator of Buddhist classics and traveler of Tang Dynasty (618-907).[239] According to Paul J. Lin's statistics in 1997, *Lao Tzu* had at least 44 different English versions, and will gain at least one new English translation every year in the future.[240]

According to a Dutch sinologist - Knut Walf's statistics, the translated versions of *Lao Tzu* in Western languages were up to 17 European languages, among which 83 were in English, 64 in German, and 33 in French. It is said that the distribution numbers of *Tao Te Jing* is only secondary to *The Shakespeare Anthology* in the West, and the numbers of its English translation versions are only secondary to that of the Bible.[241] Another piece of information reads that the distribution numbers of *Lao Tzu* is only secondary to that of the *Bible* in the West according to a statistics from UNESCO (United Nations Educational, Scientific and Cultural Organization). Anyway all shows the popularity of *Lao Tzu* in the West.

In 1884, the first English version of *Lao Tzu* got published in London with the title of "*Taoists Texts: Ethical, Political, Speculative*". Hereafter are some other English translations of *Lao Tzu*:

Paul Carus, Daisetz Teitaro. Trans. *The Canon of Reason and Virtue: Being Lao-Tzu's Tao The King* (Chinese-English), Chicago, London: The Open Court Publishing Co.,1898; 1913; 1927; 1945; 1974; By BiblioLife in 2009.

L.W. Heysinger. Trans. *Light of China, The Too Teh King of Lao Tsze.* Peter Reilly, Philadelphia: Research Publishing Co., 1903; 1913; 1922; 1939.

Walter Gorn Old. Trans. *The Simple Way, Laotze, The "Old Boy": A New Translation of the Tao-Teh-King*. London: Philip Welly; London: Rider;

---

239 But no evidence or proof has been found to confirm whether the translation transmitted to India or not although *Jiu Tang Shu* or *The Old Tang History*, *Xin Tang Shu* or *The New Tang History*, and *Biography of Xuan Zang* of *Biographies of Eminent Monks of Song Dynasty* all have this record that Xuan Zang translated *Tao Te Ching* into Sanskrit. See Ji Xianlin. *The Counterflow of Buddhism* (Vol.1). Nanchang: Jiangxi Education Press, 1998: 412-422. The fact is that Chinese culture has almost no influence on Indian culture.

240 Huang Hong. Comments on Stephen Mitchell's English Translation of *Tao Te Ching*. In Cheng Yuzhen (ed.). Colloquia of Language and Culture [C]. Beijing: Foreign Languages Teaching and Research Press, 2000: 50.

241 Wang Rongpei, Wang Hong. *English Translation of Chinese Classics*. Shanghai: Shanghai Foreign Language Education Press, 2009:57.

Philadelphia: McKay. The 1st Ed. 1904; The Popular Ed. 1905; The 3rd Ed. 1913, Reprinted in 1922.[242]

C. Spurgeon Medhurst. Trans. *Tao Teh King: A Short Study in Comparative Religion.* Chicago: Theosophical Society, 1905; Reprinted with the title of *"The Tao Teh King"* by Theosophical Pub. House in Wheaton in 1972; 1979; 1989.

Lionel Giles. Trans. *The Sayings of Lao Tzu.* London: John Murray, 1905; 1906; 1908; 1909; 1911; 1917; 1922; 1926; 1950; 1959. This version classifies the sayings of Lao Tzu into 10 categories, and is very helpful for beginners to know Lao Tzu's ideas.

Isabella Mears. Trans. *Tao Teh King.* London and Glasgow: Theosophical Publishing House, 1916; 1922; 1949.

Arthur Waley. Trans. *The Way and Its Power: A Study of the Tao Te Ching and Its Place in Chinese Thought.* [243] London and New York: The MacMillan Co., 1934; London: George Allen & Unwin, 1934; Boston: Houghton Mifflin Co., 1935; 1936; 1939; New York: Grove Press, Evergreen Book, 1958.

Chu Ta-Kao. Trans. *Tao Te Ching.* London: Allen and Unwin, The Buddhist Society of London, 1937, 1939; 1942; 1945; 1948; 1959.

John C. H. Wu. Trans. *Lao Tzu's The Too and Its Virtue.* In *T'ien Hsia Monthly* (Nov. 1939 - Jan. 1940); In Shanghai: *Journal of Oriental Literature,* Vol. IV, 1951; Oriental Literature Society, University of Hawaii, Honolulu; New York: St. John University Press, 1961; Boston and London: Shambhala Publications, Inc. *Shambhala Dragon Editions*, 1989.

Witter Bynner. Trans. *The Way of Life according to Laotzu: An American Version.* New York: John Day Co., Perigree, 1944; 1986.

Lin Yutang. Trans. *The Wisdom of Laotse.* New York and London: Random House, 1948; 1949. Included into "*The Wisdom of India and China*", pp. 583-624, New York: Random House; into "Modern Library Editions" in 1942; and into "*The Wisdom China*, pp. 23-65, Michael Joseph, London. 1944; 1948; 1949; 1950; 1954; 1956; 1969.

Holmes H. Welch. Trans. *The Parting of the Way: Lao Tzu and the Taoist Movement. Boston:* Beacon Press, 1957; London: Methuen and Co., Ltd., 1958; 1965; Renamed as *Taoism: The Parting of Way* in 1966; The 6th Ed. in 1972.

Archie J. Bahm. *Tao Teh King by Lao Tzu, Interpreted as Nature and Intelligence.* New York: Frederick Ungar Publishing Co., 1958.

Amitendranath Tagore. Trans. *To-Te-Ching.* New Delhi: Sahitya Akad, 1960.

Chan Wing-tsit. Trans. *The Way of Lao Tzu.* Indianapolis and New York: The Bobbs-Merrill Co., Inc., *Library of Liberal Arts*, 1963.

---

242 Before this his "*The Book of The Path of Virtue, or a Version of the Too Teh King of Lao-tsze*" was published in Madras by Theosophical Publishing Society in 1894.

243 This translation had been very influential in the English speaking world, and it had been reprinted 8 times since it first came out in 1934 until 1968.

Feng Gia-fu, Jane English. Trans. *Lao Tzu: Tao de ching, A New Translation.* New York: Vintage Books（a division of Random House）, Alfred A. Knopf , 1972; 1979; 1989. With introduction and annotations from Joseph Needham.

Paul J. Lin. *A Translation of Lao Tzu's Tao Te Ching and Wang Pi's Commentary.* Ann Arbor: Center for Chinese Studies, *Michigan Papers in Chinese Studies, No. 30*, 1977.

Chen Guying, Author; Rhett Y. W. Young, Roger Thomas Ames, Trans. *Laozi: Text, Notes, and Comments. San Francisco:* Chinese Materials Center Publications, 1977.

Chen Ellen Marie. *The Tao Te Ching: A New Translation with Commentary.* New York: Paragon House, 1989.

Ursula K. Le Guin. *Lao Tzu: Tao Te Ching: A Book about the Way and the Power of the Way.* Boston and London: Shambhala Publications, Inc., 1990.

Alan Kam-Leung Chan. *Two Visions of the Way: A Study of the Wang Pi and the Ho-shang Kung Commentaries on the Lao tzu.* New York: The State University of New York Press, 1991; 1998.

Michael LaFargue. *The Tao of the* Tao-te-ching*: A Translation and Commentary.* New York: The State University of New York Press, 1992.

Michael LaFargue. *Tao and Method: A Reasoned Approach to the Tao Te Ching.* New York: The State University of New York Press, 1994.

Joseph Needham**.** *The Tao Chia [Taoist] and Taoism.* In *Science and Civilization in China Series Volume 2: History of Scientific Thought.* pp 33-164. Cambridge: Cambridge University Press, 1956.

Since the Mawangdui silk manuscripts of *Lao Tzu* were unearthed at Mamangdui Han Tomb, over 10 translations based on them came out. Hereafter are several important ones:

D. C. Lau. Trans. *Lao Tzu: Tao de ching*, Translated with an Introduction, The Pengwin Classics I/3, edited by E. V. Rien. Printed in Great Britain by Cox and Wyman Ltd. London; Harmondsworth, Middlesex, England; Penguin Books, 1963; 1969; Hong Kong: The Chinese University Press, 1982; 1989. It consists of two parts: the 1st part the revised translation of the 1963 version, and the 2nd part translations of Mawangdui manuscripts of *Lao Tzu*. Sarah Allen with Lau's translations as references authored *Introduction, Lao Tzu Tao de ching: Translation Based on the Ma Wang Tui Manuscripts*, *Everyman's Library. New York:* Alfred A. Knopf, 1994.

Robert G. Henricks. Trans. *Lao-tzu Te-tao ching: A New Translation Based on the Recently Discovered Mawang-tui Texts, Translated, with introduction and commentary.* New York: Random House, Ballantine Books, The MacMillan Co., 1989; London: The Bodley Head, 1990; London: Rider, 1991; New York: Random House, Ballantine Books, 1992; New York: Modern Library Editions, 1993.

Victor H. Mair. Trans. *Tao Te Ching: The Classic Book of Integrity and the Way*. New York: Bantam Books, 1990.

In Oct. 1993, bamboo slips with *Lao Tzu's* texts were discovered at No.1 Chu Tomb of the Guodian village, Jing Men, Hubei province, which were identified as works of the middle Warring States Period. Since then studies on different editions of *Lao Tzu* achieved a big progress, but most of the translators have not fully applied the related research outcome to their translations, thus influencing their academic values. Here it is suggested to retranslate the Mawangdui silk manuscripts of *Lao Tzu* with reference to and help of the Guodian texts after making a comparative study and analysis among the popular version, the Mawangdui silk manuscripts and the Guodian texts on bamboo slips.

4.3.2 English Translation and Dissemination of *Chuang Tzu* in the West

Chuang Tzu was translated into English until the end of the 19th century. Frederic Henry Balfour (1846-1909) was the first person who did this, but the translation had long been out of print. Herbert Allen Giles (1845- 1935) said that there were a lot of mistranslations in it due to Balfour's lack of understanding the original texts. Up till today more than 20 English translations of *Chuang Tzu* have got published at both China and other countries. Hereafter is a list of some famous ones.

Herbert Allen Giles. Trans. *Chuang Tzu: Mystic, Moralist, and Social Reformer*. London: Bernard Quaritch Ltd and contributors, 1889; Revised Ed. *Chuangtzu, Taoist Philosopher and Chinese Mystic*. 1926.

James Legge. Trans. *The Writings of Kwang-Kau*. 1891.

James R. Ware. Trans. *The Sayings of Chuang Chou*. 1963.

Burton Watson. Trans. *The Complete Works of Chuang Tzu*. New York: Columbia University Press, 1968.

Victor H. Mair. Trans. *Wandering on the Way: Early Taoist Tales and Parables of Chuang Tzu*. Bantam Books, 1994; Second Printing, 1998.

Wang Rongpei. Trans. Zhuangzi. Jointly Published by Changsha: Hunan People's Publishing House and Beijing: Foreign Languages Press, 1999.

Martin Palmer. Trans. *The Book of Chuang Tzu*. London: Penguin Classics, 2006.

Nina Correa. Trans. Zhuangzi: Being Boundless. 2008.

Besides there are still several selected translations by famous scholars, such as "*A Taoist Classic: Chuang-Tzu*" (1931) translated by Fung Yu-Lan, Lin Yutang's *Introduction to Chuangtse: Mystic and Humorist* (1942), and "*Chuang-Tzu: The Inner Chapters*" (1974) by Gia-Fu Feng and his wife Jane English, etc.

English translation of *Chuang Tzu* has gone through over 120 years. As time goes by, translations have paid more attention to its readability and interpretation of classical Chinese culture. Studies on different translations are usually integrated with the development of Taoist School, and are conducted from the perspectives of philosophy, literature, and religion.

4.4 Taoist Philosophy: the Philosophical Foundation of Chinese Medicine

4.4.1 Tao: The Way of the Nature and Chinese Medicine

"Therefore, Tao is great.
Heaven is great.
Earth is great.
Man is great.
In the universe, there are four great things, and man is one of them.
Man abides by the earth.
Earth abides by the heaven.
Heaven abides by Tao.
Tao abides by the nature". (Chapter 25 of *Lao Tzu)*

"Of all things in between the heaven and the earth, nothing is more precious than man." (*Huang Di's Inner Classic*• Basic *Questions*. *Great Discourse on Yin Yang Corresponding to Images*)

"Man lives on the *Qi* in between the heaven and the earth, and grows in accordance with the law of the seasons."(*Huang Di's Inner Classic*• Basic *Questions*. *Discourse on Protecting Life and Preserving Physical Appearance*)

"Man is the most valuable being in between the heaven and the earth." (*The Origin of Chinese Characters*• *Man Part*)

Thereby, it can be seen from the above quotations that "Heaven", "Earth", and "Man"are independent from and closely related to each other, and they compose a whole system, in which man plays the leading role; and that the thinking way of the "heaven-earth-man" in *Lao Tzu* embodies the thinking way of the universe, which is specified in the *Huang Di's Inner Classic* as the thinking way of the eco-medicine, which shows that the great progress of natural philosophy in the aspect of the nature replacing the God. That is also where the holistic approach of Chinese medicine comes from. In *Lao Tzu*, Tao abides by the nature; In the *Inner Classic*, medicine abides by the Tao; In essence, medicine abides by the nature.

4.4.2 Theory of "Tao-Qi" and Chinese Medicine

It is *Lao Tzu* that discusses Tao as an abstract concept and endows it with a philosophical meaning of embracing all, which shows the generation of all things in the universe from Tao, Non-Being or "*Wu* 无" to myriads of beings, Being or "*You* 有". That is to say, Tao is the origin of all things in the universe and the Way which must be observed by all. It reads that

"Tao begets one,
The one begets two,
The two begets three,
The three begets all things in the universe.

Everything in the universe bears **yin** and embraces **yang**, where the central and harmonious ***qi*** makes them in harmony." (Chapter 42)

Lao Tzu has more than 5,000 sinograms, but only here *Qi* is addressed.

Tao is unnamable and the way of the nature; Tao is Non-being which begets Being.

The One is the Great Ultimate or *Qi*.

The Two is Yin and Yang.

The Three is Yin, Yang and *Qi*.

Three is of vital significance in classical Chinese philosophy. It can stand for the number "three" and its derived relations, the penetration and interdependence of the two opposites, and the unity "One" of integration of the opposites as well. In between the yin and yang and in the process of yin-yang begetting the myriads of beings, *Qi* functions as the bridge of the communication, interaction and mutual transformation between yin and yang.

The Origin of Chinese Characters • Qi Part states that "*Qi* refers to thin, floating clouds. The sinogram 气 is a pictograph". The sinogram 气 was written as "  " in oracle inscriptions, which resembles air current, evaporating and rising, whose image is just like cloud, will disappear very soon and become invisible. *Qi* at this moment referred to air or vapor. Therefore, *qi* is invisible and formless, exists everywhere, can be gathered into a form, for instance, *qi* can be condensed into water.

Soon afterwards, the *qi* which surrounds and congests the space of the human being was abstracted into the *qi* which bears a material meaning in philosophical sense. Philosophers of the Spring Autumn and Warring States Period (770-221B.C.) believed that *qi* is the basic substance constituting the world, and that everything in the universe comes into being by the movement and mutation of *qi*. For example, *The Book of Changes* states that "everything is transformed and generated by the enshrouding [*qi*] of the heaven and the earth".

The Book of Changes establishes *Tian Ren He Yi* 天人合一 or Universe and Man Uniting and Resembling Each Other by making a farfetched comparison between them. *Tian Ren He Yi* actually indicates that the Universe and the Man constitute in the same way, i.e. being composed of the same ingredient – *Qi* in the same order. Therefore, *Qi* becomes the foundation of *Tian Ren He Yi*.

Jiaxia school of the middle stage of the Warring States Period made the theory of *Tao-Qi* mature, which mainly reflects in the chapters entitled *Xin Shu* or *Technique of Heart* 心术, *Bai Xin* or *Whitening the Heart* 白心, and *Nei Ye* or *Inner Working* 内业 of *Guan Tzu*. Their most important creation was the Theory of Essential Qi. The chapter of *Inner Working* states that "Essence is the essential part of Qi". It is the essential *qi* that transforms everything in the universe. The chapter of *Inner Working* reads that

"The *Jing* is the essence of all things. It is with it that the Tao begins to give life. It gives life to the five grains down on the earth, and the stars up in the sky. When the Essence *Qi* drifts between the Heaven and the Earth, it is called the ghost and the divine. When stored in the bosom of a particular human being, this man would become a sage."

"What I mean by the Essence is the essential part of *Qi*, with which the Tao starts to beget life".

Therefore, you see, ontologically, the Tao preceded the Essence *Qi*, which should be created by the Tao in order to beget myriad of beings.[244]

That is to say, Essence forms everything in the universe, including man.

"Man comes into being by integrating the essence from the heaven and the shape from the earth. Harmony makes it happen, while disharmony fails in so-doing". (The Chapter of *Inner Working* of *Guan Tzu*)

"Man is born on the earth, hanging his life to the heaven. The union of *qi* of the heaven and the earth makes up a man. Man can adapt himself to the seasons for the Heaven and the Earth are his parents". (Chapter 25 of *Nei Jing Su Wen*)

It can be seen that ancient Chinese medical experts introduced "*qi*" into the medical field at the right moment. And then, "*qi*" became a medium or bridge between the natural philosophy of the Pre-Qin Days (i.e. before 221 B.C.) and Chinese medicine. The concept of "*qi*" gradually formed in Chinese medicine.

In the time of *Huang Di's Inner Classic*, "*qi*" is regarded not only as the basic substance constituting the world, but also as the basic substance constituting the human being, which can be transformed into blood, essence, and body fluid, etc., and the normal functional activities of the life which is governed by "*qi*" is known as *Shen* or spirit. For example, *Su Wen • Bao Ming Quan Xing Lun* or *Basic Questions • Discourse on Protecting Life and Preserving Physical Appearance* states that "Man is generated by qi of the heaven and the earth, and is completed by the law of the four seasons"; and that "The union of *qi* of the heaven and the earth gives birth to man". Actually, there are abundant accounts of *qi* in the *Su Wen* or *Basic Questions.* Only the monosyllabic word "*qi*" appears 1,176 times in *Basic Questions*. Almost all the 79 existing chapters of the *Su Wen or Basic Questions* discuss *qi*. All the theories and skills of the *Su Wen or Basic Questions* are related to *qi*. And there are various *qi* with a multitude of names in the *Basic Questions*, such as yin *qi*, yang *qi*; clear *qi*, turbid *qi*; heaven *qi*, earth *qi*; right *qi* or healthy *qi*, evil *qi* or pathogenic *qi*; nutritive *qi*, defensive *qi*; seasonal *qi*, visceral *qi*, meridian *qi*; and so and so forth.[245]

Qi is the foundation and one of the three treasures (i.e. Essense, Qi, and Shen) of Chinese medicine. For example,

Outside the man, the six kinds of weather conditions in the nature under normal circumstances, i.e. wind, cold, summer-heat, damp, dryness, and fire, are termed together as Six *Qi*, which are also possible pathogenic factors; Inside the

---

244 Shen, Vincent. Dao, Qi, and Body/Mind-Huanglao Daoist Methodology of Nurturing Life. In Wallner F.G., Lan FL, Jandl M.J.(eds.). The Way of Thinking in Chinese Medicine: Theory, Methodology, and Structure of Chinese Medicine. Frankfurt am main: Peter Lang, 2010: 12.

245 Lan Fengli. The Influence of *Huang Di's Inner Classic* on *The Origin of Chinese Characters*[J], Chinese Journal of Medical History, 2006, 36(4): 201-205.

man, Blood and *Qi* are both symbols of life which are indispensable to the being's physiological activities - *Qi* is the commander of the blood, which means *Qi* engenders, moves, and contains the blood; while blood is the mother of *Qi*, which means they together flow endlessly in the vessels around the whole being, enabling it to grow, develop, and fulfil its metabolic and physiological activities. We can differentiate them, but they are inseparable; they complement each other and are dependent on each other.

All kinds of *Qi* which lead to disease are termed as Evil *Qi* or Pathogenic *Qi*; The *Qi* which keeps man in a healthy state is termed as Upright *Qi* or Healthy *Qi*; Disease or health is determined by the relative strength of healthy *Qi* and pathogenic *Qi*; As for treatment, supporting the healthy *Qi* and dispelling pathogenic Qi is one of the most important general principles of treatment. And so and so forth.

According to *Jian Ming Zhong Yi Ci Dian* or *A Concise Dictionary of Chinese Medicine*, *qi* in Chinese medicine bears the following meanings:[246] ① nutritious, essential substance flowing inside the body, such as food *qi*, breathed air; ② functional activities of the *zang-fu* organs in a general sense, such as visceral *qi* (i.e, the functional activities of the *zang-fu* organs); *qi* can also be classified into original *qi*, nutritive *qi*, defensive *qi*, pectoral *qi*, etc. according to its source, distribution, and function; ③ the second location or stage of pattern identification of warm diseases.[247]

It is thus clear that *qi* was no longer air or vapor long ago. And then, what is *qi* in Chinese medicine? Energy? Vital energy? Atmosphere? Or influence? For *qi* implies so many meanings and no translation can convey all the cultural connotations of *qi*, and therefore, I believe *pinyin* transliteration *qi* is the best choice. But more important, the presupposition of *pinyin* transliteration is that you should know the origin, development and cultural connotations of *qi*.

It is thus clear that *Qi* in philosophy of Chinese medicine is to make man become man, and the logic function implied in the *Wei* (Defence) – *Qi* – *Ying* (Nutrient) – Blood Pattern Identification for treatment of warm diseases is the condition of processes and activities of life, i.e. *Qi* is the condition for what it is conditioned, which is similar to Plato's ideas. Plato's ideas are the conditions of the understanding of things and of the beings of the things. Some conceptual aspects of *Qi* have the same argumentative function as Plato's theory of ideas.

Be aware, ancient Chinese philosophy regards *Qi* as the ontology of the universe, and stresses *Qi*'s material characteristics - the basic ingredient

246 Li Jingwei, Ou Yongxin, Yu Ying'ao, et al. 2001: 173.

247 Wei-Qi-Ying-Blood Pattern Identification for Warm Diseases originated from *Huang Di's Inner Classic*, was developed by Ye Tianshi 叶天士 (1666-1745) of the Qing Dynasty. It reflects the general rule of the progression of the four different stages of warm diseases, associates the pathological changes of the four stages with corresponding organs, and advances the corresponding therapeutic principle for each stage.

constituting the universe; while in philosophy of Chinese medicine, *Qi* is the unification of material aspect and functional activities – *Qi* is not only the basic ingredient constituting the Man, but is also used to expound the dynamic processes and functional activities of the life.

Here is worth to note that the concept of *Qi* in Chinese culture is radically different from the concept of material in Western culture, a Chinese misinterpretation. *Guan Tzu* states that "*Qi* can be limitedlessly small and limitedlessly big". Therefore, *Qi*, the origin of the universe and life, is formless without any boundaries or any separation of two opposites (dichotomy). So man can feel *Qi* for man is a being of the integration of the body and the mind, of the subject and the object, of the material and the function. The concept of material in the Western culture must be something with a form even with the rapid development of understanding the structure of materials. Materialism is a philosophical foundation of Western natural science, which stresses the separation and opposition of the body and the mind, of the subject and the object, and greatly promotes the development of modern Western science.

It's necessary to know that Yin-Yang, the five phases, and the eight trigrams are all the subdivisions of *Qi* of different levels from the viewpoint of *Qi*, which indicates a gradual generating and evolving process from *Qi* to Yin-Yang then to the Five Phases then to the Eight Trigrams. *The Book of Changes* states that "the changes have *Tai Ji* (the Supreme Ultimate, the Absolute in ancient Chinese cosmology, presented as the primary source of all created things, i.e. *Qi*), *Tai Ji* generates yin and yang, yin and yang generate the four images, i.e. the greater yang, the greater yin, the lesser yang, and the lesser yin, and the four images generate the eight trigrams". That is to say, *Qi* can be transformed into yin and yang, yin and yang can generate and be transformed into the five phases which are composed of two pairs of yin and yang (water and fire, wood and metal) plus one middle soil. Actually, the four images and the eight trigrams indicate the five phases although the term "five phases" does not appear in this quotation: The four images can be regarded as four phases, i.e. water, fire, wood, and metal; the eight trigrams can be regarded as water (yin), fire (yang), wood (yin wood and yang wood), metal (yin metal and yang metal), and soil (yin soil and yang soil).

Therefore, the formless *Qi* explains the ontology of philosophy of Chinese medicine, i.e., in the structure of Chinese philosophy, *Qi* has the corresponding place of the Western ontology, and is also the foundation of the model of *Qi*, Yin-Yang, and the Five Phases.[248]

---

248 Lan Fengli. *Intercultural Philosophy and Chinese Medicine: Reflections of Philosophy of Chinese Medicine in Chinese Language*. In Wallner F.G., Lan FL, Jandl M.J. (eds.). *The Way of Thinking in Chinese Medicine: Theory, Methodology and Structure of Chinese Medicine* [C]. Frankfurt am main: Peter Lang, 2011: 14-33.

4.4.3 Health Cultivation: Following the Way of the Nature

4.4.3.1 *Lao Tzu*: Discarding the Excessive, the Extravagant, and the Extreme

How to preserve life and avoid harm and danger in the human world? According to *Lao Tzu*, the answer would be

To be meek - the way to preserve your strength and so be strong;

To be humble - humility is the direct opposite of arrogance, the way to make you advance;

To be easily contend - safeguards one from going too far, and therefore from reaching the extreme.

Therefore, the Chapter 29 states that "The sage, therefore, discards the excessive, the extravagant, and the extreme".

4.4.3.2 *Chuang Tzu:* Enlightenments of Carving up an Ox for Health Cultivation

In the chapter of *Yang Sheng Zhu* or *Essentials for Health Cultivation*, it records a story of "Carving up an Ox", which reads that

A cook was butchering an ox for Duke Wen Hui. The places his hand touched, his shoulder leaned against, his foot stepped on, his knee pressed upon, came apart with a sound. He moved the blade, making a noise, that never fell out of rhythm. It harmonized with the Mulberry Woods Dance, like music from ancient times.

Duke Wen Hui exclaimed: "Ah! Excellent! Your skill has advanced to this level? "

The cook put down the knife and answered:

"What I follow is Tao, which is beyond all the skills. When I started butchering, what I saw was nothing but the whole ox. After three years, I no longer saw the whole ox. Nowadays, I meet it with my mind rather than see it with my eyes. My sensory organs are inactive, while I direct the mind's movement.

"It goes according to natural laws, striking apart large gaps, moving toward large openings, following its natural structure. Even places where tendons attach to bones give no resistance, let alone the larger bones!

"A good cook goes through a knife in a year, because he cuts. An average cook goes through a knife in a month, because he hacks. I have used this knife for nineteen years. It has butchered thousands of oxen, but the blade is still like it's newly sharpened. The joints have openings, and the knife's blade has no thickness. Apply this lack of thickness into the openings, and the moving blade swishes through, with room to spare! That's why after nineteen years, the blade is still like it's newly sharpened.

"Nevertheless, every time I come across joints, I see its tricky parts, I pay attention and use caution, my vision concentrates, and my movement slows down. I move the knife very slightly. Whump! It has already separated. The ox doesn't even know it's dead, and falls to the ground like mud. I stand holding the knife, and look all around it. The work gives me much satisfaction. I clean the knife and put it away."

Duke Wen Hui said："Excellent! I listen to your words，and learn how to cultivate my health."

Hereafter are two questions to consider:

Why were the cook's carving-up skills so excellent?

How to preserve or cultivate health?

The cook's carving-up skills were so excellent because he

Sought for "Tao"- the rules for carving up ox as his goal, not only the skills;

Explored the rules based on repeated practices and experiences, and then applied the rules in his practices;

Kept being cautious to carefully observe the rules, and never being careless or arrogant.

What are the enlightenments of Carving up an Ox for health cultivation or How to preserve or cultivate health?

"What I follow is Tao, which is beyond all the skills." That is to say, following the way of a thing itself and the nature and avoiding getting entangled by the disputes and contradictions are keys to cultivate health. To sum up, "Essentials for Preserving and Cultivating Health" are to follow the way of the nature and live until one's allotted natural life span.

4.4.3.3 *Lao Tzu, Chuang Tzu* and *Huang Di Nei Jing Su Wen*

The huge numbers of different translations and distributed prints of *Lao Tzu* and *Chuang Tzu* show that westerners admire "Tao" and are fascinated by "Tao". Chinese medicine abides by Tao and follows the nature, which might be one reason for the needs for Chinese medicine in the West.

Huang Di Nei Jing, also known as *Nei Jing*, comprising *Su Wen* or *Basic Questions* and *Ling Shu* or *Miraculous Pivot*, is the earliest systematic and complete Chinese medical classic extant in China, one of the most important classics of Taoism, an important work to study history of Chinese civilization and medicine, and the highest authority on Chinese medicine. It is not only the breeding ground of the fundamental theories of Chinese medicine, but also an important component part of excellent cultural heritage of China. It has been guiding the development of Chinese medicine for over 2,000 years. Until today, it is still regarded as the prime classic of "the Four Great Classics"[249] of Chinese medicine, and is a required course for Chinese medical learners. As Donald

249 Now the academia of Chinese medicine generally regards *Huang Di Nei Jing* or *Huang Di's Inner Classic*, *Nan Jing* or *Classic of Difficult Issues*, *Shang Han Za Bing Lun* or *Treatise on Cold-induced and Miscellaneous Diseases,* which was later systematized into two monographs: *On Cold-induced Diseases* and *Synopsis of the Golden Chamber*, and *Shen Nong Ben Cao Jing* or *Shengnong's Classic of Materia Medica* as the "Four Great Classics" on Chinese Medicine.

Harper said, it is "the essential reference for ancient Chinese medicine and a valuable to research on early Chinese civilization".

Su Wen or *Basic Questions,* written in the form of a discourse between Huang Di and his ministers, contains a wealth of knowledge, including etiology, physiology, diagnosis, treatment and prevention of disease, as well as an in-depth investigation of such diverse subjects as ethics, psychology, astronomy, meteorology, chrono-biology, and cosmology. All of these subjects are discussed in a holistic context that says life is not fragmented, as in the model provided by modern science, but rather that all the pieces make up an interconnected whole.

Su Wen or *Basic Questions* came out in the Western Han Dynasty (206 B.C.-A.D. 24), during which "Huang-Lao's Learning" were prevailing. And therefore it was mainly influenced by the Taoist philosophy. Or we can say the Taoist philosophy is the underlying foundation of Chinese medicine.

4.4.3.3.1 Tao in *Lao Tzu* and Tao in *Su Wen*

It is *Lao Tzu* that discusses Tao as an abstract concept and endows it with the philosophical meaning of embracing all. It states that "Tao is great, Heaven is great, Earth is great, and Man is also great. ... Man abides by Earth, Earth abides by Heaven, Heaven abides Tao, and Tao abides by the nature.", and that "Tao begets one; The one begets two; The two begets three; The three begets all the things in the universe. All the things bear yin and embrace yang, where the central and harmonious *Qi* makes them in harmony". That is to say, Tao is the first cause of the universe; Yin-Yang begotten by Tao is in command of all the things in the universe, i.e. Tao abides by the nature.

Su Wen or *Basic Questions* holds that Tao of the yin-yang, the five phases, and the four seasons are the Tao of the heaven and the earth. As *Tian Yuan Ji Da Lun* or *The Comprehensive Discourse on Arrangements of the Principal Qi of the Heaven* states that "The five periods and yin-yang are the Tao of the heaven and the earth". Actually, the general idea of *Su Wen* or *Basic Questions* is that "Medicine abides by Tao", which abides by the nature, that is to say, "medicine abides by the nature". This thinking way is specified as the eco-medical thinking way of "Heaven – Earth - Man" in *Su Wen* or *Basic Questions*.

I think that Tao in the *Su Wen* or *Basic Questions* originates from Tao in *Lao Tzu,* but its meaning has already specified as "the way". Tao in *Lao Tzu* is extremely abstract, mysterious and profound, and it is the principle, the soul, and the origin of all things in the universe, as stated that "Tao begets all things in the universe. While Tao in *Su Wen* refers to a kind of concrete, sensible Tao with the meaning of "rule" or "principle". For example, *Su Wen* or *Basic Questions* states in *Yin Yang Ying Xiang Da Lun* or *The Comprehensive Discourse on Images Corresponding to Yin-Yang* that "Yin and yang are **the Way** of the heaven and the earth, the fundamental principles [governing] the myriad beings, the origin of all changes and transformations, the basis and beginning of generating and killing, the palace of spirit brilliance. Disease should be treated from its root." Besides, there are different kinds of Tao expounded in *Su Wen* or *Basic Questions* such as health-cultivating Tao, diagnosis-making Tao, and pulse-feeling Tao, etc., where Tao all means "the way", "the method".

4.4.3.3.2 Health Cultivation in *Lao Tzu* and *Su Wen*

Su Wen or *Basic Questions* is regarded as "one of the most important classics of [philosophical] Taoism" in the West partly because that the health-cultivating way in *Su Wen* or *Basic Questions* is deeply influenced by that of *Lao Tzu.* Here I want to show you some influences of health-cultivating way in *Lao Tzu* on that of *Su Wen* or *Basic Questions* with the Table 7.

Lao Tzu	***Huang Di Nei Jing Su Wen***
[The ancients] overcame cold by being active, overcame heat by keeping quiet. (Chapter 45)	[The ancients] dispelled cold by moving, avoided summer-heat by living in a cool place.(Chapter 13)
To deal with something properly before it occurs and to be well-prepared for chaos before it appears. (Chapter 64)	The sages did not treat those already ill, but treated those not yet ill (or to take preventive treatment before an illness begins); They would like to be well-prepared for chaos before it appeared. (Chapter 2)
Suppress what goes perversely upward, lift what prolapses, reduce what is in excess, and supplement what is in deficiency. The Tao of the universe is to reduce what is in excess, supplement what is in deficiency. (Chapter 77)	Suppress what goes perversely upward, lift what prolapses, and lose what is in excess, supplement what is in deficiency."(Chapter 74)
Content oneself with one's food, clothing, home, and customs (chapter 18)	Content oneself with one's food, clothing, and customs. (Chapter 1)

Table 7 A Comparison of Some Quotations from *Lao Tzu* and *Huang Di Nei Jing Su Wen*

4.4.3.3.2 Health Cultivation in *Chuang Tzu* and *Su Wen*

Chuang Tzu carries on the essentials of health cultivation of *Lao Tzu* – To conform to the nature for man lives in between the heaven and the earth. The chapter of *Si Qi Tiao Shen Da Lun* or *Comprehensive Discourse on Regulating the Spirit in Accordance with the the Four Seasons* of *Su Wen* states that "Therefore, yin-yang and the four seasons are the beginning and the ending of everything, the root of death and life. To go against them harms life; to go with them prevents illnesses from arising, which means 'achieving the Way of cultivating health'. Only the sages follow the Way while the fools violate it", which forms the core of health-cultivating theory in *Su Wen* or *Basic Questions*.

Concretely speaking, *Su Wen* or *Basic Questions* elaborates health-cultivating ways of the true men, the accomplished men, the sages, and the exemplary men, which are connected with those of *Chuang Tzu,* and the way of regulating spirit to cultivate health.

Shang Gu Tian Zhen Lun or *Discourse on the True [Qi Endowed by] Heaven in High Antiquity* of *Su Wen* or *Basic Questions* states that[250]

Huang Di:
"I have heard,
In high antiquity there were true men.[251]
They upheld [the patterns of] heaven and earth and
They grasped [the regularity of] yin and yang.
They exhaled and inhaled essence qi.[252]
They stood for themselves and guarded their spirit.
Muscles and flesh were like one.
Hence,
they were able to achieve longevity, in correspondence with heaven and earth.
There was no point in time when [their life could have] come to an end.[253]
Such was their life in the Way.

At that time of middle antiquity,
there were the accomplished men.
They were of pure virtue and they were entirely in accord with the Way.
They adapted themselves to [the regularity] of yin and yang and
they lived in harmony with the four seasons.
They left the world and they departed from the common.[254]
They accumulated essence and preserved their spirit.
They roamed between heaven and earth and
their vision as well as their hearing went beyond the eight reaches.

---

250 Translation and notes of the following paragraph are from: Unschuld Paul U., Tessenow Hermann. Trans. Huang Di Nei Jing Su Wen (Vol.1). 2011: 42-44.

251 Wang Bing: "True men are those who have attained the Way." For classic definitions of the "true men" see 庄子, 大宗师, and 淮南子, 本经训, as well as 史记, 始皇本纪.

252 " 'Exhaling and inhaling essence qi' is one of the ancient methods of nourishing life. Another name is 行气, 'to move qi.' " See also 庄子，刻意篇.

253 Wang Bing: "Their body paralleled the Way and their longevity paralleled the Way. Hence, they were able to live for an endless time in that their long life lasted through the entire [existence of] heaven and earth."

254 Gao Shishi: "With their body they were part of the customs of their days; with their heart they transcended the customs of their days."

This way, they added to their lifespan and were strong.
They, too, may be counted among the true men.

Next, there were the sages.
They lived in harmony with heaven and earth and
they followed the patterns of the eight winds.[255]
They accommodated their cravings and their desires within the world and the common and their heart knew no anger.
In their activities they had no desire to disassociate themselves from the world;
in their <clothing and> bearing they had no desire to be observed by the common people.
Externally, they did not tax their physical appearance with any affairs;
Internally, they did not suffer from any pondering.
They made every effort to achieve peaceful relaxation and
they considered self-realization as success.
Their physical body did not deteriorate and
Their essence and their spirit did not dissipate.
They, too, could reach a number of one hundred [years].

Next, there were the exemplary men.
They took heaven as law and the earth as rule;
their appearance resembled sun and moon.
They distinguished among and arranged the stars
[on the basis of their] movements contrary to or following [the movements of]
yin and yang.
They distinguished among the four seasons.
They went along with high antiquity and
they acted in complete union with the Way.
They, too, were able to add to their long life and
to have their full time."

Ogyu Sorai (1666-1728) with Butsu Sorai as his pen name, a Japanese Confucian philosopher, commented that "What Huang Di said here were written by others, and are not relevant to the foregoing paragraphs. Discussions on the sages, the accomplished men, and the true men are from teachings of *Chuang Tzu* and *Lie Tzu*"[256].

---

255 A concept referring to winds originating in the eight cardinal point East, South, West, North, East-North, East-South, West-South, and West-North.
256 Guo Aichun. 1999: 7.

Su Wen or *Basic Questions* inherits the spirit-cultivating way from *Chuang Tzu* – "being indifferent to worldly fame or gain". The chapter of *Shang Gu Tian Zhen Lun* or *Discourse on the True [Qi Endowed by] Heaven in High Antiquity* states that "The sages of the remote antiquity taught the common people who would follow that they should avoid *xu xie zei feng* or the external pernicious influences in time, and should be indifferent to fame or gain or anything else in order to keep the true *qi* flowing smoothly and freely and maintain the spirit staying inside the body. Then, where does illness come from?"; The chapter of *Yin Yang Ying Xiang Da Lun* or *The Comprehensive Discourse on Images Corresponding to Yin-Yang* states that "Therefore, the sages have effortless actions, and content themselves with being indifferent to any fame or gain."; The chapter of *Yi Jing Bian Qi Lun* or *Discourse on Moving Essence and Changing Qi* states that "In the setting that any person is indifferent to any fame or gain, the evils or pathogens cannot get way to attack the man."

Here I want to show you some influences of health-cultivating ways in *Chuang Tzu* on that in *Su Wen* or *Basic Questions* with the Table 8.

Chuang Tzu	***Huang Di Nei Jing Su Wen***
Follow the principles of the universe, practice the five virtues, react according to the [changes] in the nature, then regulate [one's activities] according to the seasons, and thus myriad of beings are living harmoniously in accordance with the alternate changes of the seasons. (Chapter "Tian Shi 天适")	Therefore, yin-yang and the four seasons are the beginning and the ending of everything, the root of death and life. To go against them harms life; to go with them prevents illnesses from arising, which means "achieving the Way of health cultivation". Only the sages follow the Way and the fools violate it. (Chapter 2)
One should be indifferent to fame or gain or anything else in order to prevent the sufferings or pathogenic agents from invading him and to preserve his body, spirit, and virtue. (Chapter of "Ke Yi 刻意")	The sages of the remote antiquity taught the common people who would follow that they should avoid disease-causing factors in time, and should be indifferent to fame or gain or anything else in order to keep the true *qi* flowing smoothly and freely and maintain the spirit staying inside the body. Then, where does illness come from? (Chapter 1)
One should be indifferent to fame or gain or anything else in order to prevent the sufferings or pathogenic agents from invading him and to preserve his body, spirit, and virtue. (Chapter of "Ke Yi 刻意")	Therefore, the sages have effortless actions, and content themselves with being indifferent to any fame or gain. (Chapter 5) In the setting that any person is indifferent to any fame or gain, the evils or pathogens cannot get way to attack the man." (Chapter 13)

Table 8 A Comparison of Some Quotations from *Chuang Tzu* and *Huang Di Nei Jing Su Wen*

4.4.4 Medical Ethics: Being Expert in Medical Skills and Sincere to the Patients

4.4.4.1 Understanding Tao, Perfecting Skill

Medicine is supposed to save lives. If a doctor is not good at arts of healing, patients will be delayed and may miss an opportunity to be cured. Sometimes, malpractice may lead to death.

Tao is the most important concept of Lao-Chuang's philosophy. Tao is the origin of the universe, the laws and rules in the nature, society, and medicine as well. *Lao Tzu* states that "The tree which fills the arms grew from the tiniest sprout; the tower of nine storeys rose from a small heap of earth; the journey of a thousand *li* (miles) commenced with a single step" (Chapter 64). Hence, you should take unceasingly efforts by having effortless actions (i.e. following the natural laws of things) in order to gradually understand Tao. Sun Simiao (581-682) exhorted medical practitioners in his "*Da Yi Jing Cheng* or *Medical Morality*" to investigate thoroughly the origin of medicine by reading extensively and diligently, and warned them against following the hearsays. As a doctor you must always seek for the Tao in medicine by continuously refining on your knowledge and skills.

4.4.4.2 Valuing Life, Equaling All

Lao Tzu holds that man is as great as Tao, Heaven, and Earth, which embodies the thinking of valuing life.

"Therefore, Tao is great.
Heaven is great.
Earth is great.
Man is great.
In the universe, there are four great things, and man is one of them.". (Chapter 25 of *Lao Tzu)*

"Of all things in between the heaven and the earth, nothing is more precious than man." (*Huang Di's Inner Classic• Basic Questions. The Comprehensive Discourse on Images Corresponding to Yin-Yang*)

"Man is the most valuable being in between the heaven and the earth." (*The Origin of Chinese Characters• Man Part*)

Valuing life is the basic moral requirements for medical practitioners. Both superb medical skills and lofty medical moralities result from treasuring life. Zhang Zhongjing (150-219) "blamed current medical practitioners who did not care and explore the arts of healing to treat the monarch and parents' illnesses in the upper, relieve the poor and lowly's sufferings in the lower, and to preserve their own health and prolong their own life in the middle", and then "regretted the lost lives from unnatural death in the past", and then "sought frequently old maxims and collected good formulae and methods from all quarters"[257], and finally accomplished the master piece *Treatise on Cold-Induced and Miscellaneous Diseases*. Sun Simiao (581-682) gave his monumental medical work the title *One Thousand Gold Prescriptions for Emergencies* or *Invaluable Prescriptions for Emergencies* for he thought that "life is more valuable than a thousand gold".

Chuang Tzu proposes "equaling all the beings". That is to say, the lives are all equal to each other without discrimination of high and low or great and small or gentle and simple. Medical practitioners are supposed to relieve patients' sufferings, and so should treat all the patients without discrimination. As Sun Simiao said that "When patients come to seek for help, they (i.e. medical practitioners) should not treat them differently by seeing whether they are rich or poor, old or young, beautiful or ugly, enemy or friend, Chinese or foreigner, foolish or wise. They should treat all the patients like their closest relatives. When treating patients, they should not think over and over for themselves and pay too much attention to the protection of their own lives. Being qualified doctors, they should regard the patients' suffering as their own and have deep sympathy for them".

4.4.4.3 Being Modest, Respecting Fraternity

Lao Tzu holds that water bears the most modest qualities: tending to be the lowest position, and soft. The chapter 8 of *Lao Tzu* reads that "The highest excellent persons or things are just like water. They benefit all things instead of contention. They stay at the lowest place which all men dislike. So this kind of persons and things are very close to 'Tao'". It is true that water nourishes and moistens all the beings, but is willing to be the lowest place. One of Lao Tzu's three treasures is "shrinking from taking precedence of others", which can make him become "a chief of all the vessels" like a leader with the highest honour (Chapter 67).

Chuang Tzu implies that every one should be modest and keep a very low profile for no matter how strong you are there is always someone stronger by telling such a fable story in the chapter of *Autumn Floods*:

At the time of autumn floods when hundreds of streams poured into the Yellow River, the torrents were so violent that it was impossible to distinguish an ox from a horse from the other side of the river. Then the River God was overwhelmed with joy, feeling that all the beauty under the heaven belonged to him alone. Down the river he travelled east until he reached the North Sea. Looking eastward at the boundless expanse of water, he changed his countenance and signed to the Sea God, saying, "As the popular saying goes, 'There are men

257 See the preface of the *Treatise on Cold-Induced and Miscellaneous Diseases* by Zhang Zhongjing.

who have heard a lot about Tao but still think that no one can surpass them.' I am one of such men. Upon hearing people belittle Confucius's learning and humiliate Bo Yi's righteousness, I simply could not believe a word they said. Now that I have seen your boundless expanse, I realize that I would have been in danger if I had not come to you. I would always be sneered at by those who are well-versed in Tao."

The God Sea said, "You cannot discuss the sea with a frog at the bottom of a well because it is confined to its dwelling place; you cannot discuss ice with a summer moth because it is limited to one season; you cannot discuss Tao with a bookworm because he is restrained to the book knowledge. Now that you have left the riverside and seen the vast sea, you are aware of your insignificance. Thus it is possible now to discuss Tao with you; Of all the waters under the heaven, nothing is greater than the sea. It receives the endless flow of ten thousand rivers but it is never full. It is leaking endlessly but it is never empty. It does not change with spring or autumn; it does not know flood or drought. It holds so much more water than the Yangtzu River and the Yellow River that it is absolutely beyond measure. Yet I am never conceited about the amount. I assume my shape from the heaven and the earth, and accumulate my vigour from yin and yang. I stay here between the heaven and the earth, just like a small stone or a small tree on a huge mountain. How can I overestimate myself when I know that I am so insignificant! Don't the four seas between the heaven and the earth resemble small holes in a large swamp? Don't the central states within the four seas resemble grains of millet in a large granary? There are hundreds and thousands of things in the world; humanity is but one of them. Human beings live in regions where grains grow and where boats and carts come and go; an individual man is but one of them. Compared with the hundreds and thousands of things, isn't an individual man but a tiny down on a horse? The succession of the five kings, the strife between the three emperors, the worries of human gentlemen, and the efforts of the capable officials – all is no more than this. Bo Yi gained fame by refusing to accept the throne; Confucius displayed his learning by lecturing all around. Isn't this self-lauding very much the same as what did not long ago about your water?"[258]

Almost all doctors of high renown in the past time were modest and respected their fraternity. Bian Que 扁鹊, a famous doctor of the Warring States Period (475-221 B.C.), was surnamed Qin and named Yueren. He said after he cured the prince of the Guo state of his syncope, which others believed that he was dead, "I certainly cannot resuscitate the dead. In fact the prince was not really dead, what I can do is just to cure his illness". Sun Simiao 孙思邈 (581-682) said that "The way of being a qualified doctor is that he should never talk nor laugh uproariously, gossip or sow discord, speak about others, show off his own

258 This part is translated by Wang Rongpei.

reputation, calumniate other doctors, or boast his own morality."[259] Every one has his strong and weak points, and should draw on each other's merits and raise the medical level together.

Besides, *Lao Tzu* and *Chuang Tzu* advocate that a doctor should be indifferent to fame and gain but be devoted himself to relieve people's sufferings.

---

259 See *Da Yi Jing Cheng* or *A Great Doctor Should Be Expert in Medical Skills and Sincere to His Patients*, from the first volume of *Bei Ji Qian Jin Yao Fang* or *The Invaluable Prescriptions for Emergencies*.

Yin and yang are
the Way of the Heaven and the Earth,
the fundamental principles [governing] the myriad beings,
the origin of all changes and transformations,
the basis and beginning of generating and killing,
the palace of spirit brilliance.

-Huang Di's Inner Classic Basic Questions• Comprehensive Discourse on Images Corresponding to Yin-Yang

5 The Theory of Yin and Yang

There is no way available to investigate when the concepts of "yin and yang" were transmitted to the West. Let's take a look at how Ilza Veith translated "yin-yang" in *Huang Di' s Inner Classic* in the 1940s[260]:

"Yin and Yang [the male and female elements in nature];
Yang, the element of light; Yin, the element of darkness;
Yin and Yang, the negative and positive principles in nature;
The element of light; the element of darkness;
Yang, the lucid element of life; Yin, the turbid element of darkness;
Yang, the male element; Yin, the female element;
Yin and Yang [the two elements in nature];
Yang, the lucid element; Yin, the turbid element;
Yin and Yang [the two opposing principles];
Yang (the male principle of light and life); Yin (the female principle of darkness and death);
…"

It is thus clear that the Westerner did not fully understand the meanings of "yin and yang" at Veith's time: yin-yang was occasionally translated into the element of light and the element of darkness; in most cases, yin-yang was pinyin transliterated with a concrete explanation.

You see, long before, "yin" had been translated into the female or feminine, negative, inactive, dark, or turbid principle or element, and "yang" into the male or masculine, positive, active, bright, or lucid principle or element in the West. As time went by, people came to find out that no such a pair of opposites available can cover all the philosophical meanings implied in "yin-yang", finally accepted the two loan words: yin and yang. Actually, the words "yin and yang" have already been included as word entries into English dictionaries such as Webster's, Longman and The Oxford Dictionaries, etc. For example,

Longman Dictionary of Contemporary English: "yin, the female principle in Chinese PHILOSOPHY which is inactive, dark, negative, etc. and which

260 Veith Ilza. 1949; 1966, 1972: 97-253.

combines with YANG (= the male principle) to form the whole world"; "yang, the male principle in Chinese PHILOSOPHY which is active, light, POSITIVE, etc. and which combines with YIN (= the female principle) to form the whole world."[261]

Webster's Encyclopedic Unabridged Dictionary of the English Language: "Yin and Yang (in Chinese philosophy and religion) two principles, one negative, dark and feminine (Yin), and one positive, bright, and masculine (Yang), whose interaction influences the destinies of creatures and things."[262]

Actually, yin and yang have already gone beyond concrete meanings and have become philosophical concepts with broad and abstract senses. Then what are the original meanings of yin and yang?

5.1 The Original Meanings of Yin and Yang

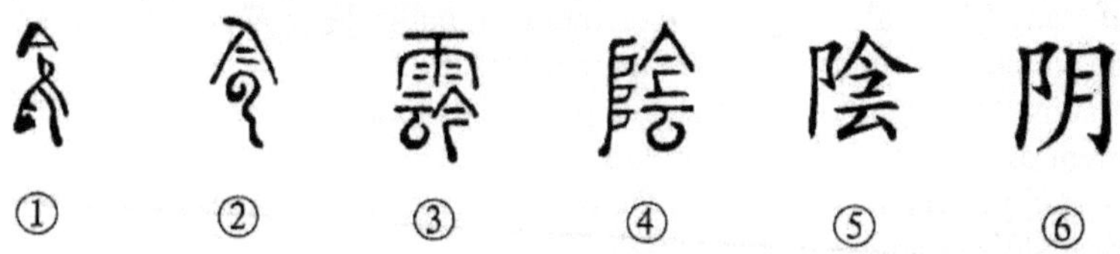

Illus. 19 The Sinogram "Yin 阴" from Oracle to Simplified Regular Script

The sinogram "阴 Yin" was originally a pictophonetic.

The first one is the writing form in the oracle script with the upper as "今" for pronunciation and the lower as "隹（鸟） bird" for the shape, which means it is going to be cloudy and the bird is unceasingly crying;

The second one is the ancient writing form in *The Origin of Chinese Characters* with the lower part changed into "云 cloud", which is still very reasonable for being cloudy indicates that there must be dense clouds;

The third one, the lesser seal script, is composed of three parts "雨 rain", "今 Jin" – the phonetic part, and "云 cloud", which apparently shows the intimate relationship between "阴 Yin" and "雨 rain";

The fourth is a variant writing form of the lesser seal script;

The fifth is the original complex writing form in regular script;

And the sixth is the simplified writing form of the sinogram.

The Origin of Chinese Characters interprets "yin 陰" as "dark", "the northern side of a mountain or the southern side of a river"; interprets "yin 霒" as "clouds covering the sun". Now there is just one sinogram "阴" for both. The

261 Longman Dictionary of Contemporary English. 1998: 1789, 1787.
262 Webster's Encyclopedic Unabridged Dictionary of the English Language. 1994: 1656.

original meaning of "阴 Yin" is cloudy. "The northern side of a mountain" and "the southern side of a river" are termed yin for they shelter from the sun. *Han Fei Tzu · Shuo Lin Shang* states that "夏居山之**阴**", which means "In the summer [it is advisable to] live at **the northern side** of a mountain". *Lie Tzu · Tang Wen* states that "达于汉**阴**", which means "Arrive at **the southern side** of Han(shui) River".

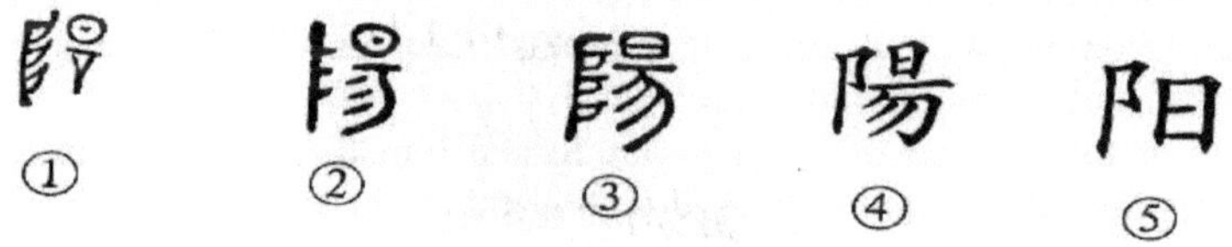

Illus. 20 The Sinogram "Yang 阳" from Oracle to Simplified Regular Script

The sinogram 阳 Yang was originally an associative compound and a pictographic character as well.

The first one is the writing form in the oracle script with the left as "阜 fu", which means "going up"; with the right as a bright lamp, which means "extreme bright";

The second is the writing form in the bronze script, which is similar to that in the oracle script, supplemented with the three left falling strokes at the lower left part to indicate "the light glittering in all directions";

The third is the writing form in the lesser seal script, which is identical with that in the bronze script;

The fourth is the original complex writing form of Yang in regular script, and the fifth is the simplified writing form of the sinogram yang in regular script.

The Origin of Chinese Characters interprets yang as "high bright". It is later extended to refer to "the sun", as stated in *The Classic of Poetry· Xiao Ya ·Zhang Lu* that "匪阳不晞", which means "if without the sun [it] would not have dried"; Then it is extended to mean "warm", as stated in *The Classic of Poetry· Bin's Tone ·July* that "春日载阳，有鸣仓庚", which means that "Spring days are warm, yellow warblers are singing". "The southern side of a mountain" and "the northern side of a river" are generally facing the sun and thus warm, so are termed as "Yang". *The Book of Documents ·Yu Gong* states that "岷山之**阳**，至于衡山", which means "from the southern side of Minshan mountain to Hengshan Mountain". *The Classic of Poetry· Qin's Tone ·Weiyang* states that "我送舅氏，日至渭**阳**", which means "I see my uncle, to the northern side of Wei(shui) River in the daytime".

Yin and Yang referred to directions of a mountain or a river in the nature. And then, the meanings of yin and yang are summarized as "the side facing the sun being yang and the reverse side being yin".

5.2 Exploring the Origin of Yin-Yang in Chinese Medicine

It was "Bo Yang Fu 伯阳父" of the last years of Western Zhou Dynasty (ca. 1100-771 B.C.) that first used the words of yin and yang, gave them the abstract meaning of opposition, and used them to explain natural phenomena. He believed that "Yang hides [inside] and can not come out, yin is forced and can not ascend, and then earthquake ensues" (*Guo Yu •Zhou Yu*). Fan Li 范蠡 (536-448B.C.) of the last years of Spring Autumn Period (770-476 B.C.) said that "Yang in its extreme becomes yin, and yin in its extreme becomes yang; the sun in the end rises again, and the moon in the full wanes" (*Guo Yu •Yue Yu*), which was the first and earliest formulation of waxing-waning and transformation of yin and yang. *Lao Tzu • the 42nd Chapter* states that "All things in the universe bear yin and embrace yang, where the central and harmonious *qi* makes them in harmony". This quotation affirms that the contradictory qualities of yin and yang are intrinsic attributes of everything.

The Book of Changes further advances that "One yin and one yang makes Tao", which abstracts yin and yang to the extensive universality and regards yin and yang as the fundamental rule of the universe for the first time. *The Book of Changes* also uses yin-yang to make a comparison with social phenomena, and yin-yang has by extension come to imply the relationship between upward and downward, monarch and ministers, wife and husband, etc. Joseph Needham (1900-1995) believed that yin and yang as definite philosophical terms appear in *The Book of Changes*. The *Chun Qiu Fan Lu* or *Luxuriant Dew of Spring-Autumn Annals* by Dong Zhongshu 董仲舒 (179-104 B.C.) states that "The heaven has yin and yang, the man also has yin and yang. Yin qi of the heaven rises and yin qi of the man will respond it to rise, while yin qi of the man rises and yin qi of the heaven will respond it to rise too. The principles or ways are the same".

Chinese medicine inherits and develops the ideas of yin-yang in *The Book of Changes*. Not all the yin-yang in ancient medical texts is abstract in the philosophical sense. For example, among the medical books unearthed from the Mawangdui Han Tomb[263], *Shi Wen* or *Ten Questions* discusses the way of

---

263 The medical manuscirpts unearthed from the Mawangdui Han Tomb in December 1973, Changsha, Hunan Province, include 11 silk manuscripts and 4 written on bamboo slips. The time of the tomb is 168 B.C. The manuscripts were copied around 3 B.C., and were the oldest documents on Chinese medicine extant in China. Most of them are stray fragments of text without a title, and then they were entitled according to their contents by modern Chinese scholars: *Prescriptions for 52 Diseases*, *Classic of Moxibustion with 11 Meridians of Arm and Foot*, *Classic of Moxibustion with 11 Yin-Yang Meridians*, *Methods of Pulse-Taking*, *Manifestations of Yin-Yang Pulse Indicating Death* (with one volume of silk manuscript); *Que Gu Shi Qi* 却谷食气, *Classic of Moxibustion with 11 Yin-Yang Meridians* (B ed.), *Illustrations of Taoist Breathing Exercises* (with one volume of silk manuscript); *Methods for Cultivating Health*, *Miscellaneous Therapies*, *On Obstetrics* (with one volume of silk manuscript); *Ten Questions* (bamboo slips), *Methods of Integrating Yin and Yang* (bamboo slips), *Miscellaneous Contraindications* (wood slips), and *Supreme Way of the Land under Heaven* (bamboo slips). The first five manuscripts and related research outcome were published with the title *Prescriptions for 52 Diseases* by Cultural Relics Publishing House in 1972.

meeting yin [the female's genitals]; *He Yin-Yang Fang* or *Methods of Integrating Yin and Yang* on the methods of copulation of the male and the female; *Tian Xia Zhi Dao Tan* or *The Supreme Way of the Land under Heaven* on harms and benefits of sexual intercourse; *Yang Sheng Fang* or *Ways of Cultivating Health* and *Za Liao Fang* or *Miscellaneous Therapies* on functions of sexual intercourse and antenatal instructions.

The theory of yin-yang is easy to tally with the male and the female in the sexual intercourse. So, it is very natural to use the principles of yin-yang to explain the sexual intercourse or even use yin-yang as a synonym or euphemism of the sexual intercourse in the above-mentioned works. These works on sexual intercourse press close to the philosophy of yin-yang on one end and to the medical life on the other, so yin-yang can be regarded as a bridge between philosophy and medicine. Thus, it is very common in ancient Chinese medical texts to adopt yin-yang to represent male and female or sexual intercourse as stated in the Mawangdui medical books.

Moreover, ancient Chinese medical classics have applied yin-yang theory extensively into the medical field in accordance with thinking way of *Qu Xing Bi Lei*, or taking images and analogizing. For example, yin-yang in concrete medical texts may refer to some specific medical meanings, such as the male and the female, sex or sexual activity, yin-yang meridians, yin-yang pathogens, yin-yang *qi*, *cun* pulse and *chi* pulse, etc.

In *The Book of Changes*, yin-yang is mainly used in the field of natural philosophy; while in Chinese medicine, yin-yang is used not only in the philosophical field, but also in the medical field, and yin-yang is an ingenious unification of philosophical and medical senses. *Huang Di's inner Classic* makes a more systematic and definite expression on the ideas of interdependence, waning-waxing, transformation, counterbalance and harmony of yin-yang implied in *The Book of Changes*, develops these ideas by integrating them with the medical practice, and thus makes yin-yang theory become the guiding theory of Chinese medicine.

5.3 Understanding Yin-Yang in the Way of *Qu Xiang Bi Lei*

As a pair of philosophical concepts, yin-yang in essence is to summarize the dynamic images of things or phenomena. Generally speaking, things that are mobile, external, upward, ascending, warm, hot, bright, hyperactive, or pertaining to functional activities can be classified as *Yang*; those that are unmoving, internal, downward, descending, cold, dull, hypoactive, or pertaining to materials (or structures) can be classified as *Yin*. (See Table 9)

	Yin	Yang
Examples From The Nature To The Man	the earth	the sky
	the moon	the sun
	Water	Fire
	Night	Day
	Cloudy	Clear
	dark (dull)	Bright
	cold (cool)	heat (warm)
	Heavy	Light
	Still	Move
	Internal	External
	Downward	Upward
	Hypoactive	Hyperactive
	structure (material)	Function
	Negative	Positive
	Descending	Ascending
	Female	Male
	Death	Life
	Abdomen	Back
	Blood	Qi
	Five zang organs	Six fu organs

Table 9 Examples of *Yin-Yang*

Based on different characteristics of images of *Yin* and *Yang*, all things in the universe can be classified as one or the other in accordance with the way of *Qu Xiang Bi Lei*. The attribute of yin or yang has nothing to do with concrete materials or shapes, but is only determined by their dynamic functions, actions and relationships instead. For example, water pertains to yin for the image of water being cool, moistening and flowing downwards corresponds to yin; fire to yang for the image of fire being warming and rising corresponds to yang. Heaven pertains to yang for the image of the heaven *qi* being light, lucid, ascending and floating corresponds to yang; earth to yin for the image of the earth *qi* being heavy, turbid, descending and sinking corresponds to yin.

Similarly, Chinese medicine often regards *qi*, which has a propelling and warming function, as *Yang;* blood, which has a nourishing and moistening function, as *Yin*. The organic structure, the physiological functional activities of the body, as well as the signs and symptoms of pathological changes, can all be differentiated on the basis of the characteristics of the images of *Yin* and *Yang*. See Table 10.

Yang Pattern	*Yin* Pattern
1. Fever, perspiration, hyperfunction	Chills or aversion to cold, hypofunction
2. Raised basal metabolic rate	Reduced basal metabolic rate
3. High temperature	Low temperature
4. Profuse perspiration	Reduced perspiration
5. Raised systolic blood pressure	Low systolic blood pressure
6. Raised diastolic blood pressure	Low diastolic blood pressure
7. Increased gastric peristalsis	Reduced gastric peristalsis
8. Sympathetic hyperactivity	Parasympathetic hyperactivity
9. Intolerance of heat	Intolerance of cold
10.Red or rosy complexion	Pale complexion
11.Desire for cold drink and food	Desire for hot drink and food
12.Dry tongue , with thirst	Moistened tongue, without thirst
13.Yellow urine	Clear urine
14.Normal quantity of saliva, normal salivation	Much saliva, hyper-salivation
15.Constipation	Diarrhea

Table 10 Pattern Identification According to Yin and Yang[264]

Therefore, in short, the meanings of Yin and Yang are extremely simple, yet very profound. One can seemingly understand them on a rational level, and yet, continually find new connotations or expressions of them in the theoretical system and clinical practice of Chinese medicine, and, indeed, in life as well for the concepts and theory of yin-yang have formed and will continually gain their new connotations in accordance with the way of *Qu Xiang Bi Lei* or Taking Image and Analogizing, as stated in the *Huang Di's Inner Classic · Basic Questions• Comprehensive Discourse on Images Corresponding to Yin-Yang* states that "**Yin and yang** are the Way of the Heaven and the Earth, the fundamental principles [governing] the myriad beings, the origin of all changes and transformations, the basis and beginning of generating and killing, and the palace of spirit brilliance".

5.4 Translation of Yin-Yang in Classical Chinese Medical Texts[265]

In classical Chinese medical texts, yin-yang bears rich and varied meanings. Since the specific meanings of yin and yang depend highly upon the linguistic context in which they appear, it is ill-advised to consistently use their pinyin transliterations in rendering the two concepts into other languages. To be adequate, their translation should accord with the actual contextual meanings they have acquired. Here I give you some examples:

264 Quoted from a secondary source. See Li Lei. New Century TCM English Course. 2006: 18.
265 Lan Fengli. The Origin of Yin-Yang as Chinese Medical Terms and Their Translation [J]. Chinese Translators Journal. 2007, 28(4): 69-72.

5.4.1 Original Text: 丈夫八岁，肾气实，发长齿更；二八，肾气盛，天癸至，精气溢泻，阴阳和，故能有子。(《素问·上古天真论》)

Translation: In the male, at the age of eight the boy's kidney qi is abundant, his hair grows and his baby teeth are replaced by permanent ones. At the age of 16 the *tian gui* or sex-stimulating essence matures, he begins to secrete semen; if at this point the male and the female unite in harmony, a child may be conceived.

Note: Here, "yin-yang" refers to female and male. "实" should be "盛". "肾气盛" is redundancy. "和" should be "和合", i.e. unite in harmony.

5.4.2 Original Text: 冲任之脉既起于胞内，阴阳过度，则伤胞络，故风邪乘虚而入于胞，损冲、任之经，伤太阳、少阴之血，致令胞络之间，秽液与血相兼，连带而下。(《诸病源候论·妇人杂病诸候·带下候》)

Translation: The controlling and thoroughfare vessels both originate from the uterus. Excessive sexual activities harm uterine network vessels, and then pathogenic wind invades the uterus, impairing the two vessels, damaging blood of Taiyang and Shaoyin, causing turbidity and blood in the uterine network vessels, together with vaginal discharge, flowing down out of the body.

Note: Here, "yin-yang" refers to the sexual activity.

5.4.3 Original Text: 百病之始生也，皆生于风雨寒暑、阴阳喜怒、饮食居处、大惊卒恐。(《灵枢·口问》)

Translation: Various diseases are caused by exposure to wind, rain, cold or summer-heat, or excess sex, or a lack of harmonious emotions, or improper diet, or a lack of regularity in lifestyle, or great fear or sudden fright.

Note: Here, "yin-yang" refers to excessive sexual activities or excess sex.

5.4.4 Original Text: 粗工治之，亟刺阴阳，身体解散，四支转筋，死日有期。(《素问·疏五过论》)

Translation: A careless doctor treats it by pricking the yin and yang vessels time and again, thus causing the patient getting emaciated, having crumps in the limbs and coming closer to the death day.

Notes: Here, "yin-yang" refers to yin *Jing* and yang *Jing*. The standardized translation for "经脉" approved by WHO（World Health Organisation) is meridian, which implies a two-dimensional grid. Seeing that "*Jing Mai* 经脉 " can carry and move qi and blood and so must be a three-dimensional tube, and that "Channel", a popular translation in the West indicating a three-dimensional tube, is a polysemant, whose meaning is not clear and definite, and that "*Jing Mai*" and "*Luo Mai*" are further divisions of "*Mai* or Vessel", "Vessel" can refer to a three-dimensional tube of the human being and therefore is a strict and proper translation for *jing mai* worth to be popularized in the future.

5.4.5 Original Text: 夫阴与阳，皆有俞会，阳注于阴，阴满之外，阴阳匀平，以充其形，九候若一，命曰平人。夫邪之生也，或生于阴，或生于阳，其生于阳者，得之风雨寒暑；其生于阴者，得之饮食居处、阴阳喜怒。(《素问·调经论》)

Translation: The yin and yang vessels possess acupuncture points, where transportation and convergence of *qi* and blood occur. Blood and *qi* of the yang meridians will transport to the yin meridians. Blood and *qi* then fill the yin meridians and flow to other parts of the body. Then yin and yang are balanced, the body becomes robust, the nine indicators of the body's pulses will also be concert. This occurs in a normal, healthy person. The pathogens may attack the body. There are internal damages caused by yin pathogens and external contractions caused by yang pathogens. The external contractions caused by yang pathogens may result from exposure to rain, wind, cold, or summer heat; while the internal damages caused by yin pathogens may arise from improper diet, a lack of regularity in lifestyle, excessive sexual activities, or a lack of harmonious emotions.

Note: "Yin and yang" in "夫阴与阳" refers to the yin and yang vessels; "yin-yang" in "阴阳匀平" refers to the abstract yin-yang in general sense, thus should be pinyin transliterated into "yin and yang"; as to "yin and yang" in "或生于阴，或生于阳", Zhang Qi 张琦 said that "there are internal damages caused by yin pathogens, and there are external contractions caused by yang pathogens"; "yin-yang" in "阴阳喜怒" refers to "the female and the male", or "the sexual activity", here refers to excessive sexual activities. Undoubtedly, such explanation is correct in view of medical principles.

5.4.6 Original Text: 蘖木， 味苦，寒。主治五脏、肠胃中结热；黄疸；肠痔；止泄痢；女子漏下赤白；阴阳伤；蚀疮。(《神农本草经卷三·中品》)

Translation: Phellodendri Cortex (Huang Bai), bitter in flavor and cold in property. Indications: accumulated heat in the five *zang* organs, the stomach and intestines; jaundice; perianal abscess; arresting diarrhea and dysentery; spotting with red or light-colored discharge in women; hypersexuality; sores resistant to healing.

Note: Here, "yin-yang" refers to female's and male's genitals. The sinogram "伤" is interchangeable with "壮". "Yin-Yang Shang 阴阳伤" refers to "the sexual desire of female's and male's genitals being exuberant", i.e. both the female and the male having strong lust for sex, i.e. hypersexuality. In the quotation "望卿走，自投井死，昭信出之，椓杙其阴中" from *Han Shu* or the *History of the Former Han Dynasty* (《汉书·景十三王传·广川惠王刘越》), yin refers to the female's genitals; in the quotation "囝生南方，闽吏得之乃绝其阳" from *Nan* or *Boys*, by Gu Kuang of the Tang Dynasty (唐·顾况《囝》), yang refers to the boy's genitals. *Guang Ya* (《广雅·释诂四》) states that " 壮 is 伤". Yu Xinwu 于新吾 explains "伤 in the quotation "带甲婴马害歌於行伍，使人身伤" from *Xun Tzu* (《荀子·乐论》) as "壮".

5.4.7 Original Text: 伤寒之脉，阴阳俱盛而紧涩；热病之脉，阴阳俱浮，浮之而滑，沉之散涩。(《难经·五十八难》)

Translation: The pulse of cold-induced diseases: both *cun* and *chi* pulses are strong, tense, and choppy. The pulse of febrile disease: both *cun* and *chi* pulses are floating; the pulses are slippery when felt slightly, and scattered and choppy when felt heavily.

Note: Here, "yin-yang" refers to *chi* portion and *cun* portion of the pulse respectively for *chi* pertains to yin and *cun* pertains to yang.

5.4.8 Original Text: 阴阳相搏，名曰动。阳动则汗出，阴动则发热。(《伤寒论》)

Translation: When yin *qi* and yang *qi* wrestle with each other, the pulse is throbbing. When the *cun* pulse is throbbing, sweating results; when the *chi* pulse is throbbing, fever ensues.

Note: "Yin-yang" in "阴阳相搏" refers to "yin *qi* and yang *qi*"; "yang" in "阳动" refers to "the *cun* pulse", and "yin" in "阴动" refers to "the *chi* pulse".

Undoubtedly, ancient Chinese medical texts are of vital importance to study Chinese medicine. In the modern society, most of the readers of these ancient texts are practitioners of Chinese medicine who want to draw on Chinese medical knowledge from the texts and apply the knowledge to clinical practice. So I advocate that translators should choose and follow what is good about the existing critical commentaries and various annotations made through the ages on the texts to make the translation reflect a generally recognized reasonable explanation; and that "yin-yang" can not all be pinyin transliterated, its translation should be determined by its concrete and specific meanings in the different contexts.

5.5 The Application of Yin-Yang Theory in Chinese Medicine

The Yin-Yang Theory runs through almost every aspect of Chinese medicine - it is applied to explain the organic structure, physiological activities, and pathological changes of the human body in the theoretical system, and to guide diagnosis and treatment of dieases as well in the clinical practice.

5.5.1 Yin-Yang Theory is used to analyze the organic structure.

"The physical appearance of human life cannot go without yin and yang." (*Su Wen. Bao Ming Quan Xing Lun* or *Basic Questions. Discourse on Protecting Life and Preserving Physical Appearance*)

"Yin is in the inner body and protects yang; yang is in the outer body and moves yin." (*Su Wen. Yin Yang Ying Xiang Da Lun* or *Basic Questions. Comprehensive Discourse on Yin-Yang Corresponding to Images*)

Chinese medicine sees the human body as a whole[266], the component parts of which may all be analyzed in terms of yin and yang. As *Su Wen. Jin Gui Zhen Yan Lun* or *Basic Questions. Discourse on the True Words from the Golden Chamber* states that

"As to the yin and yang of the human body, the outer part is yang and the inner part is yin. As to the trunk, the back is yang and the abdomen is yin. As to the organs, the *zang* organs are yin whereas the *fu* organs are yang. The liver, heart, spleen, lungs, and kidneys are yin; while the gallbladder, stomach, large intestine, small intestine, bladder, and *San Jiao* are yang".

5.5.2 Yin-Yang Theory is used to analyze physiological activities.

Yin and yang provide a general method of analyzing the functions and activities of the human being, which can be seen in terms of ascending, descending, exiting and entering movements. Ascending and exiting are yang, while descending and entering are yin. These movements serve to explain the interactions between blood and *qi*, and the organs and the meridians. The normal life activities result from the counterbalance in between yin and yang. For example, functions pertain to yin, while materials pertain to yang. The life activities are based on materials. There would be no physiological functions if without materials. And physiological functions promote metabolism of materials as well. As *Su Wen. Sheng Qi Tong Tian Lun* or *Basic Questions. Discourse on How the Generative Qi Beats as One with Heaven* states that "If one keeps yin even and yang firm, one's spirit will be in order; If one's yin and yang fail to communicate, his essential qi will be exhausted."

5.5.3 Yin-Yang Theory is used to analyze pathological changes.

In Chinese medicine, morbidity (unhealthy states) is explained in terms of yin-yang imbalance, relative predominance or decline of yin or yang. The occurrence and development of illnesses relate to two aspects, i.e. healthy qi and pathogenic factors. Both healthy *qi* and pathogenic factors can be analyzed in terms of yin and yang - Healthy *qi*, the body's health-maintaining force, comprises two aspects, yang *qi* and yin humor; There are both yin and yang pathogenic factors, e.g. among the six external pernicious influences, pathogenic cold and damp being yin; while pathogenic wind, summer-heat, heat or fire, and dryness being yang. The process of illnesses is actually the process of the healthy *qi* fighting against pathogenic factors.

"When yin prevails there is cold, when yang prevails there is heat; when yang is deficient there is cold, when yin is deficient there is heat", which can be regarded as the general principle of pathogenesis of Chinese medicine.

---

266 Chinese medicine is a holistic medicine, which treats the whole person, not just the diseased part. In other words, Chinese medicine is based on holistic approach, or holism.

5.5.4 Yin and Yang are the general principles of diagnosis.

Imbalance of yin and yang accounts for the emergence and development of diseases. The essential nature of any disease may be analyzed in terms of yin and yang, despite the infinite number of possible clinical manifestations, as *Su Wen. Yin Yang Ying Xiang Da Lun* or *Basic Questions. Comprehensive Discourse on Yin-Yang Corresponding to Images* states that "Proper diagnosis involves inspecting the appearance and feeling the pulse, first differentiating yin and yang."

As regards to pattern identification, yin and yang form the basic principles of eight-principle pattern identification - exterior, heat and excess disorders being yang; interior, cold, and deficiency disorders being yin.

As regards to the color and luster, being bright and lustrous is yang; while being dark and gloomy is yin.

As regards to breathing and speaking sounds, being loud, sonorous, talkative, and restless is yang; while being low, weak, and silent is yin.

As regards to pulse image, *cun* is yang, while *chi* is yin (location); being rapid is yang, while being slow is yin (the number of beats); being floating, surging, flooding, and slippery is yang, while being sunk, small, thin, and choppy is yin.

All in all, the four examinations should take differentiating yin and yang as the primary task.

5.5.5 Yin and Yang are the foundation of treatment and medication.

Because imbalance of yin and yang accounts for the emergence and development of diseases, treatments must involve restoring the balance between yin and yang. *Su Wen. Zhi Zhen Yao Da Lun* or *Basic Questions. Comprehensive Discourse on Essentials of Diseases and Therapies* states that "One must carefully observe the positions of yin and yang, and apply proper treatment until they are balanced".

The general treating principle is to reduce what is in excess and to supplement what is in deficiency. Besides, yin-yang is also used to generalize properties, flavors, and actions of Chinese medicinal agents.

As to the properties, cool and cold are yin, while warm and hot are yang; As to the flavours, sour, bitter and salty are yin, while acrid, sweet and bland are yang; As to the actions, astringing, descending and sinking actions are yin, while dispersing, ascending and floating actions are yang.

To sum up, for the purpose of treating an illness, the treating principle should be determined first, and then corresponding medicinal agents are chosen according to their properties, flavors, and actions to correct the imbalanced state of yin and yang, and finally cure the illness.

5.6 Yin-Yang Diagram and Dichotomy

How do you appraise the Yin-Yang theory? You must be very familiar with these two illustrations. One is *Tiao Ji Tu* 太极图 or Yin-Yang Diagram, one of the vital philosophical foundations of Chinese medicine, while the other is one of the vital philosophical foundations of Western science – Dichotomy.

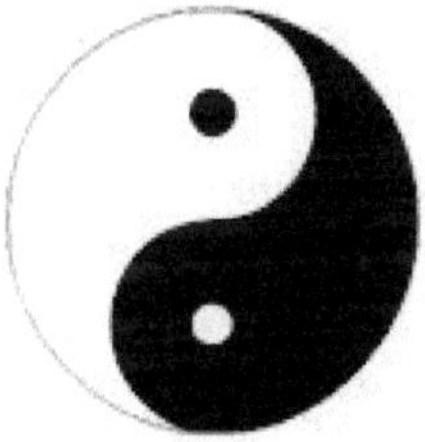

Yin-Yang Diagram

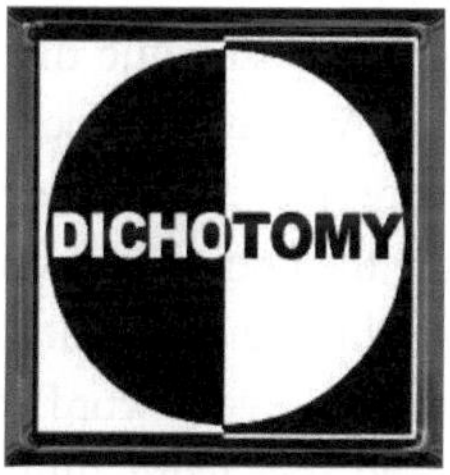

Illus.21 Yin-Yang Diagram and Dichotomy

As you know, a dichotomy is any splitting of a whole into exactly two non-overlapping parts. In other words, it is a bipartition of elements which are mutually exclusive, nothing can belong simultaneously to both parts, and everything must belong to one part or the other. Dichotomy is directly applied in mathematics, philosophy or linguistics. For example, if there is a concept A, and it is split into parts B and not-B, then the parts form a dichotomy: they are mutually exclusive, since no part of B is contained in not-B and vice-versa, and they are jointly exhaustive, since they cover all of A, and together again give A.[267] In the anthropologic field of theology and in philosophy as well as in the Western medicine, dichotomy is the belief that humans consist of a soul or mind and a body, which is a vital cultural presupposition of Western medicine. Western medicine focuses on studying the human body from a system to separate organs, to cells, to genes, and so on, therefore is good at treating body diseases; it views the body like a machine, and so surgery, even organ transplantation, is so advanced; but as regards to psychosomatic diseases it cannot achieve satisfactory therapeutic effects.

Tiao Ji Tu or Yin-Yang Diagram shows that in Chinese thinking everything in the universe has two facets: one yin aspect and one yang aspect; yin contains the seed of yang, and vice versa; yin and yang create, counterbalance (or wax and wane), transform into each other. The illustration of dichotomy is like "1", while that of *Tiao Ji Tu* or Yin-Yang Diagram is like "S", much more complicated than dichotomy, therefore more exact and fitting to the complicated living system. You know Chinese medicine is constructed under the guideline of *Tian Ren He Yi*, and

267 http://en.wikipedia.org/wiki/Dichotomy

the object of Chinese medicine is human being, composed of the body, mind and other aspects. Chinese medicine can usually achieve desired therapeutic effects in treating psychosomatic diseases. You know now why Chinese medicine is more exact than Western science in this sense.

Here I could make this much clearer by another example. For Western medicine the body is a cooperation of genes, cells, organs, tissues, systems, and so on; For Chinese medicine the living system is just like a text, like a composition of words and every word can be understood by the other words. And you cannot understand one word fully if you don't know all the other words; You cannot understand the meaning of the text if you just check the letters and words. You must care the relations among them for the purpose of understanding the text. Now you can see the source of the exactness of Chinese medicine. The text offers so much knowledge, information, much more than the stabilized objects of Western medicine.

In Western medicine – referring to the example – the lungs are an object which is clearly defined by its place and its functions, and there are some diseases possible which are clearly defined and all other things are uninteresting. For example, in Chinese medicine, constipation caused by the heat in the lungs can be effectively relieved by the therapeutic method of clearing the heat in the lungs; but in Western medicine, constipation is not associated with and treated through treating the lungs. This reduces so much the possible information that a living system can offer. In a difficult text in the field of Philosophy or Poetry you can understand a word only if you understand the full text. You must go always around. You cannot read the full text at the beginning, you must read word by word and then you must find out what is the meaning of the word of this text.

"We think this is fascinating. This is the motivation for us to study Chinese medicine because it is incredible fascinating – what can be done in interpreting a text".[268]

268 Wallner FriedrichG., Lan Fengli. Researching Chinese Medicine: Methods and Problems. In Wallner F.G., Lan FL, Jandl M. J. (eds). Chinese Medicine and Intercultural Philosophy: Theory, Methodology and Structure of Chinese Medicine [C]. Frankfurt am main: Peter Lang, 2011: 171-182.

The five phases are the root and source of the Creator[269], the endowment and beginning of the human relations. Emergence, change, and extinction of all the qualities result from the inter-actions among them. … Therefore, Heaven has the five phases to reveal *Xiang* or Images, Earth has the five materials available to use, and Man has the five constant virtues – benevolence, righteousness, propriety, knowledge (or wisdom), and sincerity (or faith) to show his moral integrity. The myriads of beings take five as the limit. Beyond five, the essence of the numbers changes.

- The Preface of *The Great Connotations of Five Phases*[270]

6 The Theory of Five Phases

In actual fact, the concept and theory of five phases were put forward earlier than that of *qi* and yin-yang as first stated in the *Shang Shu· Hong Fan* or *The Book of Documents · The Fundamental Principles*, which comes from observing and taking the images of the five materials: wood, fire, soil, metal and water in the nature, and analogizing.

6.1 The Origin and Background of *Wu Xing*

The concept of five phases in classical Chinese philosophy evolved from the ancient concepts: "five directions" and "five materials". Now let us take a look at the background of the unique five phases in China:

Firstly, the land of China has been vast with clear definition of the five directions. According to the records of oracle inscriptions of the Yin-Shang Dynasty 殷商 (ca. 16th-11th century B.C.) on the tortoise shells or animal bones, the people of Yin Dynasty 殷人 termed the Shang's territory "Center Shang", being juxtaposed to "East Land", "South Land", "West land", and "North Land". Thereby, the whole territory was divided into five parts, and then the concept of "five directions" formed.

Secondly, China is located in the North Temperate Zone with clear division of the four seasons - hot summers, freezing winters, and regular floods. If the location of China were in/around the Equator or the Polar Regions, terribly hot or freezing cold all year round, how could the ancient Chinese develop the system of the five phases – generating in spring, growing in summer, transforming in the late summer, reaping in autumn, and storing in winter?

Thirdly, in the remote antiquity, China had quite well developed agriculture and metallurgical engineering, which resulted in philosophical understanding of

269 Creator refers to the Nature.

270 *Wu Xing Da Yi* 五行大义 or *The Great Connotations of the Five Phase* is the most important work on five phases of the middle ancient times written by Xiao Ji 箫吉 in 594 for his emperor, a comment from Joseph Needham (1900-1995), which not only epitomized the thoughts on five phases theory before its time, but is also a must for studying the entire developing course of the five phases theory in China.

the five materials – wood, fire, soil, metal, and water. In the late period of Western Zhou Dynasty and Spring-Autumn Period (ca.1100-476 B.C.), theory of "the five directions" was followed by the theory of "the five materials". Shi Bo 史伯 of the late period of Western Zhou Dynasty said that "the metal, wood, water, fire and soil are mixed to generate one hundred items"（*Guo Yu • Zhen Yu*）. Zi Han 子罕 of the Spring-Autumn period said that "the heaven gives birth to the five materials. People use them together. Either can not be disposed with"（*Zuo Zhuan • The 27th Year of Xiang Gong's Reign*）.

Fourthly, China had been in relative isolation - bounded by Pacific, Himalayas, deserts. Hence Chinese thinking is quite conservative, and the theory of five phases independently evolved from the concepts of "five directions" and "five materials", thus being radically different from the Greek system of the four elements from the beginning. The Greek system of the four elements was abolished in Greek medicine as the Greek culture has been continuously exchanged with and influenced by other cultures.

Fifthly, as we know, Chinese characters or sinograms are logographic writing. The two sinograms 五行 embody cultural connotations of the five phases:

, the oracle script of *Wu* 五. *The Origin of Chinese Characters* interprets that "[It refers to] the *wu xing*. [It] follows 二, indicating that yin and yang interact in between the heaven and the earth. All of the fives follow it." "二" is interpreted by Xu Xuan 徐铉 (916-991) as "the heaven and the earth".

, the oracle script of *Xing* 行; , the Lesser Seal Script of *Xing* 行. It is a pictographic sinogram, and originally means "the way to talk".

The writing record of the generalization from the concrete material concept "five materials" to the philosophical concept "five phases" starts with *Shang Shu• Hong Fan* or *The Book of Documents · The Fundamental Principles*, which states that "The five phases: the first is water, the second is fire, the third is wood, the fourth is metal, the fifth is soil. Water is moistening and downward flowing. Fire is flaming upward. Wood is bending and straightening. Metal is transforming and changing. Soil, then, is sowing and reaping. Moistening and downward flowing generates salty [flavor]. Flaming upward generates bitter [flavor]. Bending and straightening generates sour [flavor]. Transforming and changing generates acrid [flavor]. Sowing and reaping generates sweet [flavor]". It is thus clear that the five phases do not refer to the concrete five materials any more, but to five kinds of functional attributes which are the distillation of the five materials, becoming five kings of symbolic images or imagery symbols, thus belonging to the category of image.

In the late Warring States Period (475-221 B.C.), Lu Buwei, 吕不韦, the prime minister of the Qin Kingdom, compiled *Lu Shi Chun Qiu* or *Lu's Spring and Autumn Annals*, , which continued to use the thinking way of *Hong Fan* or *The Fundamental Principles*, affirmed that many things in the world could be attributed to the five phases according to their qualities, and related the system of five phases to flavors, sounds or tones, colors, seasons, directions, internal organs, insects and domestic animals, and grains, and universalized the attributes of the five phases as well. So, the concept of five phases in philosophical sense had formed.

Pang Pu 庞朴 (1928-) pointed out that "almost all of the thinkers of the Pre-Qin Days talked about *wu xing* from the record of the five directions on oracle inscriptions of the Shang Dynasty (ca. 16th-11th century B.C.) to *Lu Shi Chun Qiu • Shi'Er Ji* or *Lu's Spring and Autumn Annals • Twelve Periods* where a huge system of *wu xing* was established. The only difference lies in weight or significance and special aspects of *wu xing* in their writings." [271]

As regard to Zou Yan 邹衍 (ca.305-240 B.C.), a philosopher of the late Warring States Period, Joseph Needham said, Zou Yan might not be the founder of the *wu xing* theory, but, undoubtedly, it was he who systematized and stabilized the thinking system that had been spread for over a century[272].

6.2 Introduction of the Five Phases into Chinese Medicine

The concept of the five phases had been used in medicine as early as the Spring-Autumn and Warring States Period to explain the attributes of internal organs and relationships among them. That is to say, introduction of the philosophical five-phase theory into Chinese medicine is undoubtedly earlier than the time of *Huang Di's Inner Classic*. A quite systematic five-phase theory has already formed in the *Huang Di Nei Jing Su Wen* or *Huang Di's Inner Classic · Basic Questions*, and all of the fives in the book evolved from the five phases, such as the five *zang* organs, five flavors, five colors, five *qi*, five essences, five spirits, five diseases, five excesses, five deficiencies, five methods, five grains, and so and so forth. For example, *Jin Kui Zhen Yan Lun* or *The True Words from the Golden Chamber* states that "The east and the green color correspond to the liver. The liver opens into the eyes, and the essence is stored in the liver. Illness may manifest on the head. The flavor is sour, the plant is tree/wood, the animal is chicken, the grain is wheat, the planet is Sui/Jupiter, the number is 8, the smell is foul, the season is spring, which all pertains to the wood in *wu xing*. And the area affected is the tendons".[273] That is to say, the direction east, the color green, the flavor sour, the plant wood/tree, the animal chicken, the grain wheat, the planet Jupiter, the number 8, the smell foul, the season spring, and the *zang* organ liver, etc. are all attributed to the wood in the five phases by the way of *Qu Xiang Bi Lei*. See Table 11.

271 Pang Pu. *A Corpus of Meditation*, Shanghai: Shanghai People's Publishing House. 1982: 219.

272 Translated from Chinese translation. See: Translator: Department of History of Sciences of Shanghai Jiao Tong University; Author: Needham, Joseph. 2001: 149.

273 The translation accords with the interpretation and commentaries by Guo Aichun, See Guo Aichun. 1999: 26.

NATURE	TONES	JUE	ZHI	GONG	SHANG	YU
	Flavors	Sour	Bitter	Sweet	Acrid	Salty
	Colors	Green	Red	Yellow	White	Black
	Transformations	Generate	Grow	transform	reap	store
	Climatic factors	Wind	Heat	Dampness	Dryness	Fire
	Directions	East	South	Center	West	North
	Seasons	Spring	Summer	Late Summer	Autumn	Winter
Five Phases		**Wood**	**Fire**	**Soil**	**Metal**	**Water**
MAN	**Zang Organs**	Liver	Heart	Spleen	Lung	Kidney
	Fu Organs	Gallbladde r	Small Intestine	Stomach	Large Intestine	Bladder
	Sense Organs	Eyes	Tongue	Mouth	Nose	Ears
	Tissues	Tendon	Vessel	Flesh	Skin & Hair	Bone
	Emotions	Anger	Joy	Anxiety	Sorrow	Fear
	Sounds	Shouting	Laughing	Singing	Crying	Groaning
	Movements	Grasping	Worrying	Vomiting	Coughing	trembling

Table 11 Relating the Nature and Man to the Five Phases

6.3 How to Translate *Wu Xing* into English?

How do we translate *wu xing* into English? There are several different translations available for *Wu Xing*: the five elements, the five phases, the five agents, and the five elemental phases.

"*Wu xing*" has long been mistranslated into the five elements, which is very possibly influenced by the Greek System of the Four Elements. That is to say, translator adopts the strategy of "domestication" in order to make the translation more acceptable to the Western readers. Now let us first take a look at how the word "element" was translated into Chinese.

6.3.1Element, *Yuan-Xing*, and *Yuan-Su*

The modern concept of a chemical element as a "substance that cannot be split up by any known means into something simpler" did not exist in classical Chinese natural philosophy.

When the concept of the four elements was introduced into China in the late Ming dynasty (1368–1644), the translation *yuan-xing* 元行 (original-phase) for the term "element" was influenced by the theory of *Wu Xing*. There are five *xing* (phases) in China, namely, metal, wood, water, fire, and soil, which have an interdependent cyclic relationship. In the Chinese view of the nature, fire represents not only the real fire, but also the substances and qualities bearing characteristics of fire.

Although there were different Chinese translations for "element" in the 19th century, those terms are mostly forgotten nowadays. Only the word *yuan-su* 元素 (original-element), which is derived from the Japanese language and was introduced into China after the Sino-Japanese war (1894–95), is still in use today.

As we know *Wu Xing* evolved from the "five materials", but were not five concrete materials any more, and therefore they are not five elements.

6.3.2 Five Phases and Four Elements

In fact, "five phases" is the most popular translation for *Wu Xing* in the literature published in the West. Ted J. Kaptchuk commented that "The Five Phases are not in any way ultimate constituents of matter. This misconception has long been embodied in the common mistranslation 'Five Elements' and exemplifies the problems that arise from looking at things Chinese with a Western frame of reference. The Chinese term that we translate as 'Five Phases' is *wu xing*. *Wu* is the number five, and *xing* means 'walk' or 'move', and, perhaps most pertinently, it implies a process. The *wu xing*, therefore, are five kinds of processes; hence the Five Phases, and not the Five Elements. The theory of Phases is a system of correspondences and patterns that subsume events and things, especially in relationship to their dynamics".[274]

The mistranslation "Five Elements" exemplifies the problems that arise from looking at things Chinese with a Western frame of reference. Here "a Western frame of reference" actually refers to the Greek System of the Four Elements, which was advanced by Empedocles (504-433 B.C. or 490-430 B.C.) , an ancient Greek philosopher. He believed that the four elements, i.e. fire, water, soil, and air, were the basic constituents of things and objects, related the four elements to four categories like four basic properties, four humors, etc., and he also advocated that the continual change among the four elements was unceasing.[275]

Hippocratic Corpus applied the Greek System of the Four Elements to medicine, which became the system of the four humors. *Hippocratic Corpus* corresponds the four humors to the four elements (soil, air, fire, and water), the four seasons, the four specific properties (hot, cold, damp, and dry), the four stages of human age, and the four dispositions, which was used to explain the human body and pathogenesis of some diseases.[276]

274 Kaptchuk, Ted J. 2000: 437.

275 Teaching and Research Section of History of Foreign Philosophy, Department of Philosophy, Peking University. 1957: 73-91.

276 Translated from Chinese. Zhang Daqing, Translator; Porter, Roy, Author. 2000: 90.

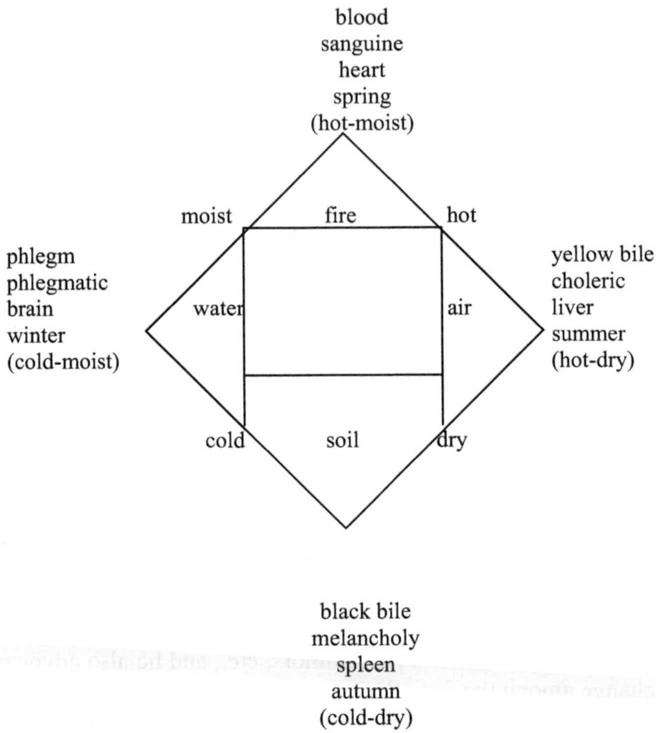

Illus. 22 The Greek System of the Four Elements

As regard to the concrete medical theory, the five-phase theory in the *Su Wen or Basic Questions* and the four-humor system in the *Hippocratic Corpus* share some similar viewpoints. But the attributes of five phases in the *Su Wen or Basic Questions* are much wider in range than that of the four-humor system in the *Hippocratic Corpus;* Integrated with *qi* and yin-yang theory, with the backing of visceral image and vessel theories, the five-phase theory runs through every link from physiology, pathology of the human being to diagnosis and treatment of diseases, thus forming a broad, circular, self-contained, integrated, and systematic theoretical system of Chinese medicine. While the four-humor system in the *Hippocratic Corpus* is far from bearing comparison.

6.3.3 Five Agents

Donald Harper, Paul U. Unschuld, and several other scholars propose to translate *wu xing* into "five agents". Unschuld comments that:

"Given the development of notions of cyclical recurrences or phases of activity of the five *xing*, a reading of 'five phases' has become popular in Western literature. In our translation we follow Harper who in his translation and discussion of the Mawangdui manuscripts adopted Marc Kalinowski's suggestion to translate *wu xing* as 'five agents'.

"The word *agent* maintains, as Harper points out, some of the material aspects of the *xing* as they are used in accounts of natural processes. A good medical example is the account of gestation in the Mawangdui medical text *Tai chan shu* 胎产书 where the bestowal of Water, Fire, Metal, Wood, and Earth/Soil on the fetus in the fourth through eight months of gestation enables blood, *qi*, muscles, bones, and skin to form"[277].

6.3.4 Comments on Different Translations

The *wu xing* theory, originating in China, is unique. The formation of the theory is related to the vast land of China with clear and definite five directions, clear division of the four seasons due to China's location in the North Temperate Zone, as well as rising and flourishing of the agriculture and metallurgy in the Yin-Shang Period (殷商, ca. 16th-11th century B.C.) and continual stable development afterwards. Therefore, the *wu xing* theory thrives and does not decline.

We have known that *wu xing* originates from the five materials, but are not the five materials whatsoever. The textbook of *The Basic Theories of Chinese Medicine* (5th ed.) states that "*Wu xing* refers to the movement of the wood, fire, soil, metal, and water". As regard to the content of the *wu xing* theory, it does not discuss the specific properties of the five materials in isolation, but "has by further extension come to mean that everything in the universe comes into being by movement, change, and transformation of the five essential materials, i.e. wood, fire, soil, metal, and water", and "that engendering and restraining among *wu xing* are used to expound the relationship among things".[278]

In view of the above-mentioned facts, I suggest to translate *wu xing* into five phases, five agents, or five elemental phases for "five phases" is the most popular translation in the West, and "five agents" and "five elemental phases" maintain some of the material aspects of *wu xing* and can reflect the evolution process of the term to a certain extent. Moreover, the translation "five elemental phases" is more comprehensible to the lay mind.[279]

277 Unschuld, Paul U. 2003: 84.
278 Yin Huihe. 1984: 18.
279 Lan Fengli. Use the Translating Experiences of Other Countries for Reference to Bring about An Advance in Translation of Chinese Medicine in China [J]. *Chinese Journal of Integrated Traditional and Western Medicine*. 2003, 23(8): 627-28.

6.4 Understanding the Engendering and Restraining Cycles in the Way of *Qu Xiang Bi Lei*

The engendering and restraining relationship among the five phases also come from direct observation and experiences of the phenomena among the five materials. As regards to the formation of the engendering relationship among the five phases, *Wu Xing Da Yi · Lun Xiang Sheng* or *The Great Connotations of the Five Phases· On Engendering* states that "Wood engenders fire for wood is warm in nature, fire is latent inside it and makes its way out of it and burns; Fire engenders soil for fire can burn wood, resulting in ashes, ashes can be [regarded as] a kind of soil; soil engenders metal for metal is usually found in a mountain which is composed of soil; metal engenders water for the metal can be melted into fluid, [which can be regarded as a kind of water]; water engenders wood for water can nourish wood and make it grow".

The restraining relationship among the five phases was established through observing the following natural phenomena among the five materials: water can extinguish fire, fire can melt metal, metal (such as sword and axe) can cut trees (wood), tree (wood) can take its root into soil, and dykes and dams (soil) can prevent flooding (water) from occurring.

6.5 Application of Five-Phase Theory in Chinese Medicine

In Chinese medicine, the five-phase theory is mainly used to explain the physiological functions, pathological changes of the internal organs and their relationships, formulating therapeutic principles according to the engendering and restraining relationship among the internal organs, thus bearing practical significance in the clinical sense.

6.5.1 Five-Phase Theory and Visceral Image Theory[280]

All of the knowledge related to *zang fu* organs in Chinese medicine were summarized and systematized as the theory of *Zang Xiang*, which is usually mistranslated into "visceral manifestation". In actual fact, *xiang* refers to image, which can be easily known by understanding the four concepts indicating the progressive process of *Qu Xiang* or *Taking Image*. Therefore, "*zang xiang* 藏象" should be translated into "the image of the viscera" or "visceral image", reflecting the integration of the *zang-fu*'s external images and the subject's deep understanding of them, which were gained by means of metaphorizing on the basis of the idea of *Tian Ren He Yi*.

The formation of the Visceral Image theory was a process of integrating knowledge on the man and classical Chinese philosophy: first anatomical

280 Lan Fengli. Metaphorizing: The Way to Bridge *The Book of Changes* and Chinese Medicine. In Wallner F.G., Schmisberger F. & Wimmer F.M.(eds). Intercultural Philosophy: New Aspects and Methods [C]. Frankfurt am Mein: Peter Lang, 2010: 177-192.

knowledge, then the attributes of the organs to the yin-yang and five phases in the way of *Qu Xiang Bi Lei* or metaphorizing guided by the idea of *Tian Ren He Yi*, which then underwent the process of proving and modifying the theory in the clinical practice.

Huang Di Nei Jing Ling Shu · Jing Shui or *Huang Di's Inner Classic Miraculous Pivot ·Rivers and Vessels* states that "Regard the body of an eight *chi* (feet) man; when alive, take his measurement, feel his pulses; when dead, dissect his body and regard the strength of his *zang* organs, the size of his *fu* organs, the volume of the trunk cavity and the organs within it, then the length of the vessels, the clarity of the blood and the state of the *qi* … All are shown to conform to a standard". The ancient Chinese people had got a rough idea on the positions of the organs of the body. For example, the lungs were analogized as "canopy" for their uppermost position inside the body in the *Huang Di's Inner Classic*. The ancient drawings on the organs also show the almost correct positions of the organs in the body such as the liver at the right side and the spleen at the left side.

Huang Di Nei Jing Su Wen · Ci Jin Lun or *Huang Di's Inner Classic Basic Questions ·Discourse on Contraindications in Acupuncture* started with Huang Di's question "Can you tell me the areas that are contraindicated in acupuncture?" Qi Bo answered that "The five *zang* organs are the vital parts of the body, so you should be very careful in acupuncture treatment as so to avoid damaging them. The liver grows at the left, the lung stores at the right". It is clear that they discuss the areas contraindicated in acupuncture, so the positions of the organs should be their real locations in the body. But why here is quoted as "the liver at the left and the lung at the right"?

There were two versions as regards to the attributes of the five *zang* organs to the five phases in the ancient times. One is recorded in *Lü Shi Chun Qiu. Shi Er Ji* or *Lu's Spring Autumn Annals. Twelve Periods* 吕氏春秋 · 十二纪, which attributes the spleen to wood (east, left), the lungs to fire (south, upper), the heart to soil (middle), the liver to metal (west, right), and the kidneys to water (north, lower). The other is the same as stated in the *Huang Di's Inner Classic*, which attributes the spleen to soil (middle), the lungs to metal (west, right), the heart to fire (south, upper), the liver to wood (east, left), and the kidneys to water (north, lower). In the two versions, only the attributes of the kidneys to water are identical with each other. Then some scholars believe that the positions of the five *zang* organs in the *Huang Di's Inner Classic* do not refer to their real positions but imagery positions instead. But *Huang Di's Inner Classic Basic Questions · Discourse on Contraindications in Acupuncture* talks about which areas should be avoided in acupuncture, so the positions of the five *zang* organs in it should refer to their actual positions in the body.

Li Ding 李鼎 (1929-) holds that the former version accords with their actual positions of the back view which was arranged according to the order of animals' internal organs in the offer sacrifices to the gods or ancestors; While the latter accords with their actual positions of the front view for the doctor sits face to face to the patient when diagnosing and treating him. Therefore the left and the right in the formulation "the liver grows at the left, the lung stores at the right" do not conform to the patient's left and right hand respectively, but refer to their opposites. The "*He Tu* 河图" and "*Luo Shu* 洛书", the two mysterious patterns of numbers of the Bearings of the Eight Trigrams (*Li* 离-South, *Kan* 坎-North, *Zhen* 震-East, *Dui* 兑-West) also takes the East as the left and the West as right.[281] I agree with the explanation. That is to say, the theory of *Zang Xiang* established in the *Huang Di's Inner Classic* first of all is based on the ancient anatomical knowledge; then, on the attributes of the organs to the yin-yang and five phases in the way of *Qu Xiang Bi Lei* or metaphorizing guided by the idea of *Tian Ren He Yi*, and then has been proved and modified in the clinical practice.

Take the spleen as an example. The spleen is located in the middle *jiao* (the center) and below the diaphragm. According to its central position and its yellow color[282], Chinese medicine attributes the spleen to the soil in the five phases. Soil is the sowing and reaping, corresponding to the late summer in the seasons and dampness in the climate, representing the features of receiving, generating, transforming, and supporting. Therefore, the spleen's function in Chinese medicine is metaphorized as transforming the water and grain into essence, then moving and sending the essence to the whole body; thereby, the spleen is regarded as the foundation of postnatal existence, the source of the formation of *qi* and blood, is interrelated with the flesh, governs the limbs, opens into the mouth, manifests its brilliance in the lips, and so on. Finally, a spleen system is formed. The common symptoms of spleen diseases such as abdominal pain or distension, poor appetite, loose stool, diarrhea, jaundice, fatigue or weakness of the limbs, edema can be successfully relieved by treating the spleen in Chinese medicine. It is clear that the spleen in Chinese medicine does not refer to any concrete organ, maybe not the organ spleen at all (according to its central position and the yellow color, this organ may be the pancreas, which was not perceived by Chinese medicine in the ancient time), but to a functional system by applying the five-phase theory in the way of *Qu Xiang Bi Lei* guided by the idea of *Tian Ren He Yi*.

In the same way, the other four organ systems have been formed. See "Table 10 Relating the Nature and Man to the Five Phases", each of the vertical columns composes a complex organ system with the attribute of five *zang* organs to the five phases as the focus, and all together make up five complex organ systems.

"Wood is the bending and the straightening," having the characteristics of growing, upbearing and developing freely; while the liver thrives by orderly

281 Li Ding. 1998: 99-191.

282 Soil is the center of the five phases, working as the link among them.

reaching, governs free coursing (or ensuring smooth free flow of qi and blood), upbearing and stirring, and is like the sprouting of "trees and plants in spring". Therefore, it is attributed to wood. Besides, the liver stores the ethereal soul, opens at the eyes, governs the sinews, its brilliance manifests in the nails, is interrelated with anger in the seven affects[283], and stands interior-exterior relationship with the gallbladder through the homing and netting connections of the meridians of the two organs[284]. Thus a complex liver system, including the ethereal soul, the eyes, sinews, nails, anger, gallbladder, spring, wood, green-blue, etc., forms in this way.

"Fire is the flaming upwards," having the quality of warming, heating and rising; while the heart governs the blood and the vessels, has the function of propelling qi and blood to warm and nourish the whole body, which is then likened to the heat of the summer, when the whole of creation thrives. Hence the heart is attributed to fire. Besides, the heart stores the spirit, opens into the tongue, its brilliance manifests in the face, is interrelated with joy in the seven affects, and stands in interior-exterior relationship with the small intestine through the homing and netting connections of the meridians of the two organs. Thus, a complex heart system, including the spirit, tongue, face, joy, small intestine, summer, fire, red, etc., forms in this way.

"Metal is the working of change," having the qualities of purifying, cleaning, and reforming; while the Lungs thrive by purifying and govern downbearing. They are likened to the clear fresh air and purifying first frosts of autumn, when the nature is withdrawing into itself. Therefore the lungs correspond to metal. In Chinese medicine, the lungs store the corporeal soul, govern qi and perform respiration, regulate the waterways, open at the nose, govern the skin and body hair[285], is interrelated with melancholy in the seven affects, and stands in interior-exterior relationship with the large intestine through the homing and netting connections of the meridians of the two organs. Thus a complex lung system, including the corporeal soul, *qi*, waterways, nose, skin, body hair, melancholy, large intestine, autumn, metal, white, etc., forms in this way.

"Water is the moistening and downward flowing," having the qualities of moistening, downward moving and cooling; while the Kidneys are located in the

---

283 Joy, anger, melancholy, anxiety, sorrow, fear and fright are the seven affects or seven emotions, which are natural human responses to the environment. Chinese medicine regards the seven affects as capable of influencing the functions of the *zang fu* organs under certain conditions, which is known as "internal damage by the seven affects". Especially vulnerable is the free coursing function of the liver. And so, the liver's function can be summarized as "prefering to function freely and disliking depression".

284 Besides, the secretion and discharge of bile is controlled and regulated by the liver's function of free coursing.

285 It is also known as "The brilliance of the lungs manifests in the body fair". In other words, the Lungs regulate the secretion of sweat, the moistening of the skin, and resistance to the six external pernicious pathogenic factors, i.e. pathogenic wind, cold, summer-heat, damp, dryness and fire.

lower *jiao*, store essence and govern fluid metabolism. It is associated with the bitter cold of winter, when the nature is dormant. For this reason, the kidneys are attributed to water. Besides, the kidneys store will, are responsible for growth, development, and reproduction (or maturation), govern the bones and engender marrow, open into the ears and the two private parts: the urethra and anus, their brilliance manifests in the hair of the head, are interrelated with fear and fright in the seven affects, and stands in interior-exterior relationship with the urinary bladder through the homing and netting connections of the meridians of the two organs. Thus a complex kidney system, including the will, essence (growth, development and maturation), water metabolism, ears, urethra and anus, head hair, fear and fright, urinary bladder, winter, water, black, etc., forms in this way.

6.5.2 To Explain the Inter-Organ Relationships and Prognosis

Both of the Engendering and restraining cycles have two aspects: engendering and being engendered (like that between mother and child); restraining and being restrained. The relationships of each organ to the other four of the five zang organs can be explained by these aspects. Let's take liver as an example.

Liver (wood) engenders heart (fire), and is engendered by the kidneys (water); Liver (wood) restrains the spleen (soil), and is restrained by the lungs (metal). The liver relies on kidney water for nourishment, which is known as "water moistening wood"; If the kidneys fail to fulfill this function, this condition is known as "water failing to moisten wood".

The five-phase theory can also be used in disease prognosis. Generally speaking, if a condition spreads in the order of engendering cycle, i.e. the condition of disease of the mother organ involving the child organ, the prospects for a good recovery are favorable and the disease can be considered minor; If, on the contrary, a condition spreads in the opposite order of engendering cycle, i.e. the condition of disease of the child organ affecting the mother organ, the prospects are unfavorable and the disease is serious. If a condition spreads in the order of restraining cycle, the condition is more serious when over-restraining than counter-restraining.

6.5.3 To Determine Therapeutic Principles and Methods

Based on the five-phase theory, the general principle of treatment is "to reinforce the mother-organ in case of deficiency, and to reduce the child-organ in case of excess". Hereafter I give you some examples formulated according to the engendering cycle of the five phases:

"Banking up earth to engender metal" actually refers to the therapeutic method of fortifying the spleen to treat disorders of the lungs, which is applied in cases of lung deficiency that occur in conjunction with spleen-stomach deficiency, manifesting clinically in pale complexion, cold limbs, poor appetite, loose stool, short of breath, cough with sputum, emaciation, weak pulse, etc.

That "metal and water engender each other" actually is that "metal engenders water". This refers to a therapeutic method of enriching kidney yin, and complemented by nourishing lung yin, applied for lung-kidney yin deficiency, manifesting clinically in the following symptoms: enduring cough, night sweating, tidal fever, vexing heat in the chest, palms, and soles, aching and weak in the lumbar region and legs, nocturnal emission, etc.

"Enriching water to moisten wood" actually refers to the therapeutic method of nourishing kidney yin to subdue liver yang for hyperactivity of liver yang due to liver-kidney yin deficiency, which presents with such symptoms as dizziness, red complexion due to rising fire, and hypertension in some cases.

In the clinical practice, the five-phase theory is applicable not only to treatment of different kinds such as medication, acupuncture, psychotherapy, but also to diagnosis, prognosis, and preventive treatment of diseases. The *Nan Jing* or *The Classic of Difficult Issues* states that "When one sees a liver disease, one should know that the liver will transmit it to the spleen. Hence one prevents such a transmission by fortifying the spleen qi" (the 77th difficult issue).

One point is worth to note that the meanings of water and fire are highly dependent on their contexts for they are not only two of the five phases, but also aspects of certain organs or something else. Fire may refer to the heart or the kidney yang for the kidney yang has also been termed as "the fire of the life gate" since the rise of the life gate theory. For example, "boosting fire to engender earth" refers to a therapeutic method of warming and supplementing kidney-yang to treat spleen disorders such as clear-food diarrhea, enduring diarrhea, early morning diarrhea when caused by a spleen-kidney yang deficiency; the pathological condition of "wood fire impairing metal" does not involve three phases, actually refers to "Liver fire impairing the lungs". Water may refer to the kidneys, pathogenic water-damp, or the symptom edema. For example, "banking up earth to control water" actually means "fortifying the spleen and boosting qi to relieve edema", where the water refers to the symptom - edema.

It is worth to note that the five-phase theory is not a universal truth. It is only true under certain conditions. The five phases are used for making analogies and inferences, and sometimes broad generalization, in most cases, in the way of metaphorizing. The theory cannot fully explain the functions of the organs of the human body and the relationships among the organs alone, and just plays one of the essential roles in the formation of the *Zang Xiang* or *Visceral Image* theory. Chinese medicine is not just based on yin-yang or/and five phases, and it is also based on a correct maybe rough understanding of man, which is composed of body and mind.

In one word, the five-phase theory enriches human's understanding of the man and the universe.

Chief References

1 Department of History of Sciences of Shanghai Jiao Tong University, Translator; Needham, Joseph, Author. Science and Civilisation in China Series [M]. Shanghai: Shanghai People's Publishing House, 2001: 149.

2 Fung Yu-Lan. A Short History of Chinese Philosophy[M]. English Version. London and New York: The MacMillan Co., 1948; English-Chinese Version. Tianjin: Tianjin Academy of Social Science Press, 2007; 2010 Third Print.

3 Guo Aichun. Collations, Annotations and Modern Chinese Interpretation of *Huang Di Nei Jing Su Wen* [M]. Tianjin: Tianjin Science and Technology Press, 1999.

4 Jaspers, Karl. The Origin and Goal of History [M]. translated by Michael Bullock. New Haven, CT: Yale University Press, 1953; Reprint. Westport, Connecticut: Greenwood Press, 1977.

5 Kaptchuk, Ted J. Chinese Medicine: The Web That Has No Weaver [M]. Revised Ed. London, Sydney, Aukland, Johannesburg: Rider, 2000: 437.

6 Lan Fengli. Use the Translating Experiences of Other Countries for Reference to Bring about An Advance in Translation of Chinese Medicine in China [J]. Chinese Journal of Integrated Traditional and Western Medicine. 2003, 23(8): 627-28.

7 Lan Fengli. Cultural Connotations and English Translation of Ancient Chinese Medical Classics: Study on English Translation of *Huang Di Nei Jing Su Wen* [D]. PhD. Dissertation. Shanghai University of Traditional Chinese Medicine, July 2005.

8 Lan Fengli. The Origin of Yin-Yang as Chinese Medical Terms and Their Translation [J]. Chinese Translators Journal. 2007, 28(4): 69-72.

9 Lan Fengli, Wallner Friedrich G., and Wobovnik Claudia (eds.). Shen, Psychotherapy and Acupuncture: Theory, Methodology and Structure of Chinese Medicine[C]. 2011.

10 Li Ding. Interpretation of Difficult Issues on Acupuncture [M]. Shanghai: Shanghai University of Traditional Chinese Medicine Press. 1998: 99-191.

11 Li Jingwei, Ou Yongxin, Yu Ying'ao, et al. A Concise Dictionary of Chinese Medicine [Z]. Beijing: China Press of Traditional Chinese Medicine, 2001: 173.

12 Li Lei (editor). New Century TCM English Course. Shanghai: Shanghai Foreign Language Education Press, 2006.

13 Ma Boying. A History of Medicine in Chinese Culture [M]. Shanghai: Shanghai People's Press, 1994.

14 Ni, Maoshing. Trans. The Yellow Emperor's Classic of Medicine. Boston, Massachusetts: Shambhala, 1995.

15 Research Center of Unearthed Documents and Ancient Writings of Fudan University (ed.). Interpretation of Unearthed Documents and Classics That Will Be Handed on from Age to Age [C]. Shanghai: Shanghai Ancient Books Publishing House, 2010.

16 Teaching and Research Section of History of Foreign Philosophy, Department of Philosophy, Peking University. Philosophy of Ancient Greece and Rome [M]. Beijing: SDX Joint Publishing Company. 1957: 73-91.
17 Unschuld, Paul U. Huang Di Nei Jing Su Wen: Nature, Knowledge,Imagery in An Ancient Chinese Medical Text [M]. Berkeley, Los Angeles and London: University of California Press, 2003.
18 Unschuld Paul U., Tessenow Hermann. Trans. Huang Di Nei Jing Su Wen (Vol.1). Berkeley and Los Angeles: University of California Press, 2011: 42-44.
19 Veith, Ilza. The Yellow Emperor's Classic of Internal Medicine. 1st Ed., Baltimore: The Williams & Wilkins Co., 1949; 2nd Ed., Berkeley, Los Angeles, London: University of California Press, 1966, 1972.
20 Wallner Friedrich G., Kubiena Gertrude, Jandl Martin J. (eds). Understanding Traditional Chinese Medicine [C]. Frankfurt Am Mein: Peter Lang, 2009.
21 Wallner Friedrich G., Lan Fengli, Jandl Martin J.(eds). The Way of Thinking in Chinese Medicine: Theory, Methodology and Structure of Chinese Medicine [C]. Frankfurt am Main: Peter Lang, 2010.
22 Webster's Encyclopedic Unabridged Dictionary of the English Language (New Revised Edition) [Z], New York: Gramercy Books, 1994.
23 Wang Rongpei, Wang Hong (eds.). English Translation of Chinese Classics. Shanghai: Shanghai Foreign Language Education Press, 2009.
24 Wiseman Nigel, Ellis Andrew. Fundamentals of Chinese Medicine [M]. Revised ed.. Brookline Massachusetts: Paradigm Publications, 1996.
25 Xue Gongchen (editor). On Confucianism, Taoism and Buddhism in Chinese Medicine [M]. Beijng: Ancient Chinese Medical Books Press, 1999.
26 Yi Zhongtian. Contention of A Hundred Schools of Thought of Pre-Qin Days [M]. Shanghai: Shanghai Literature and Art Publishing Group, 2009.
27 Yin Huihe. Textbook for TCM Higher Education • The Basic Theories of Chinese Medicine. Shanghai: Shanghai Scientific and Technological Publisher, 1984.
28 Zhang Daqing, Translator; Porter, Roy, Author. The Cambridge Illustrated History of Medicine [M]. Changchun: Jilin People's Publishing House, 2000.

III The Importance of Metaphors in Chinese Medicine (180368)

Chinese medicine is the only live symbol of classical Chinese culture, philosophy, and science.

- The Author

Introduction

Traditional medicine, also known as "Complementary and Alternative Medicine" (CAM), Non-Conventional or Non-Orthodox Medicine in the West, is a comprehensive term for all traditional medical systems or various forms of indigenous medicine. For example, Chinese medicine, a traditional medical system of Chinese origin, Indian Ayurveda medicine, a traditional system of medicine from India, Arabic Unani medicine, ancient Greek medicine that has evolved within the Muslim world for the past 13 centuries, and Mapucha medicine, a traditional healing system from Chile, etc. are all traditional medical systems from different cultures.

All these traditional medical systems share at least one thing in common, i.e. they have remarkable features of their own cultures. As *Guidance for Industry on Complementary and Alternative Medicine Products and Their Regulation* by the Food and Drug Administration (FDA, DRAFT GUIDANCE, Dec. 2006) states that "The term 'complementary and alternative medicine' (CAM) encompasses a wide array of health care practices, products, and therapies that are distinct from practices, products, and therapies used in 'conventional' or 'allopathic' medicine. Some forms of CAM, such as traditional Chinese medicine and Ayurvedic medicine, have been practiced for centuries, whereas others, such as electrotherapy, are more recent in origin.", and that "NCCAM[286] describes whole medical systems as involving 'complete systems of theory and practice that have evolved independently from or parallel to allopathic (conventional) medicine.' These may reflect individual cultural systems, such as traditional Chinese medicine and Ayurvedic medicine", which shows that the general acknowledgement of cultural dependency of medical systems from FDA and NCCAM. How about Western medicine? Is it independent from Western culture?

Western medicine, also known as modern, mainstream, conventional, orthodox, heteropathic, allopathic[287] medicine or biomedicine, is an applied medicine based on Western science and technology as well as Western culture. That is to say, Western medicine is also a culture dependent art of healing for a pure objective medicine is never possible.

286 The full name of NCCAM is National Center for Complementary and Alternative Medicine.

287 The word "allopathic" comes from the Greek word "allos" (means "different) and "pathein" (means "disease, suffering"), and thus implying the use of drugs whose effects are different from those of the disease being treated. "Homeopathy", its opposite, refers to treatment of a condition by giving the patient very small quantities of a substance which, when given to a healthy person, would cause symptoms like those of the condition being treated.

China has a long-standing, unique, deep and strong non-Western tradition. The dissemination of Western science and technology in China is a great success. If you take a look at the curriculums from the elementary to the senior middle schools in China today, you will see, except the courses of Chinese language, Chinese history and English, the contents of the others like mathematics, algebra, geometry, physics, chemistry, geography, economics, Marxism, etc., are all from the West, and more or less the same as those in Europe or America. Differences may lie mainly in forms, such as the forms of teaching and learning, and language, i.e., these courses are given in Chinese in China. And thereby such an established fact has formed - almost all the subjects of classical Chinese sciences, except Chinese medicine, have been totally replaced by the corresponding subjects of Western science, and remain mainly in the stream and field of history of science with the successful dissemination of Western science in China although they had gained splendid achievements before esp. in mathematics, astronomy, and engineering. But how can Chinese medicine survive up till today?

Actually, the dissemination, education, practice, and research of Western medicine in China has been extremely successful since the 20th century. But at the same time, it affects the survival and development of Chinese medicine. For example, "Yi Xue", originally means "medicine" or "Chinese medicine" before Western medicine came to China, but nowadays, in many cases, only refers to Western medicine in China, such as "Yi Xue Yuan" or "Medical School" is a place where Western medicine is taught and studied.

Wide-ranging heated debates between Chinese medicine and Western medicine, the rise of "Integrative Medicine with Chinese at Heart but Western Where Appropriate" in the early 20th century, and queries on validity and scienticity of Chinese medicine from some scholars in the world of today, as well as long-term application of Western scientific standards on judging Chinese medicine, all result in that "science" and "Chinese medicine" can not be mentioned in the same breath. Actually whether Chinese medicine is scientific or not depends on how you define "science". Is Western science the only possible "scientific" approach?

We have to confess that the basis of science is a process of selecting and excluding certain aspects of the analyzed object guided by theory. The scientific system can be considered as an artificial and constructed system of data and propositions, a constructed "microworld", a world that selects and reduces qualities of the object in certain aspects, which are important for our thinking and our actions as well. And then the possibilities of perceiving the world are manifold, so there are many possible ways of selection and reduction, and thus many corresponding resolutions.[288]

288 Wallner, Friedrich. How to Research TCM. In Wallner F. G, Kubiena G., Jandl M.J. (eds). 2009: 22-45.

What is Chinese medicine? Is it just an indigenous art of healing of China, which is composed of effective herbal ingredients and acupuncture skills? Or is it a healing system as a natural science? Or is it an independent medical system rooted in the specific Chinese culture, philosophy, and history? My answer is: Chinese medicine originated from China, its concepts, theories and clinical explorations have been deeply rooted in and have been in perfect harmony with Chinese culture after going through thousands of years of development, and thus is another complete medical knowledge system incompatible with Western medicine.

I think Chinese medicine can be roughly classified into two parts: one part is the "Tao 道 or Way", i.e. its philosophical foundation, which needs to be understood based on its culture and philosophy; while the other is the "*Shu* 术 or Skill", i.e. its clinical application, which can be proved in rational ways and by proper methods. As the title goes, this course discusses Tao or Way of Chinese medicine - the importance of metaphors in Chinese medicine. I hope you can also find more detailed answers to the questions raised here in the following discussions.

The first thing needed is the rectification of names.

- *The Analects of Confucius*

1 Contemplating "*Zhong Yi*"

"Chinese medicine" in Chinese is "*Zhong Yi* 中醫". The book entitled *"Contemplating Zhong Yi"*, also known as "Introduction to *Shang Han Lun"*, and subtitled "Time Interpretation of Nature and Life", authored by Liu Lihong 刘力红 (1958-) and published by Guangxi Normal University Press, one of the national bestsellers in 2005 in China, has created a miracle in publication. I have always been contemplating "*Zhong Yi* 中醫" too, and share at least one common viewpoint with the author, i.e. the importance of Chinese medical classics for training qualified professionals of Chinese medicine. At the very beginning of the course, I would like to introduce you the ins and outs of "*Zhong Yi* 中醫".

1.1 Possible meanings of "*Zhong Yi* 中醫"

First, what are the possible meanings of "*Zhong Yi* 中醫"?

1.1.1 According with Medical Principles

The two sinograms showed up together as a compound in the *Han Shu. Yi Wen Zhi* or *Treatise on Literature* of *The History of the Former Han Dynasty* 漢書•藝文志 [289] for the first time, which reads that "Therefore, a proverb reads that 'Leaving a disease untreated usually accords with medical principles'". Here "*Zhong Yi* 中醫" means "according with medical principles", and "*Zhong* 中" should be pronounced as the falling tone.

1.1.2 Medicine that Accords with the Doctrine of Mean

With the rise of the "Hundred Schools of Thought", the intellectual flowering in early China, "*Zhong Yi*" has been interpreted as the "medicine that accords with the doctrine of mean".

The core value of the golden mean of the Confucian school can be summarized into the following three aspects: ① Sticking to principles in the unbiased way; ② Seeking stable and harmonious state; ③ Advancing with the times, judging the hour and seizing up the situation.[290] In one word, the core value of the golden mean is to seek the healthiest state of the development of things and beings.

---

289 Authored by Ban Gu 班固 (A.D. 32-92), with the bibliographies *Bie Lu* 别录 and *Qi Lue* 七略 based on Imperial Library catalog compiled by Liu Xiang 刘向 (77?-6 B.C.) and Liu Xin 刘歆 (50 B.C.? – A.D. 23), father and son, as the original versions.

290 Kang Zhen 康震 (1970-). Eight Great Master Writers of Tang & Song Dynasties. Zeng Gong. Lecture Room of CCTV 10, 2010.

The golden mean of the Confucianism actually refers to that man's words and deeds should accord with the middle, harmonious standard, opposing "going too far" and "not going far enough", which reflects in almost every aspect of Chinese medicine, including physiology and pathology of the human body, and etiology, treatment and prevention of diseases. "Making Harmony and Balancing Yin-Yang" has always been the Tao or Way of Chinese medicine.

1.1.3 A Common Doctor or A Doctor of the Average Level

"*Zhong Yi* 中醫" may refer to "a common doctor". Sun Simiao 孫思邈 (581-682) said that "In the ancient times, a superior doctor administers a country, a common doctor cares the human being, while an inferior treats the disease"[291]. Actually "A superior doctor administers a country" first showed up in *Guo Yu* or *Records of States* 國語[292], where it means to rid the country of sufferings and disadvantages and make it run well in order. The metaphor "Being A Good Doctor Is only Secondary to Being A Good Prime Minister" first appeared in *Mo Tzu,* and was clearly formulated by Fan Zhongyan 范仲淹 (989-1052). It has been a motto for Confucian scholars even up till today. For example, Wu Yi 吳儀 (1938-), a former deputy prime minister of the Chinese government retired in 2008, announced that she would go to learn medicine (here it refers to Chinese medicine) to be a good physician since she retired from his post as a deputy prime minister.

"*Zhong Yi* 中醫" may also refer to a doctor of the average level". *Huang Di Nei Jing Su Wen* or *Huang Di's Inner Classic Basic Questions* states that "The sages did not treat those already ill, but treated those not yet ill; They would like to be well-prepared for chaos before it appeared." (Chapter 2), where "Shang Gong or A superior practitioner 上工 treats what is not yet ill" comes from. *Nan Jing* or *The Classic of Difficult Issues* also states that "The scripture reads: The superior practitioner treats what is not yet ill; the mediocre practitioner treats what is already ill". "To treat what is not yet ill" means to take preventive treatment before an illness begins. And then Liu Zongyuan 柳宗元 (773-819) said in his *Yu Gao Huang Ji Fu* or *On Curing Diseases of Beyond Cure* 愈膏肓疾賦 that "Shang Yi or A superior doctor 上醫 takes preventive treatment before an illness shows a sign, while *Zhong Yi* or an average doctor 中醫 attacks an illness when it presents with signs".[293]

1.1.4 The Medical System of Chinese Origin: Chinese Medicine

The medical system of Chinese origin had long been named as "medicine" until around the time of the First Opium War (1840 – 1842). Most of the books on

---

291 See *Bei Ji Qian Jin Yao Fang*. *Zhen Hou* or *On Diagnosis* of *Invaluable Prescriptions for Emergencies* 备急千金要方. 诊候.

292 *Guo Yu* or *Records of States* 国语 is the earliest monograph of the history of different states from around 990 to 453 B.C. extant in China.

293 In this paragraph, I use "practitioner" for "Gong 工", while "doctor" for "Yi 医".

Chinese medicine of the Qing Dynasty (1644-1911) were still named as those on "*Yi*" or "*Yi Xue*", i.e. medicine. For example, *Yi Xue Xin Wu* or *Personal Understanding of Medicine* 醫學心悟 by Cheng Guopeng 程國彭 (1680-1733) came out in 1732, the *Yi Xue Yuan Liu Lun* or *The Origin and Development of Medicine* 醫學源流論 by Xu Dachun 徐大椿 (1693-1711) was published in 1757，and *Yi Xue San Zi Jing* or *Three-Sinogram Classic on Medicine* 醫學三字經 by Chen Xiuyuan 陳修園 (1753-1823) was published in 1804. In order to differentiate the medical system of Chinese origin from Western medicine, the Dutch East India Company gave it the name "Chinese medicine", i.e. *Zhong Yi*.

Mao Zedong 毛澤東 (1893-1976) advocated that "Chinese medicine 中醫藥學 is a great treasure house, which needs to be worked hard on and explored so as to develop and improve it". In his letter to Yang Shangkun 楊尚昆 (1907-1998) on Oct. 11th 1958, he wrote that "From now on study classes should be held for medical workers of Western medicine to learn *Zhong Yi* or Chinese medicine 中醫, which should be directed and managed by the Party committees of all the cities, provinces, and autonomous regions."[294], which bears profound and far-reaching historical and realistic significance.

In this sense, *Zhong Yi* 中醫 is the same as *Zhong Yi Yao Xue* 中醫藥學, both of which refer to "Chinese medicine". Actually, Chinese medicine is a time-honoured medical system that has evolved over the last 3,000 years. As early as in the Zhou Dynasty (ca.11th century - 256 B.C.), medicine in China had already been classified into different clinical subjects. *Zhou Li* or *Rites of the Zhou* 周礼 天官 冢宰 records that there were four types of royal doctors, i.e. dieteticians, physicians, surgeons, and veterinarians. Among them, "the dieteticians were in charge of six foods, six meals, a hundred delicacies, and eight dainties for the king"; "the physicians were responsible for diseases of ten thousands of people"; "the surgeons took care of abscesses, ulcers, wounds and fractures complicated with infections by applying ointments, scraping pus and blood, removing bad blood or bad flesh with corrodents, and thus healing the wound. When treating sores or ulcers, use the five poisonous medicinals[295] to attack them, the five kinds of *Qi* to nourish them, the five medicinals to heal them, and the five flavors to regulate them"; and "the veterinarians were responsible for treating diseases of animals. When treating animals, make them drink [the medicinal liquid] and then walk them around afterwards".

It is well known that Chinese medicine is based on the holistic concept of the universe outlined in the Taoist school, and has produced a set of highly sophisticated practices designed to cure illnesses and to maintain health and well-being. These practices include acupuncture, moxibustion, cupping, herbal

294 From *Selected Letters • To Yang Shangkun.*

295 The word "medicinal" here is used as a noun, and refers to substance with healing properties.

remedies, Chinese massage, dietary therapy, *Tai Ji Quan*, *Qi Gong* or breathing exercises, five animal exercises, etc. All of these treatments in Chinese medicine are to seek to reestablish harmony and equilibrium for each individual within his or her unique environment, which is known as "Individualized treatment based on pattern identification". Here we have the two basic characteristics of Chinese medicine, i.e. Holistic Concept (or Holism) and Individualized Treatment based on Pattern Identification (or Pattern Identification and Treatment).

1.1.5 Practitioners of Chinese Medicine

In *The Old Lady Pan and Zhong Yi* 潘老太太與中醫, the author Zou Taofen 鄒韜奮 (1895-1944) wrote that "Just in Shanghai, this port city, there are (about) 2,000 practitioners of Chinese medicine and (about) 300 shops of herbal medicine". Since then, "*Zhong Yi* 中醫" may also refer to "practitioners of Chinese medicine".

It is thus clear that the meanings of "*Zhong Yi* 中醫" rely highly on the time and its contexts.

1.2 Chinese Medicine: Being both Classical and Traditional

1.2.1 *Zhong Yi* as a Medical System: Chinese Medicine or Traditional Chinese Medicine?

The first four colleges of *Zhong Yi* established in 1956 in China changed their names into universities in the 1990s one after another, and their official English names are as follows: Shanghai University of **Traditional Chinese Medicine** since Dec. 21st, 1993, Beijing University of **Chinese Medicine** since Dec. 28th, 1993, Guangzhou University of **Chinese Medicine** since 1995, and Chengdu University of **Traditional Chinese Medicine** since 1995. The official English name of the national association of *Zhong Yi* is known as "China Association of **Chinese Medicine**". The official national administration for *Zhong Yi* is known as "State Administration of **Traditional Chinese Medicine**". And so, what is the proper translation for *Zhong Yi* as a medical system? Chinese medicine or traditional Chinese medicine?

Then, what is TCM? "The term 'TCM' is increasingly used in the West for the artificial construct generated between 1950 and 1965 by committees in P.R. China (as described by Kim Taylor in her book 'Chinese Medicine in Early Communist China'). 'TCM' is not considered a suitable term for describing Chinese medicine prior to the 20th century. We use either 'Chinese Medicine' or, in juxtaposition with 'Western Medicine': Chinese Traditional Medicine".[296]

296 Unschuld, Paul U. Personal Mail to the Author in 2008.

The making of Traditional Chinese Medicine (TCM) in the communist China and the followed dissemination of TCM to other countries result in that Chinese medicine has been gradually losing its advantages and being westernized in the whole world. "TCM, the medical system that has monopolized the practice of Oriental medicine in mainland China, and that has come to serve as the main mold for the budding profession of Oriental medicine around the globe. It exposes a system that has been conditioned by a distinctly political agenda, and reveals its logo 'TCM' (Traditional Chinese Medicine) as a grave misnomer - designating a medicine that is not at all aiming to preserve the traditional characteristics of Chinese medicine, but, on the contrary, to expurgate, reform, and control the classical and folkloric texture of the traditional record in the name of progress. Between the lines of this argument resides the warning that the progressive removal of the unique foundations of Chinese medicine is far more than just a philosophical issue. It affects the heart of our medicine itself, namely the nature of the clinical encounter and the quality and the results of therapy. It greatly diminishes, moreover, the unique edge that the traditional science of Chinese medicine has over allopathic medicine and its various offshoots. "[297]

Judged from the translation standards and the real contents of *Zhong Yi*, I think "Chinese medicine" would be a proper English translation for *Zhong Yi* as a medical system of Chinese origin.

Besides, *Zhong Yi* as a medical system has gained some other names, such as "Chinese Life Sciences" and "Chinese Medical Sciences". For example, Prof. Paul U. Unschuld is the director of Horst-Goertz Institute for the Theory, History, and Ethics of Chinese Life Sciences, Charité Universitätsmedizin; and the national research institute on Chinese medicine of China is known as "China Academy of Chinese Medical Sciences" in English. Is Chinese medicine a science in the common sense? Or is Chinese medicine scientific? I hold that, compared to natural science in the common sense, Chinese medicine goes closer to humanities. You will understand and know why after the course is over in the end.

1.2.2 The Ways of Knowing Chinese Medicine

Knowing Chinese medicine has meant acquiring profound knowledge by memorising experiences of the ancients in the texts and integrating them with one's own experiences in medical practice for many centuries up till now. But the ways of knowing Chinese medicine in the past and nowadays are somehow different.

297 Fruehauf, Heiner. Chinese Medicine in Crisis: Science, Politics, and the Making of "TCM"[J]. Journal of Chinese Medicine. No 61 Oct 1999: 1-9.

1.2.2.1 The Ways of Knowing Chinese Medicine in the Past before 1915

Before the establishment of the first modern school of Chinese medicine: Shanghai Specialized School for Chinese Medicine in 1915 by Ding Ganren 丁甘仁 (1865-1926) et. al.,[298,299] the ways of knowing Chinese medicine in the past were of mainly three patterns: one was taught by a specific person such as a local famous doctor, known as master-apprentice type; one was handed down from the older generations of the family such as his father, grandfather, or uncle; and one was self-taught, i.e., reading and studying ancient medical classics by himself. Now I would like to give you three examples to illustrate the three ways of knowing Chinese medicine in the past.

① Zhang Zhongjing 張仲景 (150?-219? A.D.): Zhang Zhongjing, one of the most influential physicians in the history of Chinese medicine, established the system of individualized treatment based on pattern identification, thus laying the foundation for clinical Chinese medicine. His work *Shang Han Za Bing Lun* or *Treatise on Cold-induced and Miscellaneous Diseases* was systematized and rearranged into "*Shang Han Lun* or *On Cold-induced Diseases*" and "*Jin Gui Yao Lue* or *Synopsis of the Prescriptions from the Golden Chamber*", which are regarded as the two of the "Four Great Classics on Chinese Medicine" (the other two are *Huang Di's Inner Classic* and *Shennong's Classic of Materia Medica*),[300] and have been the required readings and courses up till today.

Zhang Zhongjing lived in the late period of the Eastern Han Dynasty (25-220A.D.), during which tangled warfare lasted for many successive years and many natural disasters occurred. People had to give up farming, wandered from place to place, and suffered the terrible hardship of hunger and cold. "A big war or disaster must be followed by a serious epidemic", a Chinese proverb says.[301] In Zhang's time, epidemics broke out at many places of the country. It was recorded that almost every family suffered and cried for their family who died of epidemic. It was also the case with Zhang's family – 2/3 of his patriarchal clan with over 200 members died of successive years of epidemic diseases.[302] Therefore, Zhang was determined to be a doctor to save people's lives from epidemics. He followed an extremely famous doctor of his hometown named Zhang Bozu 張伯祖 to study medicine. At the same time, he advocated "seeking frequently old maxims

---

298 Yang Xinglin, Lu Ming. Introduction to the Modern Education of Chinese Medicine in Shanghai [J]. Chinese Journal of Medical History, 1994, 24 (4): 215.

299 The earliest national medical university can be traced back to 581 A.D., when "Bureau for Imperial Doctors" of Sui Dynasty was established to train doctors and practice medicine. See Fu Weikang. 2001: 48-51.

300 In the other version, "the four great classics" include *Huang Di's Inner Classic*, *The Classic of Difficult Issues*, *Treatise on Cold-induced and Miscellaneous Diseases*, and *Shen Nong's Classic of Materia Medica.*

301 Taking a sweeping view of the history, records on epidemics were indeed present much more in turbulent dynasties such as Eastern Han (25-220A.D.), Three Kingdoms (220-265A.D.), Southern Song (1127-1279), Ming (1368-1644) and Qing (1644-1911) Dynasties.

302 See the original preface of *On Cold-induced Diseases* (Shang Han Lun, 傷寒論) by Zhang Zhongjing.

and collecting good formulae & methods from all quarters", integrated the theory and practice (formulae) for the first time and accomplished the great work - *Treatise on Cold-induced and Miscellaneous Diseases* by so doing.

Seeking Frequently Old Maxims: Zhang Zhongjing had studied and summarized the theories and experiences of Chinese medicine before his time. He had carefully studied *Huang Di Nei Jing* or *Huang Di's Inner Classic,* including *Su Wen* and *Jiu Juan*[303], *Nan Jing* or *The Classic of Difficult Issues* (also know as "*The Huang Di's 81 Difficult Issues*"), *Yin Yang Da Lun* or *Comprehensive Discourse on Yin and Yang* (lost), *Tai Lu Yao Lu* or *Records of Herbal Treatments for Women's and Children's Diseases* 胎臚藥錄 (lost),[304] among which *Su Wen* or *Basic Questions* exerted greatest influence upon him. *Su Wen* or *Basic Questions* states that "all of the febrile diseases can be ascribed to cold-induced diseases". Zhang developed this theory based on his own practical experiences, classified all of the diseases into two major categories - cold-induced diseases (or febrile diseases) and miscellaneous diseases, and put forward instituting corresponding treatments for cold-induced diseases based on six-meridian pattern identification.

Collecting Good Formulae & Methods from All Quarters: Zhang Zhongjing extensively gathered all of the available effective formulae and treating methods of all the times, including folk recipes, acupuncture, moxibustion, warm pressing, medicinal massage, suppository, bathing, feet soaking, ear pouring, ear blowing, sublingual medication, artificial breathing, etc. He recorded for the first time in the world the methods of artificial breathing, enema, and how to treat biliary ascarriasis in his work: *Shang Han Za Bing Lun* or *Treatise on Cold-induced and Miscellaneous Diseases.*

Here it is worth to note that the way of "seeking frequently old maxims and collecting good formulae & methods from all quarters" is one of the most important universal and successful ways of doing scholarly work – studying carefully and seriously the former works on a specific topic or of the related academic fields, then developing your own idea or work based on your own understanding, your own academic background, your own talents, and so on. That is actually what Sima Qian 司馬遷 (145 or 135? - ca. 86 B.C.) said in his *Shi Ji* or *The Historical Records* that "To explore the relationship between Universe and Man, understand the changes through the past to nowadays, and then form an independent school of his own". In a time of globalization, a qualified scholar should also be well-informed about the cultures of his or her home and of other nations.

Zhang Zhongjin died in 219 A.D.. *Shang Han Za Bing Lun* or *Treatise on Cold-induced and Miscellaneous Diseases* lost the author's protection, and began

303 *Jiu Juan* or *Nine Volumes* was an alternative name for *Ling Shu* or *Miraculous Pivot*, also known as *Zhen Jing* or *Classic of Acupuncture,* which is generally regarded as the other part of *Huang Di Nei Jing*.
304 See the original preface of *On Cold-induced Diseases* (Shang Han Lun, 傷寒論) by Zhang Zhongjing.

its travel in the world. At that time, transmission of the books was very difficult, and could only rely on the hand copies. How has this work successfully been handed down to nowadays? A distinguished physician Xu Dachun 徐大椿（1693-1771）said "How could we have this book if without Wang Shuhe"! Then who was Wang Shuhe?

②Wang Shuhe 王叔和(A.D. 201-280): Wang Shuhe was a self-taught distinguished scholar physician of the Western Jin Period (265-316), and had been nominated as an imperial doctor because of his superb medical skills. Wang Shuhe occasionally saw Zhang Zhongjing's work: *Treatise on Cold-induced and Miscellaneous Diseases*, which was already incomplete at that time, and he was so excited when reading this amazing book. Then Wang Shuhe made use of his social status: imperial doctor, and tried his best to collect all of the available hand copies of the book. Finally, he systematized all the parts of the book into two books: one part on cold-induced diseases known as *Shang Han Lun* or *On Cold-induced Diseases*, the other on miscellaneous diseases known as *Jin Gui Yao Lue* or *Synopsis of the Prescriptions from the Golden Chamber*, which have been transmitted until today.

Wang's another major achievement lies in that he compiled the first monograph on pulse diagnosis: *Mai Jing* or *The Classic of Pulse Diagnosis*, which not only summarizes the achievements on pulse diagnosis before his time, but also records his own understanding and experiences on pulse diagnosis. This classic has been highly appreciated and observed by the medical circle of the later generations for 1,800 years. It is interesting that this classic has traveled quite far away. The classic transmitted into Japan during Sui-Tang Dynasties (581-907A.D.), into Europe through Middle East in the 11th century. In the 14th century it was transmitted into Poland. Three hundred years later it was translated into Latin by a Pole: M. Boym, whose father had been the Chief of imperial doctors of the King of the Poland Sigismon. The translation *Clavis Medica ad Chinarum Doctrinam de Pulsibus* was then spread widely throughout the Europe, thus enriching the world medical culture.[305] As I know, *Mai Jing* or *The Classic of Pulse Diagnosis* by Wang Shuhe is one of the first books on Chinese medicine which were translated into Western languages, here Latin.

③ The third example is Li Shizhen 李時珍 (1518-1593), the author of the monumental work *Ben Cao Gang Mu* or *The Compendium of Materia Medica* 本草綱目. Joseph Needham (1900-1995) compared him to Galileo Galilei (1564-1642) and Andreas Vesalius (1514-1564) of the Europe, and said he was the greatest scientist outside the Europe at that time.[306] *Ben Cao Gang Mu* or *The Compendium of Materia Medica* was appraised as "encyclopedia of China

305 Wang Jimin, Fu Weikang. 1963: 19.
306 Translated from Chinese into English. Translation. Needham, Joseph. 1990: 151.

published in 1596" by Charles Robert Darwin (1809-1882), and there exist evidences to show that this work also inspired him a lot to develop the Doctrine of Evolution. Then you see that Li Shizhen is well-known as a world famous scientist rather than a practitioner of Chinese medicine. Why and how did he grow up to such a distinguished scientist?

Li Shizhen was born out of a family of practitioners of Chinese medicine for at least 3 generations. His grandfather was a bell practitioner, who shook a bell to call on notice from patients or their families to provide medical service. His father had been a "*Xiu Cai* 秀才" by passing the imperial examination at the county level, finally became a famous Confucian scholar physician of the local region, had been promoted as an imperial doctor, and wrote several monographs on Chinese medicine. As regards to Li Shizhen's future, his father's original intention was to make him become an official by taking imperial examinations of different levels. Li Shizhen also passed the imperial examination at the county level, and thus became a "*Xiu Cai* 秀才", but failed three times in the provincial examinations for the selection of "*Ju Ren* 舉人" out of "*Xiu Cai*". Then he decided to give up the way of becoming an official, and turned to follow his father to learn Chinese medicine.

Li Shizhen's success actually resulted from two major aspects: one from his long tradition of family learning - Confucian scholar physician, the other from his own multi-disciplinary academic background, esp. rationalistic Confucian philosophical school known to the West as Neo-Confucianism, other disciplines like classical Confucianism, history, literature, as well as learnings of other different academic schools.

Li Shizhen improved ancient scientific methods based on his own practice and experiences, and successfully developed and applied the following methods: observing and doing experiments, classifying and comparing, analyzing and synthesizing, critically assimilating, and doing textual research on historical records. After 27 years of hard work and unremitting efforts, he accomplished the monumental work *Ben Cao Gang Mu* or *The Compendium of Materia Medica* in 1578, which not only makes great contribution to Chinese pharmacology, but also exerts far-reaching influences on pharmacology, botany, zoology, mineralogy, and chemistry of the whole world.

Besides, he was also an expert in pulse diagnosis and the eight extraordinary vessels, and wrote two monographs on the two topics, which have also been emphasized by practitioners of the later generations. As a physician, he had also been promoted as an imperial doctor, and he resigned one year later for he would like to take time to investigate materia medica, and to provide medical service for the common people.

By the above three examples, I want to show the three ways of knowing Chinese medicine before the 20th century, the great lasting vitality of the ancient

Chinese medical literature and their application in clinical practice until nowadays, and distinguished physicians' approaches in academic and clinical pursuits.

Actually, the ways of knowing Chinese medicine in the past result in the distinction of classical Chinese medicine and Chinese folk medicine. What the above mentioned three masters studied and practiced was classical Chinese medicine, which is based on classical Chinese philosophy and Chinese medical classics; while practitioners who only knew one formula, or one recipe, or one technique from someone somewhere to treat one certain problem can be named as practitioners of Chinese folk medicine.

1.2.2.2 The Way of Knowing Chinese Medicine Nowadays after 1915: the Westernized Professional Standard Way[307]

In mainland China, there are 24 universities or colleges or institutes of Chinese medicine, and some other schools or departments of Chinese medicine at comprehensive or medical universities, where Chinese medicine are taught, studied and practiced in a more or less similar way, i.e. the standard professional way.[308]

After the establishment of the first school of Chinese medicine in 1915, esp. of the colleges of Chinese medicine since 1956, the Westernized professional standard way of knowing Chinese medicine has been the major way to become a practitioner of Chinese medicine no matter in China or in other countries. "The Four Great Classics", and "*Yi Gu Wen* 醫古文 or Ancient Medical Chinese", which is designed for training students to be capable of reading and studying ancient medical literature by themselves, have been the required courses for majors of Chinese medicine since then. Besides, the textbooks are compiled by systematizing the knowledge contained in the ancient Chinese medical literature with reference to the textbooks of Western medicine, such as Fundamental Theories of Chinese Medicine, Diagnostics of Chinese Medicine, Chinese Herbal Medicine: Materia Medica, Formulas and Strategies, Chinese Internal Medicine, Chinese External Medicine, Gynaecology and Obstetrics of Chinese Medicine, Paediatrics of Chinese Medicine, Dermatology of Chinese Medicine, Orthopedics and Traumatology of Chinese Medicine, Acupuncture & Moxibustion, Chinese Tuina Therapy, and so on. That is to say, the core knowledge of the textbooks of Chinese medicine is from ancient Chinese medical literature.

---

307 Hsu, Elisabeth also discusses "Styles of Knowing" of Chinese medicine in her work *The Transmission of Chinese Medicine,* 1999: 225-240, where secret knowing, personal knowing, standardized knowing, non-verbal knowing and participant experience, and verbal knowing, word meaning, and social practice are discussed.

308 Note: The old ways of knowing Chinese medicine still exist in contemporary China. The government of China promotes the master-apprentice style of knowing Chinese medicine as one major way to inherit and carry on famous doctors' experiences.

Here is worth to note that the knowledge contained in the textbooks of Chinese medicine has been modified by removing the "superstitious parts" according to compilers' understanding of the "materialism and dialectics". Besides, generally speaking, the class hours of the courses of Western medicine and common required courses including English, History of China Revolution, Marxism, Philosophy, etc. occupy around 50% of the total. Therefore, graduates from colleges or universities of Chinese medicine in China can practice Chinese medicine or Western medicine or both, esp. before the 21st century.

Generally speaking, the studies on Chinese medicine nowadays can be roughly classified into three major categories, i.e. Studies on History and Literature of Chinese Medicine - approaches of sinology and history, Clinical Trials of Herbal Remedies or Acupuncture such as RCT (Randomized Controlled Trials), and Experimental Studies on Chinese Medicine such as animal experiments, extracting effective ingredients from herbal substances with modern technology, etc.. The latter two are usually conducted in accordance with Western scientific methods and evaluated with Western scientific standards. Most of the academic papers on Chinese medicine trace their research backgrounds to ancient Chinese medical texts, and discuss their research results based on quotations from ancient medical classics no matter how modern technologies have been applied in their researches or how high level such as molecular or gene level they have reached in their research results.

In one word, the way of knowing Chinese medicine nowadays results in the formation of the so called "Traditional Chinese Medicine" (TCM).

1.2.3 Chinese Medicine: Being both Classical and Traditional

We know now the ways of knowing and practicing Chinese medicine in the past and nowadays are somehow different, which results in the gap between Classical Chinese Medicine (CCM) and Traditional Chinese Medicine (TCM). Such differences are of vital importance for understanding the ins and outs as well as the further development of Chinese medicine. Table 12 shows the gap between Classical Chinese Medicine and Traditional Chinese Medicine.

Type of Difference	Classical Chinese Medicine	Traditional Chinese Medicine
Philosophical Foundation	Naturalist philosophy, e.g. philosophy of Taoist School	Pragmatist philosophy, e.g. scientific materialism, communism
Definition of the Profession	Requires broad base of knowledge due to intimate relationship to other traditional arts and sciences	A technical and highly specialised trade
Understanding of the Body	Body is treated as a microcosm that follows macrocosmic laws and is continually informed by macrocosmic influences	Body is treated as an independent entity
Diagnostic Procedure	Clinical diagnosis primarily based on "subjective" experience of the senses	Clinical diagnosis primarily informed by "objective" instrumental data

Table 12 The Gap between Classical Chinese Medicine and Traditional Chinese Medicine[309,310]

Here we have Classical Chinese Medicine, Chinese Folk Medicine, and Traditional Chinese Medicine, which are all Chinese medicine. What is the difference between them? I would like to classify them into two major groups, one is Chinese Academic Medicine composed of Classical Chinese Medicine and Traditional Chinese Medicine, and the other is Chinese Folk Medicine, which has been declining since almost all the professionals graduate from universities or colleges. The established fact is that Classical Chinese Medicine and Traditional Chinese Medicine together make up the Chinese Medicine today.

To sum up, generally speaking, no matter in the past or nowadays, Chinese medicine is leant, known and practiced in this similar way: acquire profound knowledge by memorising theories and experiences of the ancients in the texts, put these theories and experiences into practice and integrate them with one's own practice (no matter in textual research, clinical trials, or experimental studies), and develop Chinese medicine by interpreting ancient medical literature with one's own experiences and leaving one's own writings to the later generations if possible. I think, compared to memorising, understanding is much more important, which has been rarely discussed no matter in the past or nowadays.

309 Fruehauf, Heiner. Chinese Medicine in Crisis: Science, Politics, and the Making of "TCM"[J]. Journal of Chinese Medicine. No 61 Oct 1999: 1-9.

310 Wallner, Friedrich, Lan Fengli. Rationality of Acupuncture: How to Protect Acupuncture from Misunderstanding. In Lan Fengli, Wallner FG, and Wobovnik C (eds).2011: 167-188.

1.3 Understanding Chinese Medicine as Its History, a Linguistic Medical System, and a Philosophy

There are two main ways of researching Chinese medicine in the West, the way of Sinology and the way of natural sciences (especially pharmaceutics). Sinology is a geisteswissenschaft not taking into account that Chinese medicine is more than a system of signs; natural sciences, on the other hand, neglect the fact that the art of healing in Chinese medicine is insolvably connected with its cultural background. Hence, the first way of research does not pay respect to the effectiveness of Chinese medicine, and the second way actually destroys Chinese medicine by imposing its own methods on it. But Chinese medicine is a culturally dependent art of healing, i.e. a real medicine that roots in a special culture.

1.3.1 Understanding Chinese Medicine as Its History[311]

The history always becomes the past. But the history of Chinese medicine is surely an exceptional case. I would like to say "Chinese Medicine Is Its History" for the historical literature of Chinese medicine reflects itd cultural presuppositions, records its origin and development, and is the most important source of the knowledge system of Chinese medicine. The update knowledge system of Chinese medicine is the sum total of the knowledge contained in all of the literature on Chinese medicine of all the times - from Qin-Han Dynasties (221 B.C. – 220 A.D.) to the 21st century.

Historical Literature of Chinese medicine reflects its cultural presuppositions - *Qu Xiang Bi Lei* 取象比类 and *Tian Ren He Yi* 天人合一, thus weaving natural and social phenomena together with the basic correct understanding of the human being into the knowledge system of Chinese medicine.

Historical Literature of Chinese medicine is shown in the original complex writing forms, for example the "Four Great Ancient Chinese Medical Classics" (1,800-2,000 years old), i.e. *Huang Di's Inner Classic, The Classic of Difficult Issues, Treatise on Cold-induced and Miscellaneous Diseases,* and *Shen Nong's Classic of Materia Medica*. Here I have to say that the simplified forms of original Chinese characters reduce a lot of cultural information contained in them. For example, "脏腑", the current writing forms for *Zang-Fu* or viscera and bowels in the modern texts, embody the concrete thinking based on their morphological structures; while "藏府", the original writing forms for *Zang-Fu* in the four great medical classics, embody the image thinking based on *Qu Xiang Bi Lei* or Taking Image and Analogizing.

Historical Literature of Chinese medicine is the foundation for its clinical practice, and one of the most important inspiration sources for modern studies on

311 Lan Fengli. Chinese Medicine Is Its History. In Lan FL, Wallner F.G., and Wobovnik C.(eds). 2011: 289-314.

Chinese medicine. Most of the academic papers today trace their research backgrounds to ancient Chinese medical texts, and discuss their research results based on quotations from ancient medical classics no matter how modern technologies have been applied in their researches or how high level such as molecular or gene level they have reached in their research results. Here I give you 3 examples to illustrate this viewpoint.

Example 1 "Healthy *Qi*", "Immunity", and pharmacological effects of "*Qi*-Tonifying" agents: *Huang Di's Inner Classic* states that "If the Healthy *Qi* resides inside the body, then the pathogenic factors cannot find a way to invade it". Modern research results read that *Qi*-Tonifying agents such as Huangqi or Radix Astragalus can improve both the humoral and cellular immunity, strengthen leukocyte's phagocytic power, and increase the ratio of T cell and lymphocyte's transformation rate.

Example 2 "The lungs stand interior-exterior relationship with the large intestine" stated in the *Huang Di's Inner Classic*: In the clinical practice, patients with serious dysfunction of the intestinal tract are always accompanied by acute respiratory failure or adult respiratory distress syndrome (RDS); Pathological anatomical studies on dead bodies with lung diseases show that the large intestine and the small intestine are both seriously aerated, the mucous layer of the small intestine is necrotic with ulceration; Experimental studies with rabbits or rats as the objects demonstrate that ischemic dysfunction of intestinal tract is the underlying cause for damage of the lungs and that relieving constipation relates to transformation of the lung tissue from the abnormal pathological changes to the normal.

Example 3 Multi-disciplinary approaches to "the kidneys opening into the ears" stated in the *Huang Di's Inner Classic*: In the clinical practice, Kidney-Supplementing method can achieve satisfactory therapeutic effect in treating tinnitus and deafness; A series of studies have proved the relationship between the kidneys and the ears from the aspects of adrenocortical hormone (ACH), thyroid hormone and the effects of Kidney-Supplementing medicinal agents in treating tinnitus and deafness by applying modern physiological, morphological, histochemical, and pharmacological methods; Research results also suggest that applying Kidney-Supplementing method to treat toxic deafness caused by ototoxic diuretics, gentamicin, and kanamycin is a quite satisfactory method, which also provides new theoretical and clinical evidence for treating deafness with this method.

You can see the great lasting vitality of the ancient Chinese medical literature and their application in clinical practice and modern research until nowadays.

To conclude, the ancient Chinese medical literature is one of the most important inspiration sources for modern studies on Chinese medicine; Research outcome of the modern studies enrich Chinese medicine on one hand, and provide understandable evidence for people with Western scientific background on the other.

The importance of metaphors in Chinese medicine can be partly explained with this viewpoint that "Chinese Medicine Is Its History" for metaphors reveal how Chinese medicine was formed, has been developed and studied through its history up till today.

We know from the above discussion that differences in the ways of knowing and practicing Chinese medicine in the past and nowadays result in the gap between Classical Chinese Medicine (CCM) and Traditional Chinese Medicine (TCM) (See Table 11), and that both make up the Chinese medicine of nowadays. But both Classical Chinese Medicine and Traditional Chinese Medicine are different stages in its long development course. In the 21st century the most important thing for Chinese medicine is how to modernize not westernize it preconditioned that its specific advantages can be preserved.

1.3.2 Understanding Chinese Medicine as a Linguistic Medical System[312]

Compared to Western medicine, which is an applied science based on achievements of Western science and technology, Chinese medicine is a typical linguistic medical knowledge system in essence for it is formed in the way of linguistication and is recorded in self-interpreting sinograms. Therefore Chinese medicine can be regarded as a linguistic medical system being composed of its logographic language writing forms, concepts, terminology, formulations, sentences, and their logic relationships.

The core knowledge of Chinese medicine is from classical Chinese medical texts, which are written in self-interpreting characters, or more exact, sinograms. Compared to phonetic writing forms, Chinese language (logographic writing) is more stable and accumulative. In Chinese language, giving the original sinogram new meanings by the way of metaphorizing instead of creating new sinograms is the major way to reflect the changes and developments of the world and the means and process of Chinese people cognizing, understanding and stating the world. After tracing back to the original meanings of sinograms, concepts and statements are not difficult to understand in their contexts in a broad sense, which also provide us extensive but close links among different disciplines of Chinese science and culture. Therefore, etymology investigation is of vital significance for etymology of a sinogram can unify all the migrating meanings of concepts based on the one sinogram with the same etymology. The theoretical system of Chinese medicine is stated and expressed in a natural language with the two major characteristics: being polysemous and ambiguous, which can also be clarified and unified by etymology investigation and metaphor understanding.

Take fire as an example. Fire in Chinese medicine comes from the fire in the common sense or from the fire in everyday life.

---

312 Lan Fengli. Metaphor, *Qu Xiang Bi Lei* and Chinese Medicine. In Wallner F.G., Lan FL and Jandl M.J. (eds). 2010: 63-88.

① **Etymology - Fire in Everyday Life:** "Huo 火" or Fire, as stated in *The Origin of Chinese Characters* that "火 *huo*, the phase of the South, flaming upward, is a pictograph". The ancient Chinese people observed that fire is warm, hot, red, burning, and flaming, bearing the characteristics of being bright, rising and upbearing.

② **Fire in the Five Phases:** In the five phases, fire represents not only the real fire, but also the substances and qualities bearing characteristics of fire -"Fire is the flaming upward". And then the south, summer, summer-heat, red, bitter in the nature, and the heart, small intestine, vessel, tongue, sweat, joy, laugh of the human beings are all attributed to fire in the five phases.

③ **Fire as One of the Six *Qi* or Six Climatic Factors:** In the philosophical context that *qi* is the basic substance or the source constituting everything in the universe, the fire is also a kind of "*qi*", a form of object in a specific state, also known as "fire *qi*". Six *Qi* is the summarization of six kinds of weather in three categories in the nature: the flow of air - wind, or wind *qi*; changes in temperature (*qi wen*) - cold or cold *qi*, heat or heat *qi*, summer-heat or summer-heat *qi*; and moisture - dampness or damp *qi*, dryness or dry *qi*. The heat *qi* and summer-heat *qi* pertain to fire in the five phases for they all indicate being high in temperature. The *Huang Di's Inner Classic* names the "heat *qi*" "the monarch fire", "summer-heat *qi*" "the primer fire".

④ **Fire as One of the Six Excesses or Six Climatic Pathogenic Factors:** Pathogenic fire pertains to yang, flaming upward, rising, dispersing, burning, having heat manifestations, consuming liquid, damaging *qi*, harming the upper part of the human beings, tending to produce wind, stir blood, disturb the heart spirit, etch flesh, form pus, cause sores, which should be treated by reducing fire, clearing heat and resolving toxin with medicinals of bitter and cold in property.

⑤ **Fire in the Four Properties of Medicinals:** Every medicinal is said to be cold, cool, hot, or warm (the four properties). Hot and warm pertain to fire. Warm medicinals are regarded as "lesser fire", being bland in taste, can engender *qi*; hot medicinals are regarded as "vigorous fire", being rich or thick in taste, can consume *qi*.

⑥ **Fire in the Yin-Yang Theory:** In the philosophical context of *qi* and yin-yang theory, it is believed that water and fire can fully embody the most essential characteristics of yin and yang, as stated in the *Huang Di's Inner Classic* that "water is yin, fire is yang"; "water and fire are the symbols of yin and yang".

⑦ **Fire Functions as the Physiological State of Yang *Qi*:** For fire being warm, giving heat to people (the original recognition of fire and direct experience of fire), *qi* being classified into yin and yang and the abstraction of the things with yang characteristics and functions, as well as analogizing the normal state of yang *qi* with the function and characteristics of fire, Chinese medicine calls the physiological state of yang *qi* of the human being "fire" or "lesser fire". Wang Bing's 王冰 (710-804) annotations of *Su Wen* or *Basic Questions* reads that "to supplement the source of fire to eliminate the yin shading". Zhang Jiebin 张介宾 (1563-1640) regarded the heart yang as the monarch fire, the kidney yang as primer fire, which together fulfill the function of warming, activating all the organs of the human being, maintaining the flow and distribution of the essence, blood, and body fluid for all liquid substances prefer warm and dislike cold, and warm activates them to flow, while cold causes them to stagnate.

⑧ **Fire as a Pathological State when Yang *Qi* Functions Abnormally:** The *Huang Di's Inner Classic* states that "All fever with impaired consciousness and convulsion is ascribed to fire", "All trismus with shivering chills and delirium is ascribed to fire", "All disorders with upward perversion are ascribed to fire", "All states of agitation and mania are ascribed to fire", "All illnesses with swelling and aching of the instep and mental strain are ascribed to fire". Later on, Liu Wansu 刘完素 (?1110-1200) developed and enriched the pathological connotations of fire, advanced that "the six *qi* can all transform into fire", "*qi* in its surplus will become fire".

Finally, the pathological fire bears 3 connotations: the first is "vigorous fire", referring to excessive pathological conditions of exuberance of yang *qi*, also known as "excessive fire, excessive heat", which should be treated by medicinals of cold and bitter in property to clear heat and reduce fire, including such conditions as flaming upward of heart fire, flaming upward of liver fire, exuberance of stomach fire, and fire toxin of sores and carbuncles, etc; the second is the "ministerial fire", resulting from the deficient pathological condition of relative exuberance yang *qi* due to yin deficiency failing to control yang *qi*, also known as "deficient fire, deficient heat", which should be treated with enriching yin and reducing fire, mainly including "frenetic stirring of ministerial fire", manifesting in dizziness, headache, tinnitus, irritability if the liver is chiefly involved, and feverish feeling in the chest, palms of the hands, and soles of the feet, aching in the loins, and hyperaphrodisia if the kidney is chiefly involved; the third is the "yin fire", referring to the spleen heat caused by irregularities in diets and physical overstrain as well as the heart fire caused by excessive joy, anger, or anxiety.

It is thus clear that etymology investigation of "Huo 火" or Fire is of vital significance for it can unify all the migrating meanings of the related concepts based on the same sinogram.

1.3.3 Understanding Chinese Medicine as a Philosophy: Metaphorizing[313]

Chinese medicine has been developed in the framework which the "Four Great Medical Classics" established around 2,000 years ago. Historical texts of Chinese medicine are full of metaphors: from terms to sentences, to paragraphs, to texts, and even to the whole system, which reflect the imaging thinking in Chinese medicine.

Metaphor is an important field of study shared in rhetoric, linguistics and philosophy. The nature of metaphor is to understand, analyze, perceive, and describe one category of things through another. *Qu Xiang Bi Lei* or Taking Image

313 Lan Fengli. Chinese Medicine as a Philosophy: Metaphorizing. In Lan FL, Wallner FG, and Wobovnik C (eds). 2011: 315-340.

and Analogizing, the core, specific and major methodology of Chinese science and culture (including Chinese medicine), results in the formation of metaphors, and thus is the metaphorizing process. In order words, metaphorizing is the major way to form the ontological concepts, the fundamental theories, and to develop clinical explorations of Chinese medicine. And only by understanding the metaphors in Chinese medicine, we know that Chinese medicine is a different medical system incompatible with Western medicine, which weaves natural and social phenomena together with the basic correct understanding of the human being as an integrity, thus revealing its methodology "*Qu Xiang Bi Lei* or Taking Image and analogizing" under the guidance of "*Tian Ren He Yi* 天人合一 or and Universe Man Uniting and Resembling Each Other", the core idea of classical Chinese philosophy. By this way it becomes clear that Chinese medicine must not be taken as a natural science in the Western sense, but it goes closer to humanities (geisteswissenschaften).

Here it is worth to note that *Qu Xiang Bi Lei* is the core, specific and major methodology of classical Chinese science, and metaphorizations are the centre and of the most significance in Chinese scientific discourses, while induction and deduction are the core and major methodologies of modern Western science, and metaphorizations in Western scientific discourses are far away from being acknowledged compared to the so-called objective descriptive language.

The Chapter 25 of *Lao Tzu* states:

"Therefore, Tao is great.
Heaven is great.
Earth is great.
Man is great.
In the universe, there are four great things, and man is one of them.
Man abides by the earth.
Earth abides by the heaven.
Heaven abides by Tao.
Tao abides by the nature".

It is thus clear that metaphorizing is also the bridge in between the Tao (The Way) of the Nature and Medicine. "Heaven", "Earth", and "Man" compose a whole system; In *Lao Tzu*, Tao abides by the nature; In *Huang Di's Inner Classic*, medicine abides by the Tao; In essence, medicine abides by the nature.[314]

314 Lan Fengli. Metaphorizing: The Way to Bridge *The Book of Changes* and Chinese Medicine. In Wallner F.G., Schmisberger F., Wimmer F.M. (eds). 2010: 177-192.

Western medicine is an applied medicine based on achievements of modern Western science and technology, while Chinese medicine roots in classical Chinese philosophy and culture, e.g. Taoist School, and thus goes closer to humanities. But both aim to heal the same being, which is composed of body and mind.

- The Author

2 Cultural Differences between Chinese Medicine and Western Medicine

Both transmission of Chinese medicine to the West and dissemination of Western medicine in China started in the Ming dynasty (16th-17th centuries). Some missionaries taught and spread Christian or Catholic religion by practicing Western medicine; meanwhile, they introduced Chinese medicine curiously, esp. their own experiences in Chinese medicine to the West. Over 300 years passed by. At present, Chinese medicine and Western medicine actually coexist no matter in China or in the West. So, Chinese medicine is not only a special medical system with distinctive national features of China, but also a medical system for the mankind of the whole world.

A leading authority on Chinese herbal medicine, Dr. Yakazu Domei, lists the following differences between Chinese medicine and Western medicine.[315] See Table 13:

Points	**Chinese Medicine**	**Western Medicine**
1	Philosophical	Scientific
2	Synthetic	Analytical
3	Holistic	Topical
4	Internal	Surgical
5	Conformational	Heteropathic
6	Empirical	Theoretical
7	Hygienic	Preventive
8	Individualized	Socialized
9	Preventive	Bacteriological
10	Experiential	Experimental
11	Humoral	Cellular
12	Subjective	Objective
13	Natural sources	Synthetic analogy

Table 13 Differences between Chinese Medicine and Western Medicine

315 www.tcmhelp.com/Theory/3.htm

It is worth to note that, as medical systems, both Chinese medicine and Western medicine are "scientific systems of studying life processes of the human being and prevention and treatment of diseases"[316]. They share at least 3 common features: ① the same object - life processes of the human being; ② the same goal - To prevent and treat diseases; and ③ both are members of "scientific systems", which depends on how you understand "Science". But, Chinese medicine bears strong humane characteristics, and thus goes closer to humanities; while Western medicine, esp. modern Western medicine, is an applied medicine based on achievements of modern Western science and technology, and thus has typical features of modern Western science. What are the cultural differences between the two medical systems? I think that clarifying these differences will be very helpful for you to understand Chinese medicine.

2.1 Chinese Medicine Going Closer to Humanities Rather than Natural Science

There is no breakthrough but only development and enrichment in Chinese medicine since the establishment of its knowledge system about 2,000 years ago; and there is even no real development since the establishment of standardized transmission of Chinese medicine in 1956. Why?

Chinese Medicine has formed a self-contained fruitful paradigm, so can be enriched and developed in the same framework – *Qu Xiang Bi Lei* or Taking Image and Analogizing guided by *Tian Ren He Yi* or Universe and Man Uniting and Resembling Each Other established about 2,000 years ago, and survive up till today. For example, the theory of Visceral Image embodies the holistic approach of "Four Seasons - Five *Zang* Organs – Yin-Yang – Five Phases" and "Universe and Man Uniting and Resembling Each Other". While based on reductionism, mechanism and dichotomy, Western medicine takes an analytical approach, and has been continuously refreshing itself because of the application of advanced modern scientific technology and instruments (tools) to develop itself.

In contemporary China, Chinese medicine is classified as a discipline of natural science by the government of China since 1956. For example, there are two major national foundations in China, one is National Natural Science Foundation of China (NNSFC) for sponsoring research projects in the field of natural science, where Chinese medicine is included; the other is National Funds for Social Science for sponsoring research projects in the field of social science, where Chinese medicine is excluded. That is to say, researches on Chinese medicine have to be performed by applying Western scientific methods and evaluated according to Western scientific standards,[317] which inevitably results in

316 Xia Zhengnong. 2002: 2006.

317 Note: Generally speaking, the researches on Chinese medicine are mainly classified into three major categories: Studies on the History and Literature of Chinese Medicine, Clinical Trials, and Experimental Studies, of which studies on the history and literature are the most difficult to get funds and are usually separated from clinical and experimental studies on Chinese medicine, and almost all clinical and experimental studies are performed in accordance with Western scientific standards.

that there is even no real development in Chinese medicine no matter in aspect of theoretical or clinical framework. The reason is that Chinese medicine is totally different from and incompatible with Western science and it is not researched in an adequate way, and such approaches to Chinese medicine do not accord with its philosophical characteristics.

2.2 Linguistic Differences

"Language is an outcome of the culture. Language of a nation is the general reflection of the culture of the nation; but we can also say that language is a part of the culture … and that culture and language have developed together for thousands of years." (Claude Levi Strauss)

2.2.1 Logographic Writing, Phonetic Writing, and Thinking Modes

Chinese characters or sinograms, the writing forms of Chinese language and one of the most important marks of Chinese civilization, emerged independently around 6,000 years ago, which is identified by the history of Banpo Ruins of Xi'an, Shaanxi Province. *Shuo Wen Jie Zi* or *The Origin of Chinese Characters* is the first comprehensive systematic dictionary of Chinese characters (or sinograms) arranged by sections with shared components, called radicals (*bùshǒu* 部首, lit. "section headers") and finished in 100 A.D. by Xu Shen 许慎 (A.D.58? – 147?) of the Eastern Han Dynasty. It is the first dictionary which interprets the original meaning of a sinogram by analyzing its structure and gives the rationale behind it, sometimes the etymology of the sinogram as well.

Actually, *Shuo Wen Jie Zi* or *The Origin of Chinese Characters* is far beyond a dictionary, and moreover it can be interpreted from cultural and philosophical perspectives. It is indeed the case that no monograph on philosophy of Chinese language has ever been available up till today except this book. A study on the relationship between *Huang Di Nei Jing* or *Huang Di's Inner Classic* and *Shuo Wen Jie Zi* or *The Origin of Chinese Characters* shows that "The knowledge of Chinese medicine contained in *The Origin of Chinese Characters* is in direct line of succession with *Huang Di's Inner Classic*; The universal and ecomedical thinking modes of "Heaven-Earth-Man" in them are cut from the same cloth; The theories of *qi*, yin-yang, and the five phases, the theoretical foundation of *The Inner Classic*, can be traced back to their sources through *The Origin of Chinese Characters* which expounds the original meanings of them by analyzing the structures of their sinograms; *The Origin of Chinese Characters* traces back to origins of sinograms and their original meanings through analyzing their structures, therefore, it is important for us to study and read *The Inner Classic*, and to probe into the origin of Chinese medicine as well".[318]

---

318 Lan Fengli. Influence of *Huang Di's Inner Classic* on *The Origin of Chinese Characters* [J]. Chinese Journal of Medical History. 2006, 36（4）: 201-205.

Take "*Qi* 气" as an example. *The Origin of Chinese Characters • Qi Part* states that "*Qi* refers to thin, floating clouds. The sinogram 气 is a pictograph". The sinogram 气 was written as "" in the oracle inscriptions of the Shang Dynasty (ca. 16th-11th century B.C.), which resembles air current, evaporating and rising, whose image is just like cloud, will disappear very soon and become invisible. *Qi* at this moment referred to air or vapor. Therefore, *qi* is invisible and formless, exists everywhere, can be gathered into a form, for instance, *qi* can be condensed into water.

Soon afterwards, the *qi* which surrounds and congests the space of the human beings was abstracted into the *qi* which bears a material meaning in philosophical sense. Philosophers of the Spring Autumn and Warring States Periods (770-221B.C.) believed that *qi* is the basic substance constituting the world, and that everything in the universe comes into being by the movement and mutation of *qi*. For example, *The Book of Changes* states that "everything is transformed and generated by the enshrouding [*qi*] of the heaven and the earth".

Later on ancient Chinese medical experts introduced "*qi*" into the medical field at the right moment. And then, "*qi*" became a medium or bridge between the natural philosophy of the Pre-Qin days (before 221 B.C.) and Chinese medicine. The concept of "*qi*" gradually formed in Chinese medicine.

In the time of *Huang Di's Inner Classic*, "*qi*" is regarded not only as the basic substance constituting the world, but also as the basic substance constituting the human being, which can be transformed into blood, essence, and body fluid, etc., and the normal functional activities of the life which is governed by "*qi*" is known as *Shen* or spirit. For example, *Su Wen • Bao Ming Quan Xing Lun* or *Basic Questions • Discourse on Protecting Life and Preserving Physical Appearance* states that "Man is generated by *qi* of the heaven and the earth, and is completed by the law of the four seasons"; and that "The union of *qi* of the heaven and the earth gives birth to man". Actually, there are abundant accounts of *qi* in the *Basic Questions*. Only the monosyllabic word "*qi*" appears 1,176 times in *Basic Questions*. Almost all the 79 existing chapters of the *Su Wen or Basic Questions* discuss *qi*. All the theories and skills of the *Su Wen or Basic Questions* are related to *qi*. And there are various *qi* with a multitude of names in the *Basic Questions*, such as yin *qi*, yang *qi*; clear *qi*, turbid *qi*; heaven *qi*, earth *qi*; upright *qi* or healthy *qi*, evil *qi* or pathogenic *qi*; nutritive *qi*, defensive *qi*; seasonal *qi*, visceral *qi*, meridian *qi*; and so and so forth.[319]

According to *A Concise Dictionary of Chinese Medicine*, *qi* in Chinese medicine bears the following meanings:[320] ① nutritious, essential substance flowing inside the body, such as food qi, breathed air; ② functional activities of

319 Lan Fengli. The Influence of *Huang Di's Inner Classic* on *The Origin of Chinese Characters* [J]. Chinese Journal of Medical History. 2006, 36(4): 201-205.
320 Li Jingwei, Ou Yongxin, Yu Ying'ao, et al. 2001: 173.

the *zang-fu* organs in a general sense, such as visceral *qi* (i.e, the functional activities of the *zang-fu* organs); *qi* can also be classified into original *qi*, nutritive *qi*, defensive *qi*, pectoral *qi*, etc. according to its source, distribution, and function; ③ the second location or stage of pattern identification of warm diseases.[321]

It is thus clear that *qi* was not air or vapor long ago. And then, what is *qi* in Chinese medicine? Energy? Vital energy? Atmosphere? Or influence? For *qi* implies so many meanings and no translation can convey all the cultural connotations of *qi*, and therefore, I believe *pinyin* transliteration *"qi"* is the best choice. But more important, the presupposition of *pinyin* transliteration is that you should know the origin, development and cultural connotations of *qi*.

You see, the shape of a Chinese character is directly related to its meaning, and both integrate into a unity. The formation of a Chinese character, an organic whole of the shape and the meaning, is one-step made following the rule of nature, reflecting the direct communication between and integration of the subject and the object. The formation also implies an important thinking way, i.e. the imaging thinking.

Integration of the subject and the object is a thread running through classical Chinese culture and science, on the basis of which Universe and Man Uniting and Resembling Each Other (tian ren he yi, 天人合一) constitutes the foundation of the classical Chinese culture and science.

The imaging thinking is a classical Chinese thinking way, and the process, methods, and rules of which make up "Taking Image and Analogizing" (qu xiang bi lei, 取象比类), the fundamental methodology of classical Chinese culture and science[322]. Chinese characters, which have developed on the basis of the pictographic writing, and their meanings are quite stable and conservative, which promotes the development of imaging and analogizing thinking of Chinese medical experts. Then such thinking modes were set up in the *Huang Di's Inner Classic* and have greatly influenced Chinese medical experts of the later generations.

The logographic writings of yin-yang 阴阳, *wu xing* 五行, and *qi* 气, the extensive imaging and analogizing thinking modes in the *Huang Di's Inner Classic*, and criticism, proofreading, annotations for sinograms from the aspects of the "shape", "pronunciation", and "meaning" in the ancient medical classics

321 Wei-Qi-Ying-Blood Pattern Identification for Warm Diseases originated from *Huang Di's Inner Classic*, was developed by Ye Tianshi 叶天士 (1666-1745) of the Qing Dynasty. It reflects the general rule of the progression of the four different stages of warm diseases, associates the pathological changes of the four stages with corresponding organs, and advances the corresponding therapeutic principles for each stage.

322 The word "traditional" is sometimes disapproving, and means "following older methods and ideas rather than modern or different ones" (Oxford Advanced Learner's Dictionary). Chinese culture and science, including Chinese medicine, are based on classical Chinese philosophy, and so I name them "classical Chinese culture and science" and "classical Chinese medicine". They are classical but not old-fashioned or out-of-date because they are still developing in their own framwork.

made since its appearance, all demonstrate the far-reaching influences of the imaging thinking mode on Chinese medicine. For example, in *Ling Shu* or *Miracullous Pivot* of the *Nei Jing*, the chapter *Xiao Zhen Jie* or *An Explanation of Small Needles* is an interpretation of the part of "Small Needles" of the chapter *Jiu Zhen Shi Er Yuan* or *Nine Needles and Twelve Source Points*. Actually, most of the books on classical Chinese science were composed in this way, i.e. the way of annotating former classics. I think the formation of this common feature results from influences of the logographic writing and the imaging thinking way as well as the writing tradition of Confucian classics.

Phonetic writing, as opposed to logographic writing, is the most common writing form in the world. English, German, French, Spanish, Portuguese, etc. are all phonetic writings, but are different languages composed by the same Latin alphabets. Let's take English as an example.

English is a kind of phonetic writing. The shapes of English words are directly related to their pronunciations, but have nothing to do with the meanings or the external images of concrete things. That is to say, in the phonetic writing, the shape is separate and independent from the meaning, and the meaning comes from man-made prescripts outside the shape, which indicates that the formation of a word of the phonetic writing is composed of two steps: first, building its shape - spelling of alphabets; second, defining its meaning based on linguistic rules or grammar.

Understanding the meanings of words is based on the sense of hearing, thus jumping out the thinking frame of the visual sense of the concrete images of things, then providing a bigger possibility for logic thinking based on the abstraction, finally forming thinking traditions of abstract inference, conceptual thinking, categorization, and trying to make an objective judgment to the world.

The formation of phonetic writing reflects its two important characteristics: tool - alphabets and abstraction - linguistic rules. Every tool is made to have a certain function according to man's specific aim or intention, thus becoming a medium of connection between man and the nature, and so interrupting the natural direct communication between them. Tool plays a vital role in the Western culture, esp. in the natural sciences, where it is standardized and systematized, and the experimental research approach characterized by the use of various tools is set up.

Actually, the alphabet is the mother of various tools. The thinking way relating to the experimental research approach is abstraction. The rule of abstraction is logic, while linguistic rules or grammar is an embryonic form of logic. The emergence of tool reflects the relationship between the subject and the object, i.e., the separation and opposition of them - man remakes the nature. The abstraction pays more attention to being analytical, logical, and restricts imagination.

The tool and abstraction become the foundation of Western culture and science and of the natural science (including Western medicine) in particular. Western natural science manifests in two opposite ways, which have been realized by more and more people as time goes by. The two edges lie in that the environmental pollution and the ecological imbalance, the repay of the nature to the man, always accompany the process of the man conquering and remaking the nature. As regards to Western medicine, the two edges lie in that the severe side effects, drug resistance, and effect being temporary always accompany the notable therapeutic effects.

2.2.2 Chinese Medical Terminology and Western Medical Terminology

Chinese medical terminology is very different from Western medical terminology. For example, a kind of eye disease, which is caused by "pathogenic wind-fire" and marked by acute onset of redness and pain in the eye accompanied by photophobia and lacrimation, is named "wind-fire eye" in Chinese medicine. Such a disease is generally diagnosed as "acute conjunctivitis" in Western medicine, which is a kind of "inflammation of the conjunctiva" of the eye. It is interesting that Chinese medicine does not speak of "inflammation[323]" nor does Western medicine speak of "wind fire", but both can heal the same disease by different methods.

"Not only the names of diseases, not only the grouping of systems were not the same, but the fundamental perceptual codes that were applied to patients' bodies , the field of objects to which observation addressed itself, the surfaces and depths traversed by the doctor's gaze, the whole system of orientation of his gaze also varied",[324] What Michael Foucault says about medical perception in different historical periods could apply as well to these different cultural traditions.[325] These different cultural traditions of Chinese medicine and Western medicine are embodied in their specific terminologies.

Undoubtedly, no matter the language of Chinese medicine or the language of Western medicine is a kind of technical language. Modern terminologists define a "technical language" as a form of any given language that is used by people involved in a special field and that has a "terminology", i.e., a set of expressions not used in the common language or, as is often the case, expressions that are used in a different or more specific way than in the common language.

A popular misconception about technical terms is that they are words used *exclusively* by specialists. In actual fact, technical terms in most disciplines largely,

323 It is interesting that the root of the word "Inflammation" is "flame", which means "n. a hot bright stream of burning gas that comes from sth. that is on fire" and "v. to burn with a bright flame" (Oxford Advanced leaner's Dictionary).
324 Foucault, Michel. 1973: 54.
325 Kaptchuk, Ted J. 2000: 3.

if not mostly, come from the common language. Any language only has a certain number of words, and new terms are usually combinations of existing lexical items. Many terms are completely indistinguishable in form from expressions in the common language although they are more specific in meaning. The process whereby common language expressions are given more specific or metaphorical meanings in the technical contexts is called "terminologization". The modern terminological observation that technical terms are largely derived from the common language is reflected clearly both in Chinese medicine and Western medicine. Those acquainted with the language of Chinese medicine are aware that most of the sinograms they come across in Chinese medical texts are used in the common language. And most of the Western medical terms are combinations of Latin or Greek morphemes. Actually, about 10,000 Latin or Greek words came into English during the Renaissance Period and finally became a part of English vocabulary.

Actually, both Chinese medical terminology and Western medical terminology can be classified into three levels: ① words and expressions for everyday use; ② specialized terms of their own; and ③ original terms of their own.

2.2.2.1 Three Levels of Chinese Medical Terminology

Both Dr. Nigel Wiseman and Prof. Paul U. Unschuld advocated classifying the basic Chinese medical terminology into two categories: one comprises of words and expressions for everyday use, e.g., 頭 head, 腳 foot, 胸 chest, 腹 abdomen, 心 heart, 肝 liver, 血 blood; the other is composed of specialized Chinese medical terms extended from the common language and formed through metaphor or analogy, e.g., 竅 orifice, 穴 point or hole, 正 upright, 邪 evil, 營 nutrient, 衛 defense, 命門 life gate, 督脈 the governing vessel.[326]

According to my understanding of Chinese medical terminology, esp. of *The Origin of Chinese Characters*, I think that Chinese medical terminology can be classified into 3 levels:

The first level is made up of words and expressions from the common language, e.g., some body parts like 心 heart, 肝 liver, 脾 spleen, 肺 lungs, 腎 kidneys, 鼻 nose, 目 eyes, 耳 ears, 頭 head, 腳 foot, 胸 chest, 腹 abdomen, 血 blood; some disease names like 霍亂 cholera, 麻疹 measles, 麻風 leprosy, 瘧疾 malaria, 癲癇 epilepsy; some climatic pathogenic factors like 風 wind, 寒 cold, 濕 dampness, 燥 dryness, 火 fire; some symptoms like 發熱 fever, 頭痛 headache, 痛 pain, 咳嗽 cough, 心悸 palpitation, 健忘 forgetfulness, 頭暈目眩

326 Wiseman, Nigel. Translation and Transmission of Chinese Medicine in the West. Medicine and Philosophy. 2001, 22(7): 51-54.

dizziness, 嘔吐 vomiting, 噁心 nausea, 泄瀉 diarrhea, 便秘（不更衣）constipation.

The second level constitutes specialized Chinese medical terms from daily words and expressions formed through metaphorizing or analogizing process, e.g., 藏 depots or viscera, 府 palaces or bowels, 經 meridian, 絡 collateral or network vessel, 竅 orifice, 穴 point or hole, 正 upright, 邪 evil, 營 nutrient, 衛 defense, 督脈 the governing vessel, 任脈 the controlling vessel, 三焦 the *san jiao*, 命門 life gate, etc. which usually bear historical, cultural, and medical values at the same time.

The third level comprises of original Chinese medical terms, e.g., some pictophonetic characters such as 疝, 疸, 癰, 瘍, 痔, 痿, 痹, etc. in *The Origin of Chinese Characters • Disease Section.*

2.2.2.2 Three Levels of Western Medical Terminology

Dr. Nigel Wiseman[327] roughly classified the Western medical terminology into 3 levels and distinguished them as well.

The first level constitutes borrowings from the common language, e.g., fever, chill, cough, cold, hiccough, headache, pain, tenderness, soreness, palpitations, bleeding, hot flushes, forgetfulness, dizziness, vomiting, blindness, jaundice, deafness, nausea, emaciation, diarrhea, constipation, goiter, sores, corn, sty, boil, measles, mumps, and fracture. These words, commonly used by doctors, are known to all speakers and denote conditions that can be identified by most normal adults.

The second level comprises terms devised by modern medicine to describe certain technical concepts: conjunctivitis, anemia, hypertension, paranasal sinusitis, trichomoniasis, arteriosclerosis, optic atrophy, hyperchlorhydria, coronary thrombosis, glomerulonephritis hematoma, cerebrovascular ischemia. Although some of these words (such as anemia, hypertension and conjunctivitis) may be familiar to and even used by non-experts, the conditions they denote cannot be diagnosed by the non-experts with the medical precision. These terms reflect knowledge that lies at a long distance from the lay understanding.

Between these two levels is the third comprising terms of medical origin that do not require any specialist knowledge or instrumentation to understand or identify, e.g., enuresis, lochia, pharynx, larynx, dysphagia, strangury, scrofula, tumor, fistula, miliaria, macule, papule, and diphtheria.

I think that the terms of the first level are actually from words and expressions for everyday use, that of the second level are specialized terms of Western medicine, and that of the third level are original terms of Western medicine.

327 Wiseman, Nigel. The Translation of Chinese Medical Terminology. 1996: 67.

2.2.2.3 Drawing Lessons from English-Chinese Translation of Western Medicine in China

In the course of transmission and exchange of medical cultures, linguistic contact is a forerunner of the contact of different medical cultures. Language, an essential medium, is the carrier of the medical knowledge. The transmission and exchange between different medical cultures will first manifest in the terminology. The foreign terminology comes to be the "envoy" of the different medical cultures. Generally speaking, a foreign medical culture is introduced and disseminated by translating the foreign medical terminology in a proper way. The translated terminology gradually integrates into the native language, finally becomes an organic part of the mainstream medical culture of the nation proper.

The history of translation and dissemination of Western medicine in China shows that Western medical terminology and culture are very closely associated with each other, just like the shadow following the person. It also took a very long time for the formation of standard Chinese translation of Western medical terminology in China. In the early stage of translation and dissemination of Western medicine in China, for example, translation of the term "scarlet fever" had been very confusing, which had many different translations such as "紅熱症，紅疹，疹子熱病，痧病，花紅熱症，猩紅熱", etc.

It can be seen from the history and reality of translating Western medicine into Chinese that the first and third levels of Chinese medical terms have been successfully used to translate the first and third levels of Western medical terms and thus to express Western medical knowledge, and that using the second level of Chinese medical terms, which are specialized terms carring the most distinctive Chinese medical knowledge, to translate specialized terms of Western medicine, has produced serious confusions or even mistakes. Here are two examples:

① Translating "typhoid" into "傷寒" Typhoid refers to "infection of the intestine caused by *Salmonella typhi* in food and water"[328], manifesting in fever, diarrhea, even bloody stool; while "傷寒" is a specialized Chinese medical term, bears two meanings in Chinese medicine: in a broad sense, "傷寒", cold-induced disease, is a general term for various externally contracted febrile diseases, as stated in the *Basic Questions · Discourse on Febrile Diseases* (*Su Wen·Re Lun*, 素問•熱論: "今夫熱病者，皆傷寒之類也)"; in a narrow sense, "傷寒", cold affection, refers to a condition caused by cold, manifesting in chills and fevers, absence of sweating, headache, floating and tense pulse, as stated in *The Classic of Difficult Issues* (*Nan Jing*, 難經·五十八難: 傷寒有五：有中風，有傷寒，有濕溫，有熱病，有溫病，其所苦各不同"). Later on, some translators rendered "傷寒" in Chinese medicine back into "typhoid". Such a translation has confused the differences between "typhoid" in Western medicine and "傷寒" in Chinese

328 Collin, P.H. 2001: 613.

medicine, thus causing misunderstanding the both terms or even misleading the readers.

② Translating "surgery" into "外科學" Surgery refers to "treatment of a disease or disorder which requires an operation to cut into or to remove or to manipulate tissue or organs or parts"[329]; while "外科學" in Chinese medicine refers to a specialty which studies the causes, pathogenesis, and treatments of the diseases on the body surface[330]. Many majors of Chinese medicine, including undergraduates and even doctorate candidates, and some translators as well, translate "外科學" in Chinese medicine into "Surgery". Actually, "外科學" in Chinese medicine should be translated into "external medicine" for the real "surgery" in Chinese medicine declined long ago since Hua Tuo 华佗 died in 208 A.D.. So "中医外科学" should be "Chinese External Medicine" not "TCM Surgery" or "Surgery in Chinese Medicine".

We should draw some lessons from the above mentioned translation examples that the second level of Western medical terms should not be used to translate and express the specialized Chinese medical terms. For example, although "風火眼" in Chinese medicine and "acute conjunctivitis" in Western medicine actually refer to the same disease, it is ill-advised to translate "風火眼" into "acute conjunctivitis" for such a translation must confuse cultural differences between the two medical systems, and fail to produce such an association of the cause (pathogenic wind-fire) and therapeutic method (coursing wind and clearing fire) with the translation "acute conjunctivitis", thus destroying the independency, wholeness and systematicness of the theoretical system of Chinese medicine.

An interesting issue to be addressed here is that some disease names in *Su Wen* or *Basic Questions* may be of foreign origin. Here are some examples:

"*Li Lai* 癘癩": "癘", whose ancient pronunciation is *ljadh* or *rjats*, and "癩", whose ancient pronunciation is *ladh* or *rats*, the initial consonants come closer to those of the three most popular ancient European terms for *leprosy*, one might speculate about an association of *li* and *lai* with *leuke, lepra,* and *e-lephantiasis*;

"*Huo Luan* 霍亂", the compound *huo luan* does not correspond to the graphic structure of the vast majority of ancient Chinese disease terms, while its ancient pronunciation **hwak* luan* was formed to reflect in ancient Chinese the sound of the term *cholera* used along the travel routes from regions where the Greek term was in use to the Far East to designate a particularly violent type of diarrhea;

329 Collin, P.H. 2001: 571.
330 Li Jingwei, Ou Yongxin, Yu Ying'ao, et al. 2001:301.

"*Fei Xiao* 肺消", whose ancient pronunciation is **phjats*sjaw,* literally "lung wasting", could be a rendering into Chinese of the ancient Greek term *phtisis* or lung *phtisis,* which has exactly the same meaning;

"Xiao ke 消渴", wasting/melting and thirst，a label used to this day for diabetes, is a compound ideally suited to signify two obvious symptoms of the disease. An identical meaning was expressed in European antiquity by Aretaios of Cappadochia.[331]

Is it purely coincidental? Or there existed medical cultural exchange between the East and the West around the Zhou Dynasty (ca.1100-256 B.C.)? Anyway, these terms all came out far before the modern Western medicine and should be regarded as the terms of the first level. The above understanding further provides etymological evidence when translating "癘癩，霍亂，肺消，消渴" into "leprosy, cholera, lung wasting, wasting and thirst" respectively.

2.2.2.4 Learning Successful Experiences of Dissemination of Western Medicine in China

Why has Western medicine been successfully transmitted to China? The key lies in that Western medical terminology has been translated into Chinese in a complete, independent and systematic way through literal or word-for-word translation approach, e.g., "Conjunctivitis" is rendered as "結膜炎" not "風火眼"; "Acute contagious conjunctivitis" as "急性觸染性結膜炎" not "天行赤眼"; "Globus" as "球;球(狀)感", and "Globus abdominalis" as "腹(部)球(狀)感" not "癥瘕", "Globus hystericus" as "癔症球，癔病性窒息(感)" not "梅核氣".

The Chinese terms of Western medicine are so strange to the terminology of Chinese medicine and to the Chinese fraternity as well, but why do translators not adopt the terms of Chinese medicine to translate Western medical terms? Because the translator intends to preserve the systematicness, independence, and completeness (or integrity) of Western medicine, and don't want to make Western medicine in China become a Non-Chinese Non-Western Medicine or Non-Donkey Non-Horse medicine.

2.2.3 Classical Medical Chinese，Medical English and Epistemology

Ferid Murad (1936-), a Nobel Prize winner in medicine (1998), set up Murad Research Institute for Modernized Chinese Medicine, a modern research centre on Chinese pharmacology named after his name with the collaboration with Shanghai University of Traditional Chinese Medicine in 2003. At that time, he said he was seeking for a language which is able to give a scientific interpretation for pharmacological and molecule mechanisms of the therapeutic effects of Chinese herbal remedies. Chinese medicine has its own discourse, and so why do we need

331 Unschuld, Paul U. 2003: 203-204.

to look for another language to interpret it? Is it possible to find such a kind of language?

Ludwig Wittgenstein (1889-1951) believed that language is a kind of picture, which cannot be proved with facts of the real world. That is to say, we do not need to prove or interpret the logic contained in the discourse of Chinese medicine with the so-called scientific methods, what we should do is to regard it as a picture in which the discourse of Chinese medicine describes man's lifestyle - a harmonious state among man, the nature and the society, how man behaves in the daily life to preserve health, to prevent and treat illnesses, and which is like a picture of the life world.

According to Wittgenstein's idea of philosophy of language - "language games", Chinese medicine is definitely a kind of language, a language game in respect to man, its healthy state, and its connection with the Universe; Western medicine is another language game in respect to the body and its diseases; and differences between them is that Chinese medicine does not reduce its language but it enriches it by metaphors. Therefore it makes sense to say: Chinese medicine is a natural language and Western medicine is a formal descriptive technical language. Here is an importance difference for the theoretical understanding of both: Formal languages must be interpreted for getting sense; Natural languages are interpreting themselves.

It's true that the textual criticism, exegetical studies and annotations of ancient medical classics have always been an important academic field of study in Chinese medicine up till now since the era of the *Huang Di's Inner Classic*,[332] which helps practitioners of Chinese medicine of the past dynasties understand and develop Chinese medicine in both theoretical and clinical explorations.

Now, let's look at the two paragraphs about the origin of man both from the angle of genetics in Chinese medicine and Western medicine respectively:

① "人生於地，懸命於天，天地合气，命之曰人。人能應四時者，天地為之父母"（素問•寶命全形論）。

Translation: Man is born on the earth, hanging his life to the heaven. The union of *Qi* of Heaven and Earth makes up a man. Man can adapt himself to the seasons for Heaven and Earth are his parents. (*Basic Questions · Discourse on Protecting Life and Preserving Physical Appearance*)

② "Man is metazoon, triploblastic, chordale, vertebrate, pentadactyle, mammalian, eutherian, primate... The outlines of each of his principal system of organs may be traced back, like those of other mammals, to the fishes." (L.A.B.-orradaile)

332 Note: For example, the chapter of *Zhen Jie* or *An Explanation of Needles* of *Basic Questions* 素問• 針解 and the chapter of *Xiao Zhen Jie* or *An Explanation of Small Needles* of *Miraculous Pivot* 靈樞•小針解 both interpret the chapter of *Jiu Zhen Shi Er Yuan* or *Nine Needles and Twelve Source Points* of the *Spirit Pivot* 靈樞•九針十二原.

譯文：人屬於後生動物，系五趾，三胚層高級動物，屬脊索動物門，脊椎動物亞門，哺乳綱，靈長目……象其他哺乳動物一樣，他的每一個器官系統的輪廓可以追溯到魚類。[333]

It is clear that the latter is a kind of formal technical language, a typical language of modern Western science, which is only used as a tool to convey information, to identify its reference, and to express points of view. And it has become so boring and dry by the so-called theoretical and scientific formulations. While discourse of Chinese medicine is a kind of hermeneutic language full of metaphors, and it is closely related to the context of the life world - an inseparable organic whole of man, the nature and the society. It can inspire, hint, and enlighten you to know how Chinese medicine understands man in a direct and original way.

According to Wittgenstein's idea of philosophy of language, the discourse of Chinese medicine and that of Western medicine are different "language games", showing different lifestyles, and describing different "pictures" of life, and so one cannot be interpreted or proved by the other. For example, mixing the discourse of Western medicine with that of Chinese medicine will disturb the cognizing way of Chinese medicine, which is just like to coat or cover the transparent life world with the scientific formal language. Therefore, we should reconsider the current progress of researching, modernizing, or even westernizing Chinese medicine, and what we need to do is to understand the rationality of Chinese medicine from its own discourse, from the "picture" of the lifestyle in the life world its discourse describes. That is to interpret Chinese medicine with itself. I do not deny the approach to apply modern science and technology to study Chinese medicine, but such researches must be in accordance with philosophy of Chinese medicine.

2.3 Differences in Their Philosophical Foundations

Philosophy, the core of culture and the theoretical thinking of the top level, has been guiding the development of medicine and other subjects of science. Western thinking mode is known as analytical thinking, causal thinking, or conceptual thinking, on the basis of which the mechanism, reductionism, dichotomy formed and greatly promoted the development of Western medicine.

Surgery and organ transplantation medicine have developed on the basis of the mechanism which views the human body as a "machine".

On the basis of reductionist ideology or reductionism - that is, it seeks to understand a system by breaking it down into its constituent parts, experimental physiology and cellular biology were founded in the 19th century and molecular biology was founded in the 20th century; influenced by such a thinking, Western medicine has studied various systems and organs of the body down to cells, to

---

333 Hou Weirui. 1988: 278.

molecules, and to genes in the recent 2 centuries, and constructed a series branches of learning of basic medicine, thus forming the so-called "scientific" Western medicine.

Dichotomy, philosophy of a division into two opposite parts - A and Non-A, indicates the separation of the subject and object, of the nature and man, of the time and space, of the body and mind, of the ontology and epistemology, ect., and guides the treating principle of Western medicine as well which treats a condition using drugs which produce opposite symptoms to those of the condition.

Classical Chinese thinking mode is known as correlative thinking, which originated in the *Book of Changes* and is mainly characterized by explaining dynamic life processes by opposing and complementing as the Yin-Yang Diaphragm suggests. The correlative thinking sees everything in the universe as interdependent and interactive. In Chinese medicine, the correlative thinking manifests itself concretely in the yin-yang theory, the five-phase theory, and the visceral image theory, the vessel theory, etc., which evolved in the way of following the features of the heaven and the earth (nature) to the human being from concrete to abstract, from structure to function. In Chinese medicine, disease is regarded as the result of imbalance or disharmony of yin and yang, and the goal of Chinese medical treatment is to restore the balance for each individual under his or her own unique environment.

Actually, correlative thinking mode of Eastern tradition and causal thinking mode of Western tradition depend on each other and complement to each other, to some extent oppose to each other. Both together will surely make a better world for the mankind. More and more scholars of the West and the East have recognized this point.

Compared to the Western philosophical thinking mode, classical Chinese philosophical thinking mode is not inferior at all, but can be a perfect complement to the Western philosophical thinking. The two traditions should understand each other, respect each other. Only in this way, each tradition can understand its own culture more thoroughly; the two traditions can promote each other and develop together.

That is to say, there are no ranking cultures. Actually, both correlative thinking mode of Eastern tradition and causal thinking mode of Western tradition have their advantages and disadvantages, thus can complement to each other in an almost perfect way. Intercultural activities such as translation and intercultural philosophy can make them understand each other, promote each other and develop together.

I would like to reformulate Confucius's statement "Men of noble character can be harmonious but different" in this way: Culture, Philosophy and Medicine of East and West are different but together can make a harmonious world.

2.4 The Incompatible Thinking of Chinese Medicine with Western Medicine

Chinese medicine originated from China, its concepts, theories and clinical explorations have been deeply rooted in and have been in perfect harmony with Chinese culture after going through thousands of years of development. And the Table 14 shows that Chinese medicine is another complete medical knowledge system incompatible with Western medicine in ontology, methodology, way of thinking, theoretical structure, practical experiences, and knowledge system.

	Chinese Thinking	**Western Thinking**
Ontology	Phenomena: unstable, emerging, and disappearing	Unchangeable, universal basis of changing things (Plato: Being)
Methodology	*Qu Xiang Bi Lei* or Taking Image and Analogizing: Governing changes	Deduction and Induction
Way of Thinking	Circular reasoning: one point is explained by all the others (relationship)	Linear reasoning: reason and cause (causality)
Theoretical Structure	Unity and joint development of theory and practice	Separation of theory and practice; theory guiding practice
Practical Experiences	Result of interaction and unification between subject and object	A passive information reception; stressing objectivity, trying to reduce subjectivity to zero
Knowledge System	Forming a direct line of succession	Continuously renewing itself with new research findings along with achievements in modern science and technology

Table 14 The Incompatible Thinking of Chinese Medicine With Western Medicine[334,335]

Kaptchuk applied portions of clinical studies to illustrate difference between Western and Eastern perceptions. Six patients with stomach pain were all diagnosed as having peptic ulcer disease by using upper-gastrointestinal X-ray or endoscopy by means of a fiberscope. From the perspective of Western medicine,

334 Wallner, Friedrich. 2009: 12.

335 Lan Fengli. Philosophical Reflections on Standard English Terminology of Chinese Medicine [J]. Medicine and Philosophy, 2010, 31 (7): 72-73.

they suffered from the same disease; and if they were treated by this doctor they would have accepted more or less the same treatment. Then this physician sent the patients to a doctor of Chinese medicine for examination.

Upon questioning and examining the patients, the physician of Chinese medicine found that they suffered from different kinds of pain: pain that increases at touch but diminishes with the application of cold compresses; or a minor but persistent discomfort, which can be somewhat alleviated by massage and heat; or very severe cramping pain; or sharp pain, which diminishes by massaging the abdomen, but heat and cold have no effect; or extremely severe stabbing pain in the stomach that sometimes goes around to the back, etc. Besides, their outlooks, behaviours, emotions, living conditions, images of pulse and tongue, accompanied symptoms all varied. Finally they were diagnosed as having six different patterns of disharmony: “Damp Heat Affecting the Spleen”, “Deficient Yin Affecting the Stomach” (also known as “Stomach Yin Deficiency”), “Exhausted Fire of the Middle Burner” (also known as "Deficient Cold Affecting the Spleen” or “Spleen Yang Deficiency”), “Excess Cold Dampness Affecting the Spleen and Stomach”, “Disharmony of the Liver Invading the Spleen”, and “Disharmony of Congealed Blood in the Stomach”. Of course, if they were treated by this doctor they would have accepted different individualized treatment based on their specific patterns.

You see, the Western physician starts with a symptom - stomach pain, then searches for the underlying cause by the aid of instruments - upper-gastrointestinal X-ray or endoscopy by means of a fiberscope, and then gives a precise diagnosis - peptic ulcer disease, and finally will administer a treatment which zeroes in on the focus, and tries to change, control or destroy. The physician does not care conditions of other aspects of the patient.

While, the Chinese physician, in contrast, collects and relates so much information and so many phenomena happening to the patient at the same time together, including symptoms, physical signs, subjective feelings, emotional and living conditions, images of tongue and pulse, etc., then forms a pattern of disharmony, and finally institutes individualized treatment based on this specific pattern to this individual.

This case also clarifies a common misunderstanding about Chinese medicine - Chinese medicine is not so exact as Western medicine. In fact, Chinese medicine is even much more exact than Western medicine for it cares the relationships among bodily events occurring at the same time while Western medicine just cares the focus - the ulcer, the cause of the stomach pain.

2.5 Strangification: Bridging Cultural Differences between Chinese Medicine and Western Medicine

Hence, a strict intercultural and interdisciplinary approach is necessary in order to bridge cultural differences between Chinese medicine and Western medicine, to disclose the thinking structure of Chinese medicine and to understand why

Chinese medicine has been working until now. Constructive Realism developed by Prof. Dr. Friedrich Wallner in the 1980s connects a hermeneutical Philosophy of Science with a constructive Philosophy of Science, which connects interpretation with construction. Thus it is an interdisciplinary and intercultural hermeneutical philosophy of science, which offers a methodology named "strangification" to make the implicit presuppositions explicit.

Constructive Realism aims at making the manifold scientific approaches depending on different cultures understandable. In fact, studies on the manifold scientific approaches are intimately related to another proposition that modern science results from European culture under specific conditions. Prof. Wallner holds that European science is not the only rational way of constructing the world, and there are still some other reasonable ways of constructing different aspects of the world in different approaches and based on different cultures, such as classical Chinese science.

Constructive Realism stresses the importance of understanding and interpreting science, and so Prof. Wallner introduced "Strangification" as its methodology for the sake of a valid and effective interpretation of a scientific system. "Strangification" is a coined word, a translation of the German word "Verfremdung". This methodology comes from the field of hermeneutics, which is a way of interpreting and understanding. Strangification is able to show the presuppositions of a scientific system, and represents one of the core ideas of Constructive Realism. How does the procedure of Strangification go? It follows a simple strategy: Take a proposition system or a concept out of its original context and put it into another different context, then observe what happens with the proposition system. The more different the other context is the better it is for the use of this methodology.

Strangification is proposed preconditioned that a scientific system is a proposition system based on certain presuppositions. That is to say, a certain scientific proposition system is not always true but only true under certain conditions. Strangification aims to improve scientific understanding by revealing and expressing the implicit theoretical presuppositions, which are actually the foundation of the scientific theories, arguments, approaches, conclusions and results. The equality and no ranking of different cultures and sciences is an essential prerequisite to the application of this methodology. "Mutual Strangification", i.e. strangification in double directions, can promote and realize self-understanding and mutual understanding between different cultures and different sciences.

For instance, transfer a proposition system from the context of Chinese medicine to the context of Western medicine but not in the aim of direct comparison. Then observe what will happen with the proposition system of Chinese medicine.[336] Take "*Pi* 脾" or Spleen as an example.[337]

In Western medicine, the spleen refers to the organ in the top part of the abdominal cavity behind the stomach and below the diaphragm; it is the largest lymphatic organ, appears to act to remove dead blood cells and fight infection; and an adult can live normally after his spleen has been removed. But the spleen in Chinese medicine is radically different from that in Western medicine except its location: The spleen is located in the middle *jiao*[338] (the center) and below the diaphragm. According to its central position and its yellow color, Chinese medicine attributes the spleen to the soil in the five phases. Soil is sowing and reaping, corresponding to the late summer in the seasons and dampness in the climate, representing the features of receiving, generating, transforming, and supporting. Therefore, the spleen's function in Chinese medicine is metaphorized as transforming the water and grain into essence, then moving and sending the essence to the whole body; thereby, the spleen is regarded as the foundation of postnatal existence, the source of the formation of *qi* and blood, is interrelated with the flesh, governs the limbs, opens into the mouth, manifests its brilliance in the lips, and so on. Finally a spleen complex system is formed. The common symptoms of the spleen diseases such as abdominal pain or distension, poor appetite, loose stool, diarrhea, jaundice, fatigue or weakness of the limbs, edema can be successfully relieved by treating the spleen in Chinese medicine. It is clear that the spleen in Chinese medicine does not refer to any concrete organ, maybe not the organ spleen at all (according to its central position and the yellow color, this organ may be the pancreas, which was not perceived by Chinese medicine in the ancient time), but to a functional system by applying the five-phase theory in the way of *Qu Xiang Bi Lei,* the methodological principle which demonstrates the circular reasoning and phenomena as reality guided by the idea of *Tian Ren He Yi,* the ontological principle and the presupposition of Chinese medicine. The spleen in Chinese medicine suggests a complex system, which is understood based on a holistic approach and emphasis of relations and functions.

Strangification has been always a way of mutual learning and understanding. Therefore, meanwhile, it is also clear that understanding of the spleen in Western

---

336 Wallner Fritz G.How to Deal with Science If You Care for Other Cultures: Constructive Realism in the Intercultural World [M]. Wien: Wilhelm Braumuller, 1997.

337 Lan Fengli. Metaphorizing: The Way to Bridge *The Book of Changes* and Chinese Medicine. In Wallner F.G, Schmisberger F., Wimmer F.M. (eds). 2010: 177-192.

338 "Energizer" is a standard translation for "*Jiao* 焦", which is approved by World Health Organization, such as "Triple Energizer" for "*San Jiao* 三焦". Actually, "Burner" is more popular than "energizer" in the English literature on Chinese medicine published in the West. But actually both translations are misleading. Pinyin transliteration is the best but far away from well-known. See Lan Fengli. A Corpus-Based Study on Cultural Connotations and Translation of Fundamental Concepts in Classical Chinese Texts [D]. Shanghai: Shanghai Jiao Tong University, 2008.

medicine is based on Reductionist Ideology with deduction and induction as its methodologies by taking an analytic approach, emphasizing morphological structure based on experimental studies.

By this way, you see the underlying reason that Chinese understanding of the spleen is so different from Western understanding of the spleen. The underlying reason is that they are based on different cultural presuppositions. Chinese understanding of the spleen is based on the specific cultural foundation of classical Chinese science, e.g. the philosophical theories of yin-yang and five phases, the methodology of *Qu Xiang Bi Lei* or Taking Image and Analogizing guided by the idea of *Tian Ren He Yi* or Universe and Man Uniting and Resembling Each Other, etc. and thus finally forming **a spleen complex system** which involves Universe and Man but centers the spleen; While Western understanding of the spleen is based on the cultural foundation of Western science, e.g. the analytic approach based on reductionist ideology, mechanism, dichotomy, the methodology of deduction and induction, the methods of anatomy and experiments, etc. Successful practice of Chinese medicine and Western medicine demonstrates that both understandings about the spleen are true under their own specific cultural presuppositions.

Strangification is really pretty precious under the background of the current prevalence of "West-Centralism" or "Europe-Centralism" in the world, just as Prof. Vincent Shen comments, "Strangification is a miraculous cure to resolve human dilemmas and philosophical difficulties, and a driving force that suggests the willingness to go unceasingly out of oneself, to head for others and the society, for other disciplines, for other cultures, for the nature, for the ideals and the holiness. It implies the primary noble generous spirit that is willing to go out of oneself and perfect oneself by mutual enriching each other"[339].

Based on the standpoint of Constructive Realism, Prof. Wallner advocates that Chinese medicine is a scientific system with its own specific methodology, and thus is completely incompatible with Western medicine for the ways they construct their microworlds are totally different from each other; that compared to science in general sense, Chinese medicine comes closer to humanities; and that "Chinese medicine has its claims for truth".

Science depends on culture. There are different cultures in the world, such as Islamic, Indian, Chinese, and Western cultures. Hence different scientific approaches based on different cultures are possible to reveal the manifoldness of the world to the mankind. I think that Chinese culture and Western culture are two major and influential different types of cultures originated and developed in incompatible but complementary approaches, from which classical Chinese science and modern Western science have evolved and developed. Strangification is a vital method for us to learn from and understand each other, on the basis of which a harmonious sustainable world will be set up in the future.

339 Shen Qingsong (known as Vincent Shen in the West). 2005: the Cover.

Languages are metaphoric in its essence and nature. …

- Ernst Cassirer[340]

3 *Qu Xiang Bi Lei*: The Metaphorizing Process & the Way to Form Metaphors in Chinese Medicine

Modernization of Chinese medicine must be directed by scientific methodology, and scientific methodology is in the field of philosophy, esp. the field of philosophy of science. The key tone of the modern Western philosophy focuses on analysis and understanding of the language. Language analysis plays a vital role in the scientific methodology, thus promoting the development of modern logic.

What is the definition of language? Today, language is redefined as "the means and process of man cognizing, understanding and stating the world".[341] The characteristics of this definition of language manifest in the following three aspects: first, "cognizing" and "stating" instead of being "communicative" and "systematic" ; second, "means", a kind of subjective behavior and manifestation of subjectivities, instead of "tool", an object; third, emphasizing "process". It is well known that language is dynamic, constantly changing, generating new words to meet the needs of the developments and changes of the world.

The founding of philosophy of language at the beginning of the last century is another "Copernican revolution" in the history of philosophy, which has deeply influenced philosophy of science, highlighting the vital role of linguistic analysis in the scientific methodology, thus promoting the development of modern logic. Modern logic stresses the role of language, and regards a scientific theory as a language system, being composed of word items, sentences, and their logic relationships.

How is the human being understood in Chinese medicine? How is the theoretical system of Chinese medicine formed, stated and constructed? How is the Chinese herbal theory constructed? How has Chinese medicine been developed? How should Chinese medicine be modernized? My answer to these questions is but one: metaphorizing.

3.1 Metaphor West and East: Similarities and Differences

3.1.1 Metaphor West and East: Origins

The English word "metaphor" originates from the Greek word "metaphora", which means "carrying across", i.e. "from one to the other". Metaphor studies in the West can be traced back to Aristotle's works such as *Poetics* and *Rhetoric*

340 Translated into English from Chinese. Gan Yang, Translator; Ernst Cassirer, Author. 2004: 152. Its Original Version is: An Essay on Man: An Introduction to a Philosophy of Human Culture [M]. New Heaven: Yale University Press, 1944.

341 Pan Wenguo. Redefining Language: Means and Process of Man Cognizing and Stating the Genuine World [J]. (Hongkong) Chinese Philology Correspondence. 2002, 2: 33-36.

(Aristotle, 384-322 B.C.) of the ancient Greek times. Later on, many philosophers, linguists and scholars of other disciplines have developed many different theories on metaphor in different times in the West.

Metaphor studies in China have a unique and original style, including important concepts such as "word-image-idea (yan-xiang-yi, 言—象—意)" in the field of philosophy, "*fu-bi-xing* (賦—比—興)[2]" in the field of poetics, "analogy-metaphor (pi-yu, 譬—喻)" in the field of rhetoric, "implication (yin xiu, 隱秀)" and "artistic conception [qing jing, 情景 (境)]" in the field of aesthetics, etc., thus running through classical Chinese philosophy, poetics, rhetoric, and aesthetics. Compared to metaphor studies in the West, they are not inferior at all no matter in the scope or the depth. Besides, they interpret "metaphor" from another specific angle of view, embodying the distinctive cultural and national features of China.

As early as in the Pre-Qin days (before 221 B.C.) [3], the ancient Chinese people did a deep-going research on "metaphor". Actually, *The Book of Changes*, which is composed of symbols (divinatory trigram image, *gua xiang*, 卦象) and interpreting words (*gua ci*, 卦辞 and *yao ci*, 爻辞), is a remarkable piece of writing on metaphor, and occupies an immeasurable place in the metaphor studies of China.

3.1.2 Metaphor West and East: Similarities

As we know, no matter in the West or in China, metaphor is an important field of study shared in rhetoric, poetry, linguistics and philosophy. As a rhetorical skill, metaphor is given a much more extensive meaning by logic pragmatics, referring to phenomena of meaning transfer of language in the course of expression and exchange; As a basic cognitive activity, metaphor is the medium as well as the result of man's metaphoric cognitive activities, and an indispensable means by which man cognizes the world; And besides, metaphor is an indispensable feature of poetry. The poems by Tomas Tranströmer (1931-) are full of metaphors, and as we know, the author won the Noble prize for literature in 2011 "because, through his condensed, translucent **images**, he gives us fresh access to reality". Chinese poets stress particularly the expression of their feelings by different **images** too.

Language by itself contains a system of metaphor. This system is closely connected with man's thinking system. Language and symbol have formed a complete model that a nation cognizes and understands the world. Human beings have made themselves a whole. While metaphor is used, it brings back to life the image of human beings in the nature and the image of the nature of human beings as well.

3.1.3 Metaphors in Discourses of Western Science and Chinese Science: Similarities and Differences

Metaphors can be seen almost everywhere in seemingly objective scientific discourses[342] for metaphors play an absolutely necessary role in scientific

342 "Scientific discourses" here refer to "discourses of Western science".

exploration and dissemination of scientific thoughts.[343] In the recent years, studies on the essence, characteristics, methods, and principles of metaphors in Western scientific discourses have achieved important progress and gratifying outcome[344], but studies on metaphors in discourses of classical Chinese philosophy and science, which originated from *The Book of Changes*, are rarely seen. Among all the subjects of classical Chinese science, Chinese medicine remains to be the only one to survive up till today when facing the challenge from Western medicine; all the others like mathematics, astronomy, and engineering exist mainly in the field of study of history of science although they had gained splendid achievements before since corresponding Western sciences have been successfully transmitted to and disseminated in China.

What on earth is Chinese medicine? Is it just an indigenous folk art of healing, which has superficial understanding of human body and diseases and can be judged by Western scientific criteria? Or is it an independent, systematic, and complete medical system? My answer is: Chinese medicine originated from China, its concepts, theories and clinical explorations have been deeply rooted in and have been in perfect harmony with Chinese culture after going through thousands of years of development. And the Table 14 shows that Chinese medicine is another complete medical knowledge system incompatible with Western medicine in ontology, methodology, way of thinking, theoretical structure, and practical experiences.

Western medicine is an applied science based on the achievements of modern Western science and technology. Metaphors exist almost everywhere in discourses of Western science and Chinese medicine, and the essence, characteristics, methods, and principles of which are exactly no different from each other.

The significant difference lies in that: What Western scientific discourse has been always seeking is objective description, Western science takes deduction and induction as its core methodologies, and the functions of metaphors in scientific cognition and exploration has always been in a marginal position in Western science; while Chinese medicine takes *Qu Xiang Bi Lei* or Taking Image and Analogizing as its core methodology, and is metaphorical from the formation of its concepts, construction of its theoretical framework, to the development of its clinical explorations, and even to the whole system. In other words, the functions of metaphors in scientific cognition and exploration have always been in the core position in Chinese medicine. I think that is the fundamental difference in between Western science and Chinese medicine, and that study on metaphors in Chinese medicine can reveal values of classical Chinese science.

Metaphors in Chinese medicine bear specific features of classical Chinese culture and science. Chen Kui 陈骙 (1128-1203) pointed out in his *Wen Ze* or

343 Dong Hongle. 2005: Synopsis.
344 Guo Guichun. Metaphor, Rhetoric, and Scientific Interpretation [M]. Beijing: Science Press, 2007.

Writing Principles that "*The Book of Changes* has ***Xiang*** **or Image** to fully express its ideas; *The Classic of Poetry* has ***Bi*** **or Analogy** to convey its feelings; and so how could the composition writing go if without ***Yu*** **or Metaphor**?" Chen Kui showed clearly the three key elements of metaphor studies of Chinese tradition: "Image, Analogy, Metaphor", or rather, "Imaging, Analogizing, Metaphorizing". Thus Metaphor is not only a kind of formless thinking process, but also visible language forms.

3.1.4 Philosophical Foundations of *Qu Xiang Bi Lei*

The theme of Chinese philosophy is to probe into the relationship between the "heaven (universe) and man", and classical Chinese philosophy believes that "The heaven (universe) and man unit each other, and resemble (mirror) each other". The *Tian Ren He Yi* or "Universe and Man Uniting and Resembling each other" makes up the ontological presupposition of Chinese medicine.

Huang Di's Inner Classic states that "Man is born on the earth, hanging his life to the heaven. The union of *qi* of Heaven and Earth gives birth to Man. Man can adapt himself to the seasons for Heaven and Earth are his parents". It can be seen that Heaven, Earth and Man constitute with the same ingredient - *Qi* in the same way, thus Uniting and Resembling Each Other, which is abbreviated as "Heaven (Universe) and Man Uniting and Resembling Each Other".

The same constituent - *Qi* is the very basis of "Universe and Man Uniting and Resembling Each Other". The worldview determines the methodology. Chinese medicine believes that everything in the world is universally related to each other, that the world is composed of the same constituent, that the immense variety of things and phenomena in the world share some similar characteristics at different levels, different categories, and different aspects, and moreover, there exist many necessary relationships among them.

"Languages are metaphoric in its essence and nature...." "We should not content ourselves to the present state of language. We have to trace back to the origins of words if we want to discover the ties which link the words and their references". (Ernst Cassirer)

Chinese characters or sinograms are a kind of logographic writing based on pictographs, and *Qu Xiang Bi Lei* is the core methodology of Chinese medicine. Metaphor is universal in Chinese medical language from words, phrases to sentences, reflecting how basic Chinese medical concepts and theories were formed, stated, and constructed, and how Chinese medicine has been developed, determining that Chinese medicine is a metaphor system in its underlying structure. Therefore, the metaphor system formed by the way of *Qu Xiang Bi Lei* is the deep structure of Chinese medicine.

Based on the philosophical foundation of *Tian Ren He Yi* or Universe and Man Uniting and Resembling Each Other, the ontological Chinese medical concepts and theories were formed, stated and constructed, and Chinese medicine has been developed by the way of Metaphorizing, or *Qu Xiang Bi Lei* or Taking Image and Analogizing:

Introducing and constructing the theories of essential *qi*, yin-yang, and five phases to explain physiological functions and pathological changes of human being, and to guide diagnosis and treatment of diseases in the clinical practice;

Constructing the visceral image system to interpret functions of *zang fu* organs;

Inferring the flow of *qi* and blood to expound physiology of yang *qi*;

Constructing the *Jing-Luo* or Vessel theory to elaborate the amount of yin, yang, *qi* and blood in different meridian-vessels;

Constructing the theories of etiology and pathogenesis to interpret the onset and development of diseases;

Constructing the therapeutic system to interpret actions of acupoints and medicinals, and thus determining principles and methods of treatment.

3.2 Three Key Processes of *Qu Xiang Bi Lei*: Imaging – Analogizing – Metaphorizing

Qu Xiang Bi Lei or Taking Image and Analogizing is the core methodology of Chinese medicine. Its procedure "Observing Objects - Taking Image - Analogizing - Understanding Tao" runs through almost all the aspects of Chinese medicine from forming its fundamental concepts, elaborating its theories, to developing its clinical explorations, embodying the thinking process of "Imaging - Analogizing - Metaphorizing", finally forming metaphors in Chinese medicine, guiding clinical practice, and developing Chinese medicine as well. Based on the three key elements i.e. "Imaging - Analogizing – Metaphorizing" in classical Chinese metaphor studies, I advance and demonstrate that *Qu Xiang Bi Lei* or Taking Image and Analogizing is the metaphorizing process and the way of forming metaphors in Chinese medicine.

3.2.1 "*Xiang* 象": From Elephant to Imaging

Xiang is an important concept of classical Chinese culture and Chinese medicine as well. Wang Fuzhi 王夫之 (1619-1692) said in his *Zhou Yi Wai Zhuan* or *Outer Interpretation of The Book of Changes* that "What fills the world is all *Xiang*. The rhetoric *Bi* and *Xing* in *The Classic of Poetry*, the political affairs in *The Book of Documents*, a person's status in *The Spring and Autumn Annals*, the ceremonies in *The Book of Rites*, and the rhymes in *The Classic of Music* are nothing but *Xiang*, while *The Book of Changes* unites and gathers all the principles of them". Thus we can say that classical Chinese culture is a kind of *Xiang* culture, and Chinese medicine is kind of *Xiang* medicine.

Maybe some people think that the concept of *Xiang* is primitive and old-fashioned. But if we take a look at the Quantum mechanics, we will know that this is not the case. Classical mechanics believes that all the objects can be clearly classified into two categories: waves and particles. The typical example of the former is light, and the later particles compose what we name "materials". But in

1905, Albert Einstein (1879-1955) advanced interpretation of photoelectric effect with light quantum, and then people realize that the light bears double features of both waves and particles simultaneously, i.e. wave-particle duality of the light. So, the question is: what on earth is the light, wave or particle? Which on earth is the phenomenon, and which on earth is the essence? I think at the moment nobody can answer such questions because they are far beyond the scope of our knowledge.

Then, what is "*Xiang*"?

3.2.1.1 The Original Meaning of "*Xiang* 象": Elephant

The original meaning of "*xiang* 象" is Elephant, as *The Origin of Chinese Characters* states that "*Xiang* 象, with long nose and teeth, a big mammal in the Southern Yue area, will be pregnant every three years". See the Illus.6, which shows how the sinogram "象" was conceived in the way of resembling the real image of an elephant, and the Illus. 7, which shows the evolution process of the sinogram "象 *Xiang*".

In remote antiquity, the elephant had lived in the Central Plains of China. Later on, the elephant had to migrate south because of the changes in climate, so the people in the Central Plains had few opportunities to see live elephants again. Han Fei, a famous philosopher and the representative of the Legalists of the late Warring States Period (475-221B.C.), said in the chapter of *Jie Lao Pian* of *Han Fei Tzu* 韩非子·解老篇 that "people seldom see the live elephant, but has gained the skeleton of a dead one, so they can imagine what it is like after investigating the picture or image of its skeleton. Therefore, all in people's imagination is known as '*xiang*'". This quotation also reveals the mystery of the origin of the Chinese compound "*xiang xiang*" (想象， literally "thinking or imagining elephant", means "imaging or imagination"), setting off "*xiang* 象"'s "imagining" cultural connotations.

We can see that "*xiang*" originally evolved from "seeking similarities" between things from the angle of genetics, as stated in *The Book of Changes* "*xiang* refers to something being like or resembling this thing". It is well known that Chinese characters are a kind of "*Xiang Xing* 象形" writing, which literally means "resembling shape", or pictographic, logographic, or ideographic writing in English. That is to say, the sinograms are based on pictures, images, and surely suggest the imaging thinking of Chinese culture.

It is thus clear that in classical Chinese thinking, "*Xiang* or Image" and the process of "*Xiang Xiang* or Imaging" are integrated as one. While in the background of Western thinking – Dichotomy, the Westerner makes a clear-cut division between the visible "*Xiang* or Image" and man's thinking process "*Xiang Xiang* or Imaging" because the subject is completely separated from the nature.

Ontologically, Western philosophy observes one in the two aspects or in the way of dichotomy, i.e. phenomenon and essence; while classical Chinese philosophy observes one in the three aspects, i.e. Tao or Way 道, *Xiang* or Image 象, and *Qi* or Concrete Objects with Shape 器. *The Book of Changes* states that "The visible is *Xiang* 象, and the shapeable is *Qi* 器"; And that "That which lies beyond shapes and features is Tao, and all things that lie within shapes and features are *Qi* 器". Pang Pu 庞朴 (1928-) made a penetrating analysis about this: "Tao, *Xiang*, and *Qi* 器 relate to each other step by step: Tao, without Image or Shape, but can govern *Xiang* or Image; *Xiang*, with Image but no Shape, but can signify Shape; *Qi* 器, with no Image but shape, but in the shape *Xiang* and *Tao* reside."; "Therefore, we can say that in between or the middle of 'That which lies beyond shapes and features is Tao, and all things that lie within shapes and features are *Qi* 器' is 'That which lies in the middle of Tao and *Qi* 器' should be named as '*Xiang*'!"[345]

The division between phenomenon and essence, representation and reality is the outcome of artificial division between the subject and the object in the Western thinking; while such a division does not exist in classical Chinese thinking. Actually, "*Xiang*" implies all the possibilities of reality, which explains why metaphors are so important for Chinese medicine; While Language can only provide one or two possibilities, so metaphors are much richer than language. In this sense, "metaphors" are "*Xiang*" in language.[346]

3.2.1.2 *Xiang* as Reality

First, let us distinguish three types of reality or three essential and fundamental dimensions of scientific work: "Wirklichkeit", "Life World", and "Realität". "Realität" and "Wirklichkeit" both mean "Reality" in English. Actually, they are very different from each other: "Wirklichkeit" refers to the being or the existence of the universe, or "Reality as Environment and Condition for Living"; "Realität" refers to "Constructed Reality" or "Microworld"; in between is the "Life World", the world we live in.

Actually what the notions "Wirklichkeit", "Life World", and "Realität" name are three different dimensions in science and life. "Realität" describes the scientific microworld, the world that is constructed by selecting, excluding and reducing qualities of the object, a process that is guided by theory; "Wirklichkeit" describes the genuine world, the world that depicts the fundament for "Realität" and the basis for the selection, exclusion, and reduction; the "life world" describes the world the people live in, and people from different cultures have different life worlds. Both "Realität" and "Life World" take "Wirklichkeit" as the basis for their selection and reduction. The relationships among the three are different in different cultures.

---

345 Pang Pu. 1995: 231.

346 Wallner Friedrich, Lan Fengli. Ontological Ambiguity and Methodological Circularity: *Qu-Xiang Bi-Lei*. In Wallner F.G., Schmisberger F., Wimmer F.M. (eds). 2010: 163-176.

For example, Western medicine is formed by a process of selecting, excluding, and reducing qualities of the object guided by Western thinking, the same as the way Western science is formed by; and both seek universality and objectivity. Western medicine can be considered as an artificial and constructed microworld that is based on selecting, excluding and reducing a world we name "Wirklichkeit". It is quite far away from the life world of the Western people. While Chinese medicine is formed by a process of selecting, excluding, and reducing qualities of the object guided by classical Chinese thinking, which focuses on constantly changing, flowing, emerging and disappearing phenomena or image. It can be considered as another artificial and constructed microworld that is based on selecting, excluding and reducing a world we name "Wirklichkeit". But Chinese medicine goes much closer to the "life world" of the Chinese people than Western medicine goes to the "life world" of the Western people. And all artificial and constructed microworlds make up the "Realität", the part all the human beings know by different approaches, the part which is still far smaller than the "Wirklichkeit".

Then it is not difficult to understand - There is manifoldness of perceiving the world, not just one way and not just one solution. There are several and different possibilities of referring to the world, different ways of selecting, excluding, and reducing the "Wirklichkeit" and/or the "life worlds". Based on this reductive reference and the legitimate manifoldness of different references we can propose that Chinese medicine can be also considered as a scientific system that has its own and alternative reference to the world and its own approach to its object. Thus it also has a legitimate claim for truth without getting into contradiction with other different systems like Western medicine. It can also be incompatible with Western medicine for both have different ways of constructing their microworlds.[347]

Actually it is very difficult to make a strict distinction between visible phenomena and man's imagination. And therefore it is very important to understand the differences between phenomena and noumena. Western science has always pursuing objectivity, and believes that what is left after removing all the subjectivities is the real. In the Western thinking, pictures and phenomena are all illusions, and cannot replace the thing. Friedrich Schiller (1759-1805), one of the great poets and philosophers of Germany, reflected this Western thinking on picture in his famous poem – "*The Veiled Statue at Sais*" (See the poem at the end of this chapter) – Uncover the veil (phenomena) and go beyond it to the essence.

We can see from the concept of *Xiang* that *Xiang* is not representation of reality, but an offer of reality itself. *Xiang* is another "Realität" based on the same "Wirklichkeit", but goes closer to the "life world" of the Chinese people, and thus

347 Wallner, Friedrich. How to Research TCM. In Wallner F.G., Kubiena G., Jandl M.J.(eds). 2009: 22-45.

is another reality. In one word, *Xiang* is the reality in classical Chinese culture and science.

3.2.1.3 The *Xiang* Taken: Image

The key of *Qu Xiang* or "Taking *Xiang*" is "*Xiang*", which exists in the following two forms:

One is the phenomena or image the object manifests itself outwardly, which can be perceived and caught by sense organs, as Wang Bing 王冰 (710-804) said that "*Xiang* is what manifests outwardly and can be seen";

The other is moving *Xiang*, a kind of dynamic functional pattern in the world, which is constantly emerging, disappearing, and changing; it lays particular emphasis on function but not shape or material, as *The Book of Changes* states that "The changes and transformations of the heaven and the earth is what the sages follow;" "*Yao*, the line in the Eight Diagrams, follows moving images of the land under the heaven (i.e. the world)."

The whole process of *Qu Xiang* lies in observing *Xiang* and taking *Xiang*. The following four concepts indicate the progressive process of *Qu Xiang* or Taking image.

- ***Wu xiang*** 物象, refers to the appearance, phenomena the object manifests itself outwardly, and is the existing or being form of the object itself, only after it is internalized as man's conceptual image can it enter the thinking process.

- ***Zhi jue xing xiang*** 知覺形象, literally means "perceptual image", comes directly from *wu xiang*, referring to the intuition image the subject produces when the *wu xiang* acts on man's sense organs, which can not go into the thinking process for it cannot depart from the direct action of the *wu xiang* on the sense organs. But it is a necessary step in the process of internalization of the *wu xiang*. After the perception caused by the *wu xiang* disappears, there remains more or less trace of the perceptual image or *zhi jue xing xiang* in man's brain, such trace left in man's memory is known as *biao xiang* or external image.

- ***Biao xiang*** 表象, literally means "external image", is the internalized *wu xiang*, referring to the image of the object taken, stored and reflected by man's brain after repeatedly feeling, perceiving the *wu xiang* many times.

- ***Yi xiang*** 意象, literally means "imagery image" or "image in imagination", is usually translated into "image" and is defined differently by different scholars of the same or different disciplines. It is generally believed that *yi xiang* refers to the result of generalizing and abstracting the image information of the common characters of the objects of the same category, and is the rational image generalized from *biao xiang* or the external image, is the unity of the external image of the object and the subject's deep understanding of it. *Yi xiang* is the cell of the imaging thinking, running through the imaging thinking process from the beginning to the end.[348]

In fact, what is finally taken is ***Yi xiang*** 意象 or image. Wang Yuxiong 汪裕雄 (1937-) pointed out that "Image has been held in high esteem in Chinese culture, which is the so-called 'esteeming image'. This is a fact that every person gradually influenced by this culture will agree with. *The Book of Changes* applies the method of observing phenomena & image (*guan xiang*, 观象) and making instruments (*zhi qi*, 制器) to explain the origin of Chinese culture; Sinograms take 'resembling image or pictographic' as the foundation of their etymologies; Chinese medicine advocates visceral image theory; classical Chinese astronomy and calendar system stress observing phenomena & image (*guan xiang*, 观象) and issuing an official calendar (*shou shi*, 授时); Chinese aesthetic tradition takes image as its central domain, and regards full, rich image as its general appreciation of the beauty … Image, just like a huge net, encompasses all the fields of Chinese culture."[349]

3.2.2 "*Bi* 比": From "Shoulder to Shoulder" to Analogizing

The sinogram "比 *Bi*", an associative compound, follows 二 and 匕, and the 匕 also indicates pronunciation. It is written as 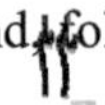 in the oracle script, which resembles the image of two persons keeping in step with each other and walking shoulder to shoulder or side by side. The shape is just like another sinogram "从 *Cong*" or to follow written as 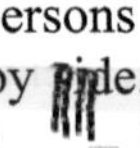 in *The Origin of Chinese Characters* but just in the opposite direction. *The Origin of Chinese Characters* reads that "Two persons make up '*Cong* 从'; Reversing '*Cong* 从' is '*Bi* 比'."The original meaning of "*Bi* 比" is "shoulder to shoulder"; "side by side".

Zhu Xi 朱熹 (1130-1200) explained "*Bi* 比", one of the three formulas for the creation of *The Classic of Poetry*, as "*Bi* is to compare that thing with this thing", which basically accords with what Huang Che 黄彻 (1093-1168) said that "*Bi* is to quote one thing with reference to other things of the same category". *Bi* in the context of *Qu Xiang Bi Lei* refers to *Bi Xiang*, i.e. to analogize with the taken image, and thus can be translated into "Analogizing". *Bi Xiang* actually refers to a method of comparing the thing which needs to be known with the image which has already taken to catch and find similarities between them, and then migrating, transferring, and inferring the knowledge from the already known image to the thing which needs to be known through metaphorizing, and so to understand its qualities or functions.

Qu Xiang Bi Lei, the core methodology of Chinese medicine, is summarized into the following four steps according to *The Book of Changes:* ① Observing the

348 Xing Yurui. 2004: 196-198.
349 Wang Yuxiong. 1996:4.

object 观物: directly observing the object or phenomenon; ② Taking image 取象: summarizing and refining the image of the object after repeatedly observing and feeling it; ③ Comparing and Analogizing 比类: comparing the things which need to understand or know with the "image (*xiang*, 象)" just taken; ④ Understanding Tao or the Way, the Rule 体道: finding the rules through the above comparing and analogizing activities.

The prominent characteristics of this methodology are as follows: ① "*Xiang*" is its foundation with observing *xiang* and taking *xiang* as key steps; ② the thinking manifests as transformation and flow of "*xiang*" as well as the contradictory movement between "*xiang*" and intuition; ③ *Bi Lei* or Analogizing is to compare, find, and catch the similarities between the two different kinds of things, then migrate and infer the knowledge of one thing to the other.

Qu Xiang Bi Lei is an immanent methodology which is given by the activity. It holds that things present themselves with phenomena or images, and abstractions and concepts which are not illustrative do not exist in classical Chinese thinking. This is similar to the core idea of phenomenology: to go back to the things.

3.2.3 "*Yu* 喻": Metaphor and Metaphorizing

"*Yu* 喻" is a signific-phonetic sinogram and originally means "to inform" as explained in *Guang Ya*[350]. The last step of *Qu Xiang Bi Lei* is "Understanding Tao". Briefly speaking, this Tao is "*Yu* 喻", which is both a gerund - metaphorizing, a formless thinking process, and a noun - metaphor, a concrete language form. Therefore, I advance that *Qu Xiang Bi Lei* is the metaphorizing process and the way to form metaphors in Chinese medicine. Specifically speaking, it manifests in the following three aspects in Chinese medicine:

① Constructing Theoretical System (Theory): Forming systematic metaphors - image-taking based nomenclature to name basic concepts, stating and constructing the theoretical system of Chinese medicine;

② Guiding Clinical Practice (Practice): Grasping the hidden essence or telling the interior through observing the external image or manifestation such as in the processes of making diagnosis and identifying pattern in the practice, which is also a metaphorizing process;

③ Gaining New Knowledge through Metaphorizing (Development): Inferring the unknown through the known image, such as developing new theories and therapeutic methods.

3.2.3.1 Constructing Theoretical System

The theoretical system is constructed by forming systematic metaphors, i.e. image-taking based nomenclature. *Qu Xiang Bi Lei* extensively embodies in the

---

350 *Guang Ya* 广雅, the earliest encyclopaedia dictionary in China with the aim to explain sinograms in ancient books, was compiled by Zhang Yi 张揖 (?-?) of the Three Kingdoms Period (220-265).

nomenclature of core concepts of Chinese medicine, which I name it as "Image-Taking Based Nomenclature to Form Systematic Metaphors" – and thus constructing the theoretical system in Chinese medicine from understanding of the human being, the onset and development of a disease, making diagnosis, to instituting corresponding treatment based on pattern identification.

For example, "*Qi* 气", originally means "cloud, a pictographic sinogram", an image taken from the nature, and is used to name "the essential nutrient substance flowing in the body"; "*Zang Fu* 藏府", originally means "depots and palaces", a pair of images taken from life and official system, and is used to name the organs of the human being; the meridians of the human being are named by metaphorizing the rivers of the earth, an image taken from the nature; the weight and graduated arm of a steelyard as well as a pair of compasses and carpenter's square are used to describe the pulse images of the four seasons, which are images taken from everyday life; "closing door to keep the invader"- e.g. administering tonics for a patient with externally contracted febrile disease will keep the external pernicious influences inside the body, and"struggle between the Upright and the Evil"- i.e. the fight between the healthy *qi* and pathogenic agents, which will determine whether a person will catch a disease or not, are named by metaphorizing events of military affairs; "Monarch, Minister, Assistant, and Envoy", images taken from political affairs, are used to name the principles and strategies of composing a prescription; and so and so forth. For the limitation of the class hours, here I just give you one detailed example, *Jing Luo* 经络.

Several translations are available for "經絡系統": "Meridian System" is the standard translation approved by WHO, but the word "Meridian" only indicates a two-dimensional grid while *Jing Luo* system is supposed to carry *qi* and blood, and thus must be a three-dimensional system; "Channel System" is the most popular translation in the English literature on Chinese medicine, but the word "Channel" is polysemous; We think "Vessel System", a translation in *Huang Di Nei Jing Su Wen* by Paul U. Unschuld in 2003 is the best translation if we take into account the origin and development of the concepts of *Mai* (脈, vessel) and *Jing-Luo* (經絡).

Based on some anatomical knowledge on *Mai* (脈, vessel) and medical practice esp. the application of acupuncture, moxibustion, *tuina* or Chinese massage, and *qigong* or breathing exercise, the concepts of *Jing-Luo* (經絡) are actually metaphors formed in the way of observing, taking images of and analogizing the water flow in the rivers under the earth and the longitudinal lines of the textiles, which are embodied in their writing forms. The chapter *Water & Earth* of *Guan Tzu* states that "Water is the *qi* and blood of the earth, running on (under) the earth just like *qi* and blood flowing in the vessels".

The simplified form of "*mai* 脉" has 4 variant original complex forms.[351]

351 Li Ding. Rationality of Acupuncture: The Origin and Development of Theories of Vessels and Acupoints. In Lan FL, Wallner F. G., Wobovnik C. (eds)2011: 191.

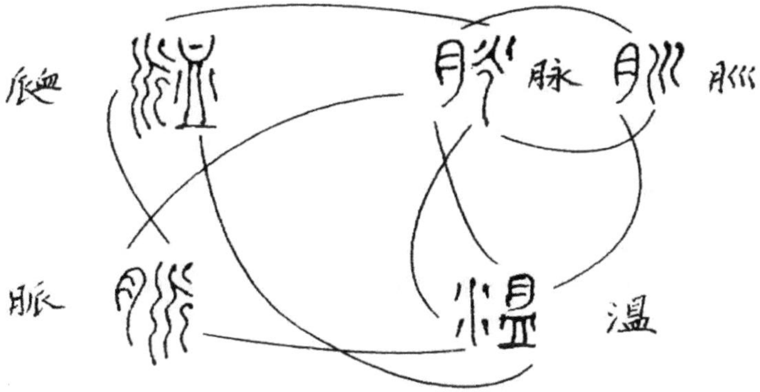

Illus. 23 Variant Original Complex Forms of "*Mai* 脉"

脈 and 衇 are its common original complex forms. Its lesser seal script is . This sinogram is a signifc-phonetic compound: the left part is the signific component 月 (flesh moon) or 血 (blood), indicating that *mai* (脈) functions to carry and move blood and is a part of the body; and the right part is the phonetic, indicating both pronunciation and meaning at the same time. In medical books unearthed from Mawangdui Han Tomb, most writing forms of "*mai* 脈" were written as "温". "水" is the variant form of " 氵 ", "目" the variant form of "flesh 肉", "皿" the variant form of "blood 血". The structure of the sinogram has clearly illustrated that the ancients analogized or metaphorized water flow with blood flow.[352] It is thus clear that "*mai*" of the early days referred to blood vessel, so "*mai* 脉" is also known as "blood vessel 血脈", as stated in *Huang Di Nei Jing Su Wen · Mai Yao Jing Wei Lun* or *Huang Di's Inner Classic ·Basic Questions ·Discourse on Subtleties and Essentials of Vessels* "the vessels 脈 are the residence of the blood"(Attention: *Qi* does not appear in this quotation).

The concepts "*jing*" and "*luo*" appeared later than "*mai* or vessel". *Jing* and *luo* are further divisions of "*mai* or vessel", i.e. "*jing*" vessel and "*luo*" vessel, which was first recorded in the *Huang Di Nei Jing Ling Shu. Mai Du* or *Huang Di's Inner Classic · Miraculous Pivot · On Vessels* "*Jing* vessels reside in the interior; their branches running transversely are known as *luo* vessels; the branches of *luo* vessels are known as grandchild vessels".

The sinograms "經 *jing*" and "絡 *luo*" share the same radical – the silk part "糸", which is originally used in the textiles. The concept "*jingmai* 經脈" is a metaphor formed in the way of *Qu Xiang Bi Lei* or taking images and analogizing. The right part of "經" is "巠"， indicating both pronunciation and meaning, which is interpreted in *The Origin of Chinese Characters* as "water vessels, following

352 Li Ding. 1998: 2-3.

（川, pictographic, indicating rivers）, under the 一; 一, refers to the earth", that is to say, "坙" refers to the water vessels running under the earth. *Jing* 經 is explained in *The Origin of Chinese Characters* as "the longitudinal lines of the textiles". The reason that "*Jing* 經" is used to name the main stems of the vessels is closely related to the origin of the character "*jing* 經", which contains two images and reflects the similarities between the longitudinal lines of the textiles, the rivers running under the earth and the running routes of the main stems of the vessels. Another part of "luo 絡" is "各", indicating both pronunciation and meaning, which is interpreted in *The Origin of Chinese Characters* as "divergence of views being different". Another interpretation of *Luo* 絡 is that "It originally meant unreeled silk, hemp, or cotton fiber, and from its association with stringy fibers came to be used in Chinese medicine as a noun that means network and as a verb that means to net".[353] Anyway, 絡 is used to name divergent branches of the vessels.

Huang Di Nei Jing Ling Shu. Ben Zang or *Huang Di's Inner Classic · Miraculous Pivot · On Viscera* states that "*Jing* vessels 經脈 function to move *qi* and blood, nourish yin and yang, moisten tendons and bones, and lubricate joints". Compared to the statement that "The vessels 脈 are the residence of the blood", quite a lot new contents were supplemented to *jing* vessels, among which the most remarkable point is that the function of moving **blood** was extended to moving ***qi* and blood.**

"*Xue mai* 血脈", "*jing* 經" and "*luo* 絡" appeared together in the *Han Shu·Yi Wen Zhi* or *Treatise on Literature* of *The History of The Former Han Dynasty* 汉书·艺文志, "Medical classics explore the origins of **blood vessels 血脈, *jing-luo*** 經絡, bone marrow, yin-yang, exterior and interior in order to treat various diseases from the root", where seemingly differentiated blood vessels from *jing-luo*.

Jing-luo 經絡 functions to carry and move *qi* and blood in the body. *Guan Tzu · Water & Earth* states that "Water is the *qi* and blood of the earth, running on the earth which is just like *qi* and blood flowing in the vessels". Judged from the cognizing order, the flow of *qi* and blood in man is analogized and inferred from the natural phenomenon of water flow in the rivers under the earth. The extensions from "vessel 脈" to "*jing-luo* 經絡" and from "blood" to "*qi* and blood" are also closely related to the application of acupuncture, moxibustion, *tuina*, *qigong*, etc, which explore the phenomenon of *qi* and blood flowing in the body, thus enriching the understanding on the "vessels".

Seeing that "*jing* 經" and "*luo* 絡" are subdivisions of "*Mai* 脉" or Vessel, i.e. *Jing* Vessel and *Luo* Vessel, *Jing-Luo* system is surely the "Vessel system" – being mainly composed of *Jing* Vessels and *Luo* Vessels.

353 Wiseman Nigel, Zhang Yuhuan. 2003: 174.

To sum up, the concepts and theory of *jing-luo* were formed first on the basis of some anatomical knowledge on "vessel 脈"; then by the way of *Qu Xiang Bi Lei*, i.e. observing and taking images of the water flow in the rivers on/under the earth and the longitudinal lines of textiles, then analogizing, enlightened by the idea of *Tian Ren He Yi*; and then have been proved and modified in the medical practice esp. the application of acupuncture, moxibustion, *tuina*, and *qigong*. That is to say, *jing-luo* or the vessels are metaphors, referring to the circular or round pathways of the living system.

Therefore, we believe that it will take forever to find any three-dimensional structure of *jing-luo* 經絡 through dissecting dead human bodies. *Jing-luo* 經絡 system or the vessel system is more like a functional concept reflecting a certain image, which is embodied in their writing forms. As stated in the *Huang Di's Inner Classic · Basic Questions · Discourse on Leaving and Uniting of True Qi and Evil Qi* (huang di nei jing su wen·li he zhen xie lun) "The sages formulated principles, which must conform to the nature. Therefore, the heaven has 365 degrees and 28 constellations, the earth has 12 *jing* rivers, and man has 12 *jing* vessels".

3.2.3.2 Guiding Clinical Practice

Lakoff and Johnson clearly pointed out in their monograph *Metaphors We Live By*[354] that metaphor is not only a rhetoric figure of speech, but rather a way of cognition or even a way of behavior deeply rooted in the thinking. They defined metaphor as using one thing to understand another, and applied existence of concept metaphors to prove this point. Man's conceptual system controls man's thinking and behaviour. So if concepts are metaphorical then thinking and action will be surely metaphorical.

The diagnosing and treating procedure, in brief, is to synthesize the information and data from the four examinations – inspection, listening and smelling, inquiry, and palpation, then to diagnose which disease the patient suffers and which pattern the patient is identified, and then to institute treatment, all of which is known as "pattern identification and treatment". Metaphor thinking or metaphorizing, intentionally or subconsciously, guides the whole process of "identifying pattern and instituting treatment", also known as "pattern identification and treatment". For example, "Insomnia. Pattern of Liver Stagnation Transforming into Fire" presents with the following symptoms as described in the 5th edition textbook of *Chinese Internal medicine*[355]: Insomnia, irritability, bad temper, no desire for food, thirsty with desire for drink, reddish eyes, bitter mouth,

354 Lakoff, George & Johnson, Mark. Metaphors We Live By [M]. Chicago: The University of Chicago Press, 1980.

355 The description of this disease pattern is taken from the textbook of the fifth edition *Chinese Internal Medicine*. See Zhang Boyu. 1989: 113-116. But the interpretation afterwards is from the author.

dark yellow urine, constipation, red tongue with yellowish coating, wiry and rapid pulse, among which the "fire" symptoms are very prominent – bitter mouth, thirsty with desire for drink, red tongue with yellowish coating, and reddish eyes are caused by "fire flaming upwards" to the mouth, the tongue, and the eyes; dark yellow urine and constipation result from "fire disturbing downward"; irritability, bad temper, wiry and rapid pulse arise for this fire is not other kinds of fire but "liver fire". Therefore, in the clinical practice, a doctor of Chinese medicine will naturally relate the above mentioned symptoms to the fire and liver fire, and thus diagnose a patient with these symptoms as "Insomnia. Pattern of Liver Stagnation Transforming into Fire" after long-term learning, studying, and practicing Chinese medicine", and then institute corresponding treatment of herbal medication or acupuncture or other kinds of treatment. In the whole process the doctor naturally or subconsciously applies the metaphorizing thinking, and here "fire" is the key metaphor to reveal the intrinsic relationships among all the pathological phenomena simultaneously happening to the patient. That is to say, metaphor reveals relationships between the phenomena - clinical manifestations and the object - patient, and makes the doctor diagnose and treat the disease properly, and thus guiding the clinical practice.

3.2.3.3 Making New Explorations

"In the beginning, metaphors in scientific discourse may be not a kind of standardized scientific language, but can produce important scientific findings or even lead to the occurrence of scientific revolutions. Metaphorization stands for an approach which frees from the shackles of a kind of literal meaning, and being divergent and being creative constitute its intrinsic essence. In the scientific activities, scientists use metaphors mainly for the purpose of theoretical innovation not out of their interest of appreciation of the beauty".[356] In Chinese medicine, *Qu Xiang Bi Lei* or Taking Image and Analogizing, the metaphorizing process, not only states, constructs its theoretical system, guides its clinical practice, but is also a very important way to develop the system. Chinese medical experts are good at taking image and analogizing, and applying metaphorizing to make new explorations so as to develop Chinese medicine. Here I give you three examples:

① *Ti Hu Jie Ga* or Carrying a Kettle and Uncovering Its Lid to Treat Dysuria

Zhu Danxi 朱丹溪 (1281-1358), a famous physician and the founder of Yin-Nourishing School of the Jin-Yuan Dynasties (1115-1368), gained inspiration from a phenomenon in daily life that uncovering the upper lid of a kettle filled with boiling water can make the water be poured out, and then inferred a treating

356 Guo Guichun. 2007: 36.

method named after this phenomenon "*Ti Hu Jie Gai*", which literally means "carrying a kettle and uncovering its lid (in order to pour out water)". What does this mean? The story reads that:

One day, a male patient with dysuria visited Zhu Danxi, who was formerly treated by other physicians with diuretics of Chinese medicine which aggravated his condition. Zhu Danxi felt that his right *cun* pulse (indicating the condition of the lungs) was quite wiry and slippery, and then treated the patient with the method of dispersing the lung *qi*, then diuresis was successfully induced, and finally the patient was cured of the disease.

Zhu Danxi pointed out that the disease was caused by accumulation of phlegm in the lungs, and that the lungs are located in the upper *jiao* and the urinary bladder is located in the lower *jiao*, and that when the upper *jiao* is blocked the lower *jiao* will surely be obstructed, just like a kettle, only after the lid is uncovered, can water be poured out. This therapeutic method is known as *Ti Hu Jie Gai* which literally means "carrying a kettle and uncovering its lid (in order to pour out water)", and actually refers to the method of dispersing the lung *qi* to induce diuresis, which is usually used to treat edema, dysuria, or anuria when the patient does not respond to the routine therapeutic methods.

② *Ni Liu Wan Zhou* or Saving the Boat in an Adverse Current to Treat Dysentery

Yu Jiayan 喻嘉言 (1585-1664), a famous physician in the early Qing Dynasty (1644-1911), created a therapeutic method termed as *Ni Liu Wan Zhou,* or saving the boat in an adverse, swift current to treat enduring dysentery. He believed that dysentery was caused by an external pathogen sinking into the interior, should be treated by lifting the external pathogen out of the exterior from the interior, just like saving a boat in an adverse and swift current to make the boat move upward. Accordingly, he formulated a formula named "Ginseng Toxin-Vanquishing Powder" to treat the disease. Afterwards, physicians of Chinese medicine usually apply this method and the formula to treat the dysentery with external pattern complicated with dampness.

③ *Zeng Shui Xing Zhou* or Increasing Water to Move the Boat to Treat Constipation

The phrase *Zeng Shui Xing Zhou* or Increasing Water to Move the Boat implies that: When the river flow cuts off for the lack of water, then boat will surely run aground; When the water is supplied and rises, then the boat will move in it easily.

Wu Jutong 吴鞠通 (1758-1836), a distinguished expert in warm disease of the Qing Dynasty (1644-1911), created the treating method termed as *Zeng Shui Xing Zhou* or Increasing Water to Move the Boat to treat constipation caused by humor insufficiency or heat drying the humor, which is just like the boat running aground for the lack of water. Accordingly, he also formulated a formula named "Humor-Increasing Decoction" to treat this condition, which has become a famous and effective formula to treat constipation of this kind.

Besides, many other effective treating methods created by the way of *Qu Xiang Bi Lei* or Taking Image and Analogizing, the metaphorizing process, have been still in use in the clinical practice, such as:

Yin Huo Gui Yuan or Conducting Fire Back to Its Origin: a therapeutic method of leading the rising fire to the kidney, used in the treatment of declining fire of the life gate with floating of deficient yang;

Fu Di Chou Xin or Taking Away firewood from under the Cauldron: a therapeutic method of clearing heat or fire by purgation;

Zi Shui Han Mu or Enriching Water to Moisten Wood, a therapeutic method of nourishing kidney yin to subdue liver yang for hyperactivity of liver yang due to liver-kidney yin deficiency, which presents with such symptoms as dizziness, red complexion due to rising fire, and hypertension in some cases.

There are still many other methods or theories in Chinese medicine created by the way of *Qu Xiang Bi Lei*. We can see that the process of constructing and understanding metaphors is a typical example for creativity. The creative nature of metaphor is to find new relationships in two or more existing concepts or phenomena so as to explore new mental spaces and advance new theories, thus developing Chinese medicine in both theoretical and clinical explorations.

3.3 Metaphors in Chinese Medicine: Revealing Relationships and an Exact Thinking

Metaphors in Chinese medicine reveal relationships, and metaphor thinking is an exact thinking.

3.3.1 Metaphors in Chinese Medicine: Revealing Relationships

As we have discussed before, metaphor is far more than a rhetoric figure of speech. Metaphor is not a description by a vivid picture but an exact description to show relations. The relations are described by the metaphor. So, metaphor does not describe objects. Metaphor reveals relations, relations done by actions. Therefore metaphor has the function of relating different phenomena. Here I give you two examples to illustrate this point of view: Tongue Diagnosis and Heart Fire Blazing.

3.3.1.1 Example 1 Tongue Diagnosis: A Metaphorizing Process

Tongue reading and pulse taking are two essential steps to diagnose a disease and identify a pattern in Chinese medicine. The tongue coating in Chinese medicine is formed by the way metaphorizing, and tongue reading is also a metaphorizing process.

As regards to the formation of the tongue coating, Zhou Xuehai 周学海 (1856-1906) said that "The coating is the result of the fuming or steaming of the stomach *qi*. All of the five *zang* organs rely on nutrients from the stomach, hence the tongue coating can be used to diagnose the conditions of the five *zang* organs, such as heat or cold, deficiency or excess". Wu Kun'an 吴坤安 of the Qing Dynasty (1644-1911) explained that "The coating of the tongue is just like the moss of the earth. The moss of the earth results from the upgoing of the dampness, while the coating of the tongue results from the upgoing of the spleen dampness steamed by the stomach. That is why it is named as *Tai* or Moss".

It is thus clear that the *Tai* 苔 or Moss or Coating of the tongue is formed by metaphorizing the moss of the earth, which is clearly embodied in the sinogram "*Tai* 苔". The sinogram "*Tai* 苔", a signific-phonetic, following 艸 (grass) and pronounced as "*Tai* 台", originally means moss, a very small green plant which grows on damp soil, or on wood or stone. Many moss plants usually grow close together in a clump.

Tongue reading is also a metaphorizing process. Illus. 24-1 shows that the tip of the tongue reflects conditions of the heart and lungs, the middle reflects conditions of the spleen and stomach, the root reflects conditions of the kidneys, and the two sides reflect conditions of the liver and gallbladder, which results from metaphorizing the locations of the organs in the body in Chinese medicine.[357] In Chinese medicine, the result of tongue inspection is usually described from the following three aspects: the body, coating, and shape of the tongue, which are collectively known as the "tongue image". The normal tongue image is usually described as "red tongue with thin whitish coating". Now let us read some tongues and practice metaphorizing thinking in this process.

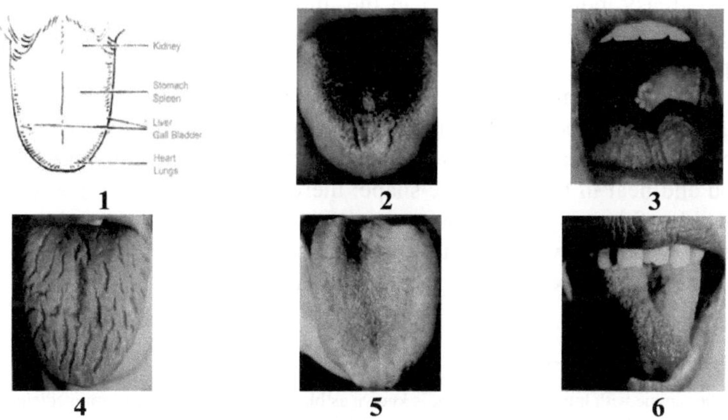

Illus. 24 Tonge Reading

The tongue image of the Illus. 24-2 can be generally described as "a pale tongue with burnt-black coating". In details, the color of the tongue proper is pale,

357 Chinese medicine views every single separate part as a part with the information of all the parts of the body. Some are significant in diagnosing and treating certain diseases while some others are not. The typical example is the ear acupuncture therapy, which is used to treat diseases of various parts of the body for the ear resembles an inverted fetus and thus has points corresponding to most imp
ortant parts of the body.

indicating blood deficiency; the shape is corpulent or swollen with tooth-prints, indicating *qi* deficiency; and the coating is burnt-black, indicating extreme fire flaming upward. So, in Chinese medicine, this tongue image usually indicates upward flaming of extreme fire and deficiency of *qi* and blood.[358]

The tongue image of the Illus. 24-3 can be generally described as “red atrophy tongue with yellowish greasy coating”. In details, the color of the tongue proper is red, quite normal; the shape is atrophy, indicating that phlegm-heat stagnates in the network vessels; and the coating is yellowish greasy, indicating accumulation of damp-heat in the body.[359]

The tongue image of the Illus. 24-4 can be generally described as “light-red tongue with fissures and little coating”. In details, the color of the tongue proper is light-red, indicating deficiency of blood; the shape: there are many longitudinal fissures distributed on the tongue, indicating flaming upward of deficiency fire; the coating is very little, indicating extreme deficiency of yin. So, in Chinese medicine, this tongue image usually indicates deficiency of yin and blood and flaming upward of deficient fire.[360]

The tongue image of the Illus. 24-5 can be generally described as “light-red tongue with white greasy coating on the edge and greenish coating in the middle”. In details, the color of the tongue proper is light-red, indicating deficiency of blood; the Shape is corpulent or swollen, indicating qi deficiency; the coating is white, greasy, but yellow-green in the middle, indicating fire-transmission from long-term cold-damp due to yang deficiency, and damp-heat retention and evaporation.[361]

The tongue image of the Illus. 24-6 can be generally described as “light-red tongue with red spots and white, light yellow, greasy coating”. As you know, the color of the tongue proper is light-red, red on the tip, indicating deficiency of blood and heat in the heart; the shape: there are many red-spots at the tip and the right side of the tongue, indicating heat-fire in the heart, lungs and stomach; the coating is full of white, light yellow, greasy coating, indicating the heat in the Nutrient phase in externally contracted febrile diseases.[362]

358 The tongue with burnt-black coating is known as black hairy tongue in western medicine, which is most often seen in acute pyogenic infections such as pyemia, gangrenous appendicitis, peritonitis, and cholecystitis, and may also occur in diseases such as chronic bronchitis and uremia. Western medicine explains that it may result from growth of bacteria after long administration of antibiotics, high fever, dehydration, absorption by the tongue coating of iron present in blood from minor bleeding in the oral cavity, etc.

359 The atrophy or shrinkage of the tongue in Western medicine can be seen in patients with pulmonary tuberculosis, or advanced carcinoma.

360 Fissures in Western medicine are chiefly associated with chronic glossitis, and 0.5% of the cases with fissures on the tongue are wholly unrelated to disease.

361 The corpulent or swollen tongue, also known as tongue enlargement, in Western Medicine, may be seen in myxedema, chronic nephritis, and chronic gastritis, and is attributed to hyperplasis of the connective tissue, tissue edema, or blood and lymphatic drainage disturbances.

362 The red spots in Western medicine result from an increase in the size or number of fungiform papillae.

You see that the tongue reading process is in essence a metaphorizing process.

Here the subjects of the five photos of the tongues are Chinese patients. It is worth to note that the result and clinical significance of tongue reading are not influenced by differences in races. If you are interested in this topic, you can read further a monograph by Giovanni Maciocia "Tongue Diagnosis in Chinese Medicine", in which 59 colored plates and accompanying case histories are from the author's own practice.

Tongue examination provides some of the most important data for pattern identification esp. of externally contracted febrile diseases, so the "Tongue Inspection and Pattern Identification Songs" by Wu Kun'an 吴坤安 says that

Exterior white, interior yellow,
Decide sweating or purgation.
Nutrient crimson, defense white,
Refine therapeutic differentiations.
Then check fluids for further information.
Moist, no damage; dry, depletion.

"Exterior white, interior yellow" refers to the color of the tongue coating: if the coating is white, this disease will be identified as exterior pattern, and thus should be treated by sweating; if the coating is yellow, this disease will be identified as interior pattern, and thus should be treated by purgation. A crimson tongue indicates that pathogenic heat penetrates to the Nutrient phase. External pathogens at the Defense phase still indicate the disease can be identified as exterior pattern. The moistness of the tongue indicates the state of the fluids.

3.3.1.2 Example 2: Heart Fire Blazing

When you see the formulation "Heart Fire Blazing", you may think it is ridiculous, and ask "How do we know there is fire in the heart?", "Is the temperature in the heart higher than that in other organs?", "How can we measure it?". Actually, fire is a metaphor, and metaphorizing is the key to understand it.

Fire is the extreme state of heat. The external pathogenic wind, cold, summer-heat, dampness, and dryness can all transform into fire when they penetrate through to the interior of the body; disorders of functions of *zang fu* organs, and internal depression of the seven affects, i.e. joy, anger, melancholy, anxiety, sorrow, fear and fright, can also transform into fire.

Fire, a yang pathogen in nature, is characterized by "flaming upward". In the case of heart fire blazing, if fire flames upward, symptoms of red complexion, thirsty, sores on the tongue or in the mouth, red tongue[363] will show up; if fire disturbs the spirit, symptoms like vexation, insomnia, manic episodes, delirious speech, and unconsciousness will show up; fire consumes fluids, symptoms like

363 "Tongue is the signal orifice of the heart".

thirsty with desire for drink, dry tongue and mouth, constipation, scanty dark yellow urine will show up; the pulse is usually rapid. Accordingly, the therapeutic principle should be "clearing the heart fire"; and then corresponding treatment of medication and/or acupuncture can be prescribed.

It is thus clear that "Heart Fire Blazing" says nothing about the temperature in the heart, but connects the concept of the heart identified in Chinese medicine with a series of phenomena of fire, such as thirsty with desire for drink, insomnia, vexation, constipation, scanty dark yellow urine, red tongue, rapid pulse, and so on. Therefore "Heart Fire Blazing" is identified by all of these phenomena which relate to each other by metaphorizing the fire and the heart.

It is thus clear that metaphors in Chinese medicine reveal relationships.

3.3.2 Metaphorizing in Chinese Medicine: An Exact Thinking

It is worth to note that, when talking about differences between Chinese medicine and Western medicine, people generally believe that Western medicine is exact, while Chinese medicine is vague. Based on the common sense and general knowledge, it is obvious that data from lab is indeed much more precise than a pattern of disharmony. But the answer is not so simple if we see this question from the perspective of metaphor cognition. We have already known that the metaphor system of Chinese medicine is the deep structure of Chinese medicine, and the key to understand Chinese medicine. In fact, metaphors in Chinese medicine not only reveal relationships, but are also a kind of exact thinking - metaphorizing. Here I give you three examples to illustrate this point of view.

3.3.2.1 Example 1: Stomach pain in 6 people

The clinical studies Kaptchuk applied to illustrate difference between Western and Eastern perceptions of medicine can also demonstrate that metaphorizing in Chinese medicine is an exact thinking. Six patients with stomach pain were all diagnosed as having peptic ulcer disease by using upper-gastrointestinal X-ray or endoscopy by means of a fiberscope. But these six patients diagnosed as having the same disease in Western medicine were identified as having six different patterns of disharmony: "Damp Heat Affecting the Spleen", "Deficient Yin Affecting the Stomach", "Exhausted Fire of the Middle Burner", "Excess Cold Dampness Affecting the Spleen and Stomach", "Disharmony of the Liver Invading the Spleen", and "Disharmony of Congealed Blood in the Stomach" by a doctor of Chinese medicine.

From the perspective of Western medicine, the six patients suffered from the same disease; and if they were treated by this doctor they would have accepted more or less the same treatment. While if they were treated by a doctor of Chinese medicine they would have accepted different individualized treatments based on their specific patterns. Obviously, six individualized treatments provided by Chinese medicine are more exact than one treatment provided by Western medicine, which is based on the same diagnosis in Western medicine - the six different patients suffer from the peptic ulcer disease.

3.3.2.2 Example 2: High Blood Pressure

"Persistently high systemic arterial blood pressure. Based on multiple readings (blood pressure determination), hypertension is currently defined as when systolic pressure is consistently greater than 140 mm Hg or when diastolic pressure is consistently 90 mm Hg or more". Hypertension, also known as high blood pressure, will be treated by antihypertensive pills of different kinds such as diuretics, beta blocker, ACE inhibitor, angiotensin receptor blocker, etc. in Western medicine. The effect can still be checked by a sphygmomanometer. If the blood pressure is lowered down and kept at the normal level, the treatment will be evaluated as effective. Generally speaking, the doctors do not care so much the other aspects of patients, or the background of the high blood pressure.

While doctors of Chinese medicine identify patients with hypertension as having different patterns such as "hyperactivity of liver fire", "yin deficiency and yang hyperactivity", "pattern of phlegm turbidity", "pattern of phlegm and blood stasis", etc., and then give them individualized treatments based on different specific patterns. Chinese medical treatments may not directly lower the blood pressure, but can be used as auxiliary treatments for relieving common symptoms of hypertension patients such as headache, vertigo, insomnia, tinnitus, and so on, in stabilizing the blood pressure, softening the blood vessels, and preventing the situation from deteriorating.

3.3.2.3 Example 3: Inflammation and Fire

Another common example is the inflammation in Western medicine and fire in Chinese medicine. Inflammation is a pathological condition in Western medicine, manifesting in local redness, swelling, pain, ulcer and dysfunction as well as fever of different degrees, leukocytosis, fatigue, poor appetite, and so on, which is usually treated by antibiotics. This pathological condition is generally known as "fire" in Chinese medicine. But you may ask what is the difference between Chinese understanding and Western understanding of the same or similar pathological condition for inflammation with the "flame" as its root is also a kind of fire?

The concept of fire in Chinese medicine comes from *Huo* 火 or Fire, as stated in *The Origin of Chinese Characters* that "火 *huo*, the phase of the South, flaming upward, is a pictographic character". The ancient Chinese people observed that fire is warm, hot, red, burning, and flaming, bearing the characteristics of being bright, rising and upbearing.

Fire as a pathological condition in Chinese medicine can be caused by eight kinds of pathological agents - warm heat, damp heat, fire toxin, yin deficiency (deficient fire caused by yin deficiency), wind cold or cold dampness, phlegm fluid (with edema), deficient cold (cold is caused by yang deficiency), stagnation of *qi* and blood (with pain). These agents are not fixed, may vary according to the progression or retrogression of the disease. But anyway, doctors of Chinese medicine prescribe different formulas to fit different patterns, i.e. identifying patterns and applying proper treatments. It is really amazing for Chinese medicine does not yield drug resistance like antibiotics do, and it works even when the agent(s) of a disease cannot be identified.

The above examples show that Chinese medicine is even more exact than Western medicine in the clinical practice. Besides, Dichotomy is like "1", while *Tiao Ji Tu* 太极图 or Yin-Yang Diagram is like "S" (See Illus. 21 Yin-Yang Diagram and Dichotomy), much more complicated than dichotomy, therefore more exact and fitting to the dynamic living system. *Tiao Ji Tu* 太极图 or Yin-Yang Diagram, one of the vital philosophical foundations of Chinese medicine, is also more exact than one of the vital philosophical foundations of Western science – Dichotomy. You know Chinese medicine is constructed under the guideline of *Tian Ren He Yi*, and the object of Chinese medicine is the live dynamic human being, composed of the body, mind and other aspects, which can explain why Chinese medicine can usually achieve desired therapeutic effects in treating psychosomatic diseases. While Western medicine is an applied science based on achievements of Western science and technology, and is practiced mainly based on understanding of the dead bodies, and has got a very detailed and precise understanding of the physical structure of the body, and thus has achieved amazing revolutionary developments in surgery, and even organ transplantation.

Metaphor thinking is an exact thinking for Chinese medicine regards the living system as a text, a composition of words and every word can be understood by the other words. And you cannot understand one word fully if you don't know all the other words. The text offers so much on knowledge, on information, on relationships among the words – its constituent parts, much more than the stabilized objects of the Western medicine. Now you can see the source of the exactness of Chinese medicine.

In Western medicine, the heart is identified by its location, functions, and some possible related diseases of the organ heart which are clearly defined, and all the other aspects or body happenings are not interesting. While in Chinese medicine, oral ulceration and frequent, difficult and painful urination with passage of dark yellow urine (which can be seen in acute urinary tract infection in Western medicine) can be both cured by clearing the heart fire with the corresponding formula *Dao Chi San* or Redness-Removing Powder.

Here to sum up, metaphor is the deep structure of Chinese medicine, and the key to understand Chinese medicine. *Qu Xiang Bi Lei* is the metaphorizing process and the Way to form metaphors in Chinese medicine.

Appendix: The Veiled Statue at Sais (Friedrich Schiller)
A youth, impelled by a burning thirst for knowledge
To roam to Sais, in fair Egypt's land,
The priesthood's secret learning to explore,
Had passed through many a grade with eager haste,
And still was hurrying on with fond impatience.
Scarce could the Hierophant impose a rein
Upon his headlong efforts. "What avails
A part without the whole?" the youth exclaimed;
"Can there be here a lesser or a greater?
The truth thou speak'st of, like mere earthly dross,
Is't but a sum that can be held by man
In larger or in smaller quantity?
Surely 'tis changeless, indivisible;
Deprive a harmony of but one note,
Deprive the rainbow of one single color,
And all that will remain is naught, so long
As that one color, that one note, is wanting."

While thus they converse held, they chanced to stand
Within the precincts of a lonely temple,
Where a veiled statue of gigantic size
The youth's attention caught. In wonderment
He turned him toward his guide, and asked him, saying,
"What form is that concealed beneath yon veil?"
"Truth!" was the answer. "What!" the young man cried,
"When I am striving after truth alone,
Seekest thou to hide that very truth from me?"

"The Godhead's self alone can answer thee,"
Replied the Hierophant. "'Let no rash mortal
Disturb this veil,' said he, 'till raised by me;
For he who dares with sacrilegious hand
To move the sacred mystic covering,
He'--said the Godhead--" "Well?"--"'will see the truth.'"
"Strangely oracular, indeed! And thou
Hast never ventured, then, to raise the veil?"
"I? Truly not! I never even felt
The least desire."--"Is't possible? If I
Were severed from the truth by nothing else
Than this thin gauze--" "And a divine decree,"
His guide broke in. "Far heavier than thou thinkest

Is this thin gauze, my son. Light to thy hand
It may be--but most weighty to thy conscience."

The youth now sought his home, absorbed in thought;
His burning wish to solve the mystery
Banished all sleep; upon his couch he lay,
Tossing his feverish limbs. When midnight came,
He rose, and toward the temple timidly,
Led by a mighty impulse, bent his way.
The walls he scaled, and soon one active spring
Landed the daring boy beneath the dome.

Behold him now, in utter solitude,
Welcomed by naught save fearful, deathlike silence,--
A silence which the echo of his steps
Alone disturbs, as through the vaults he paces.
Piercing an opening in the cupola,
The moon cast down her pale and silvery beams,
And, awful as a present deity,
Glittering amid the darkness of the pile,
In its long veil concealed, the statue stands.

With hesitating step, he now draws near--
His impious hand would fain remove the veil--
Sudden a burning chill assails his bones
And then an unseen arm repulses him.
"Unhappy one, what wouldst thou do?" Thus cries
A faithful voice within his trembling breast.
"Wouldst thou profanely violate the All-Holy?"
"'Tis true the oracle declared, 'Let none
Venture to raise the veil till raised by me.'
But did the oracle itself not add,
That he who did so would behold the truth?
Whate'er is hid behind, I'll raise the veil."
And then he shouted: "Yes! I will behold it!"
"Behold it!"
Repeats in mocking tone the distant echo.

He speaks, and, with the word, lifts up the veil.
Would you inquire what form there met his eye?
I know not,--but, when day appeared, the priests
Found him extended senseless, pale as death,

Before the pedestal of Isis' statue.
What had been seen and heard by him when there
He never would disclose, but from that hour
His happiness in life had fled forever,
And his deep sorrow soon conducted him
To an untimely grave. "Woe to that man,"
He warning said to every questioner,
"Woe to that man who wins the truth by guilt,
For truth so gained will ne'er reward its owner."

The Book of Changes deals with *Xiang Shu* (images and numbers, 象數) and their implicit meanings, while Chinese medicine talks about health and illnesses. But metaphorizing bridges them for they both actually cares the same issue in essence – life: one on the life of universe and the other on the life of man.

- The Author

4 Metaphorizing: The Way to Bridge *The Book of Changes* and Chinese Medicine

We know from the last chapter that *Qu Xiang Bi Lei* or Taking Image and Analogizing is the metaphorizing process and the way to form metaphors in Chinese medicine. In real fact, it is also the way to bridge *The Book of Changes* and Chinese medicine.

4.1 *The Book of Changes* and Chinese Medicine Being of the Same Origin: Shamans' Practice

4.1.1 The Origin of "*The Book of Changes*"

In the remote antiquity of China, shamans applied special instruments like stone, tree, tortoise or other animals to communicate with the heaven and the earth. There were many ways to communicate with the heaven and the earth, among which *bu* 卜 and *shi* 筮 were two popular ones. *Bu* 卜 with tortoise shell and *shi* 筮 with stalk of a grass, *shi* 蓍 grass, were mainly supposed to foretell good or ill luck, good fortune or misfortune in the future for the tortoise (shell) and *shi* grass not only have long lives but also bear strange shapes or patterns and thus were considered as god-created beings. The images of *gua* 卦 and *yao* 爻 were created at the inspiration of cracks on tortoise shell, while the numbers of *gua* 卦 and *yao* 爻 (nine and six) were attached to them at the inspiration of numbers of stalks of *shi* grass in divining activities. That is to say, *Xiang Shu* (images and numbers, 象數) originated from *bu* 卜 with tortoise shell and *shi* 筮 with stalk of *shi* grass respectively. Therefore, it is clear that *The Book of Changes* originates from shamans' divining activities: *bu* 卜 and *shi* 筮.

4.1.2 The Origin of Chinese Medicine

What is the origin of Chinese medicine? The circle of medical history of contempory China generally holds that Chinese medicine originated from the summarization of ancient people's living, producing and laboring experiences for such a viewpoint is believed to accord with the historical standpoint of Marxism and scientific materialism. But first of all, let's go back to the original forms of the sinogram 医 (medicine or medical practitioner): 毉 and 醫. The sinogram 毉, appearing in *Guan Tzu* and *Guang Ya* 廣雅, is composed of 医 (*yi*, medicine or medical practitioner) and 巫 (*wu*, shaman or shamans' practice), thus showing the close relationship between them. *The Origin of Chinese Characters* explains

醫 as "the practitioners who specialize in treating illnesses. The upper part means bad postures. Their treating behaviors were driven by wine (酉→酒), therefore following the wine part 酉. Wine was applied to treat illnesses. According to the records of *Zhou Li* or *The Rites of Zhou [Dynasty]* there existed medicinal wine in the Zhou Dynasty (ca.11th century-256 B.C.), and the Shaman Peng 巫彭 was one of the first medical practitioners of the remote antiquity." Illnesses are man's diseased state, as explained in *The Origin of Chinese Characters. Disease Part* (说文解字. 疒部) that "疒， leaning on or against something. Whenever man has illnesses, his posture is like leaning on something". It's interesting that shamans' extraordinary behaviors' driven by the wine could treat man's extraordinary states: illnesses. Wine may influence man's consciousness, which can be regarded as the bridge between psychotherapy and Chinese medicine. Here is an explanation of the parts to make up 毉 and 醫:

- 匸：Principles of medicine should be upright and foursquare;
- 矢：arrow; acupuncture;
- 殳：hand feeling in the water of a pond; massage;[364]
- 酉：wine;
- 巫：shaman; shaman's practice.

Besides, there are many records on witchdoctors or shamans of the remote antiquity such as in *The Classic of Mountains and Seas* (shan hai jing, 山海經)[365] and *The Historical Records* (shi ji, 史記)[366].

Actually, the formulation "medicine originates from shamans' practice" was put forward long ago in China. With the rising of anthropology in the 19th century, many scholars at abroad also insist on this point of view. This formulation includes the following three aspects: Medicine grew out of shamans' practice; the earliest medical practitioners were shamans; and shamans' practice was the earliest method to treat illnesses. This is indeed the case as regards to the origin of Chinese medicine.

364 A Chinese idiom 手到病除 relates to this sinogram, which means "Illness departs at a touch of the hand".

365 *Shan Hai Jing* or *The Classic of Mountains and Seas*, is a classical Chinese text of at least 2,000 years old. It is largely a fabled geographical and cultural account of Pre-Qin China as well as a collection of mythology.

366 *Shi Ji* or *The Records of History*, written by Sima Qian 司馬遷 (145 or 135? – ca. 86 B.C.) of the Western Han Dynasty, recounts over 3,000 years of Chinese history from Huang Di's era to his own time. As the first systematic Chinese historical text, the records profoundly influenced Chinese historiography and prose. In its effect, the work is comparable to Herodotus and his Histories.

4.1.3 *The Book of Changes* and Chinese Medicine Being of the Same Origin: Shamans' Practice

Then what is the relationship between *The Book of Changes* and Chinese medicine – one deals with *Xiang Shu* (images and numbers, 象數) and their implicit meanings, while the other talks about health and illnesses? Actually they are talking about the same issue in essence by applying metaphors: life – one on the life of the cosmos and the other on the life of man. Both are open systems, both are communicated with and related to each other, and both should be in a state of harmony in itself and with the other, otherwise problems or illnesses will ensue, which is radically different from the strict divisions between the life and the inanimate, the subject and the object, the man and the nature etc. in the Western culture. Maybe it is fantastic for the Westerners that *The Book of Changes* and Chinese medicine do not reduce life or being to something material like cells, proteins, genes, etc., instead they reduce life or being to something symbolic like *gua* 卦 and *yao* 爻, yin and yang, the eight trigrams, the five phases, the images and numbers, the visceral image, and so on.

4.2 *Qi* and *Xiang*: Fundamental Metaphors to Bridge *The Book of Changes* and Chinese Medicine

Ernst Cassirer defined man as a symbolic animal (or animal symbolicum) instead of a rational animal. He said: "Only by such a definition can we point out the specific features of man and can we understand the new way open to the man – that is the way into the culture".[367] Chinese people created specific cultural symbols like *qi* 气 and *xiang* 象, which are the fundamental metaphors of Chinese culture and medicine.

4.2.1 *Qi*: A Metaphor as Foundation of *Tian Ren He Yi*

Chuang Tzu 莊子 comments that *The Book of Changes* talks about yin *qi* and yang *qi* from the beginning to the end. Actually, the formation of the concept "*Qi*" is the process of metaphorization.

The Origin of Chinese Characters • Qi Part states that "*Qi* refers to thin, floating clouds. The sinogram 气 is a pictograph." The sinogram 气 was written as "  " in the oracle script, which resembles air current, evaporating and rising, whose image is just like cloud, will disappear very soon and become invisible. Therefore, *qi* is invisible and formless, exists everywhere, can be gathered into a form, for instance, *qi* can be condensed into water. *Qi* at this moment actually referred to air or vapor.

Soon afterwards, the *qi* which surrounds and congests the space of the man was abstracted into the *qi* which bears a philosophical sense. Philosophers of the

367 Author: Cassirer Ernst. Translator: Gan Yang. 2004: 37.

Spring Autumn and Warring States Periods (770-221B.C.) believed that *qi* is the basic ingredient constituting the world, and that everything in the universe comes into being by the movement and mutation of *qi*. For example, *The Book of Changes* states that "everything is transformed and generated by the enshrouding [*qi*] of the heaven and the earth".

Later on, ancient Chinese medical experts introduced "*qi*" into the medical field at the right moment. And then, "*qi*" became a medium to bridge the natural philosophy of the Pre-Qin Days (before 221B.C.) and Chinese medicine. The concept and theory of "*qi*" gradually formed in Chinese medicine.

In the time of *Huang Di's Inner Classic*, "*qi*" is regarded not only as the basic ingredient constituting the world, but also as the basic ingredient constituting the man which can be transformed into blood, essence, and body fluid, etc., and the normal functional activities of the life which is governed by "*qi*" is known as *Shen* or spirit. For example, *Huang Di Nei Jing Su Wen • Bao Ming Quan Xing Lun* or *Huang Di's Inner Classic· Basic Questions • Discourse on Protecting Life and Preserving Physical Appearance* states that "Man is generated by *qi* of the heaven and the earth, and is completed by the law of the four seasons"; and that "the union of *qi* of the heaven and the earth gives birth to man". That is to say, Heaven, Earth, and Man constitute with the ingredient in the same way – *Qi*. Therefore, *Qi* is the foundation of *Tian Ren He Yi* 天人合一 or Universe (Heaven) and Man uniting and resembling each other.

4.2.2 Tian Ren He Yi: Cultural Presuppostion for Metaphorizings of Chinese Medicine

The theme of Chinese philosophy is to probe into the relationship between "the heaven and the man", or the relationship between "the Way of heaven and the Way of man", regarding the heaven as man's heaven and the man as heaven's man.[368]

The Book of Changes establishes *Tian Ren He Yi* 天人合一 or Universe and Man Uniting and Resembling Each Other by making a farfetched comparison between them. *Tian Ren He Yi* actually indicates that universe and man constitute in the same way, i.e. being composed of the same ingredient – *Qi*, in the same order. That is to say, the universe is a bigger man, while the man is a smaller universe; or the universe is the macrocosm, while man is the microcosm. It states that "In the remote antiquity when Fu Xi 伏羲 ruled the country, he raised his head to observe images on the heaven, bowed his head to observe phenomena on the earth, observed images of birds and beasts and those of the earth, took near

368 Actually, "*Tian Ren He Yi* 天人合一" is the abbreviation of "*Tian Di Ren He Yi* 天地人合一". "*Tian Ren He Yi* 天人合一" can be literally translated as "Heaven and Man Uniting and Resembling Each Other", which actually implies "Heaven, Earth, and Man Uniting and Resembling Each Other", i.e. "Universe and Man Uniting and Resembling Each Other".

images from man and took far images of other things from the universe, on the basis of which he then started to make the Eight Trigrams to illustrate the phenomena", which lays the philosophical foundation for the metaphorizings of Chinese culture and medicine.

Chinese medicine believes that all things in the world are related to each other, that the world is composed of the same constituent - *Qi*, and that the immense variety of things and phenomena in the world share some similar characteristics at different levels, different categories, and different aspects, and moreover, there exist many necessary relationships among them.

The theoretical system of Chinese medicine has formed on the idea of *Tian Ren He Yi* or Universe and Man Uniting and Resembling Each Other. *Huang Di's Inner Classic ·Basic Questions· Discourse on Protecting Life and Preserving Physical Appearance* states that "Man is born on the earth, hanging his life to the heaven. The union of *qi* of the heaven and the earth gives birth to man. Man can adapt himself to the seasons for Heaven and Earth are his parents".

In one word, *Tian Ren He Yi* 天人合一 is the cultural presupposition of metaphorizings of Chinese medicine.

4.2.3 *Xiang*: A Metaphor as Foundation for *Qu Xiang Bi Lei*

Xiang 象, the most important metaphor of Chinese culture and medicine, implies the core methodology of Chinese medicine – *Qu Xiang Bi Lei* or Taking Image and Analogizing. See "7.3 *Xiang* Implies a Vital Methodology of Chinese Philosophy" of the Part One "Overview of Chinese Culture with Chinese Characters" for details.

Qu Xiang Bi Lei or Taking Image and Analogizing, the metaphorizing process and the way to form metaphors in Chinese medicine, plays a vital role in constructing and developing the theoretical system and clinical explorations of Chinese medicine.

4.3 Metaphorizing: The Way to Bridge Specific Symbols of *The Book of Changes* and Metaphors of Chinese Medicine

Metaphorizing is the way to bridge specific symbols of *The Book of Changes* and metaphors of Chinese Medicine. Let's take "—" and "- -" and yin-yang, the eight trigrams and the five phases, the five phases and the visceral image theory as examples to illustrate this point of view.

4.3.1 "—" and "- -" and Yin-Yang

The two symbols "—" and "- -" are the basic lines to compose the eight trigrams and the sixty-four hexagrams. The Fu Xi's Eight Trigrams stand for the eight basic phenomena in the nature (See Illus. 25), which are grouped into four pairs of opposites - *Qian* and *Kun*, *Kan* and *Li*, *Gen* and *Xun*, *Zhen* and *Dui*. Double the Eight Trigrams to get the Sixty-Four Hexagrams, which are used to symbolize various phenomena in the nature and the society.

- *Qian* 乾 for Heaven
- *Dui* 兑 for Lake or Marsh
- *Li* 离 for Fire
- *Zhen* 震 for Thunder
- *Xun* 巽 for Wind
- *Kan* 坎 for Water
- *Gen* 艮 for Mountain
- *Kun* 坤 for Earth

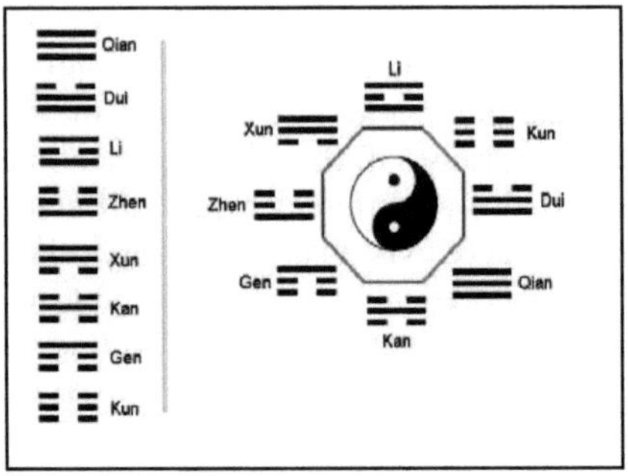

Illus. 25 Fu Xi's Eight Trigrams

There preserves a precious original manuscript in the Schlossbiliothke zu Gotha of Freistaat Thüringen in Germany, which is entitled "1 and 0, the magical origin of all the numbers, and mystical and wonderful paragons of the Nature for all comes from nowhere but the God[369]". This is Gottfried Wilhelm Leibniz's (1646 – 1716) original handwriting. But have you ever known this? His great discovery of binary system was enlightened by two illustrations of the Sixty-Four Hexagrams. The two symbols "—" and "- -" stand for "1" and "0" respectively. But then how did they evolve from?

The Book of Changes sums up the origin or ontology of man and everything in the universe as the outcome of the interaction between the heaven and the earth, yin and yang, which all apply the two symbols "—" and "- -" to stand for and interpret. The Eight Trigrams are also composed of the two symbols. Where are they from or what do they mean? Guo Moruo 郭沫若 (1892-1978) believed that they are the outcome of worshipping the male's and female's genitals. According to his understanding, the following quotation from *The Book of Changes* can be interpreted in this way: *Qian* 乾, "—", the heaven or yang, symbolizes the male's penis, which can curl up or be erectile; *Kun* 坤, "- -", the earth or yin, symbolizes the female's perineum, which can open or close. The interaction of them can produce everything in the universe.

The concepts of yin and yang are metaphors formed in the way of observing and taking the image of directions of a mountain or a river in the nature and then analogizing. Originally yin refers to the northern side of a mountain or the southern side of a river, and yang the southern side of a mountain or the northern

369 Translated from Chinese translation into English.

side of a river. Later on, the meanings of yin-yang are summarized as "the side facing the sun being yang and the reverse side being yin". Then, things that are mobile, external, upward, ascending, warm, hot, bright, hyperactive, or pertaining to functional activities can be classified as *Yang*; those that are unmoving, internal, downward, descending, cold, dull, hypoactive, or pertaining to materials (or structures) can be classified as *Yin*. Thus, yin and yang has become a pair of philosophical concepts to summarize the dynamic images of things or phenomena in the universe.

The Book of Changes advances that "one yin and one yang makes Tao", which abstracts yin-yang to the extensive universality and regards yin-yang as the fundamental rule of the universe for the first time.

The *Chun Qiu Fan Lu* or *The Luxuriant Dew of the Spring and Autumn Annals* by Dong Zhongshu states that "The heaven has yin-yang, the man also has yin-yang. Yin *qi* of the heaven rises and yin *qi* of the man will respond it to rise, while yin *qi* of the man rises and yin *qi* of the heaven will respond it to rise too. The principles or ways are the same".

On one hand, Chinese medicine discards the symbols (*gua xiang*, 卦象) and interpreting words (*gua ci*, 卦辭; *yao ci*, 爻辭) of *The Book of Changes*; on the other hand, absorbs the ideas on "—" and "- -" and yin-yang in it, and makes a systematic and definite expression on the ideas of interdependence, waning-waxing, transformation, counterbalance of yin-yang implied in it, then developing these ideas in combination with medical practice, and thus making yin-yang theory become a guiding theory of Chinese medicine.

To sum up, "—" and "- -" came from the image of the male's and female's external genitals, and *The Book of Changes* is a book on the philosophy of life or being. Then, "—" and "- -" evolved (or integrated with yin-yang) into the yin-yang theory, thus becoming a vital part of philosophy of Chinese medicine on the man.

4.3.2 The Eight Trigrams and the Five Phases

The five phases do not appear in the general version of *The Book of Changes*, but they do appear in its silk version which was unearthed in 1973 from Mawangdui Han tomb. It's generally believed that the five phases were the worldview of the people of the Yin Dynasty (ca.16th -11th century B.C.) and the eight trigrams were the worldview of the people of the Zhou Dynasty (ca. 11th century -256 B.C.). But they both were well-developed in about the same era, sharing the common and typical features and viewpoints of inland culture, expressing by means of taking image and metaphorizing, thus laying the foundation for their integration.

The Book of Changes states that, of the eight trigrams, "*Qian* 乾 is metal, *kun* 坤 is earth (soil), *zhuan* 巽 is wood, *li* 離 is fire, *kan* 坎 is water, *gen* 艮 is mountain (soil), *zhen* 震 is east (wood), *dui* 兌 is west (metal)"; and that "The heaven has 5 numbers, the earth has 5 numbers, then they integrate into five pairs", which was explained by Zheng Xuan 鄭玄(127-200) as "matching the numbers of the heaven and the earth 1, 2, 3, 4, 5 with water and north, fire and south, wood and east, metal and west, soil and middle respectively. The numbers of 1, 2, 3, 4, and 5 are regarded as solitary yin or yang, do not change, and therefore are known as generating numbers (*sheng shu*, 生數); They can generate only together with the soil, that is to say, only after they plus 5 (the number of soil), can they start to generate and transform, thus becoming round numbers (*cheng shu*, 成數). Obviously, the numbers of 8, 7, 9, and 6 are the round numbers of the wood, fire, metal and water respectively, while the soil only takes the generating number 5 not the round number 10, which is the general viewpoint of the *Xiang Shu* (images and numbers, 象數) theory. Thus, the *He Tu* 河圖 could be evolved when matching the generating numbers and round numbers with the five phases, five directions, five seasons, and so on. That is to say, the *He Tu* is the outcome of the integration of the five phases and the numbers in *The Book of Changes*.

Yin-yang, the five phases, and the eight trigrams are all the subdivisions of *Qi* of different levels from the viewpoint of *Qi*, which indicates a gradual generating and dividing process from *Qi* to Yin-Yang then to the Five Phases then to the Eight Trigrams. *The Book of Changes* states that "The changes have *Tai Ji* or the Supreme Ultimate (the Absolute in ancient Chinese cosmology, presented as the primary source of all created things, i.e. *qi*), *Tai Ji* generates yin and yang, yin and yang generate the four images, i.e. the greater yang, the greater yin, the lesser yang, and the lesser yin, and the four images generate the eight trigrams". That is to say, *qi* can generate and transform into yin and yang, yin and yang can generate and transform into the five phases which are composed of two pairs of yin and yang (water and fire, wood and metal) plus one middle soil. Actually, the four images and the eight trigrams indicate the five phases although the term "five phases" does not appear in this quotation: The four images can be regarded as four phases, i.e. water, fire, wood, and metal; the eight trigrams can be regarded as water, fire, wood (yin wood and yang wood), metal (yin metal and yang metal), and soil (yin soil and yang soil).

The theory of five phases influences almost every aspect of classical Chinese social and natural sciences, esp. Chinese medicine. The *Huang Di's Inner Classic* establishes the theory of *Zang Xiang* or Visceral Image on the basis of the five-phase theory, which is mainly used to explain the physiological functions, pathological changes of the internal organs and their relationships, formulating therapeutic principles according to the engendering and restraining relationship among them, thus constructing a dynamic model of the holistic human being, and thus bearing practical significance in clinical sense as well.

4.3.3 The Five Phases and Visceral Image (*Zang Xiang*)

All of the knowledge related to *zang fu* organs in Chinese medicine were summarized and systematized as the theory of *Zang Xiang*, which is usually mistranslated into "visceral manifestation". In actual fact, *xiang* refers to image, which can be easily known by understanding the four concepts indicating the progressive process of *qu xiang*[370]. Therefore, "*zang xiang* 藏象" should be translated into "the image of the viscera" or "visceral image", reflecting the integration of the *zang-fu*'s external images and the subject's deep understanding of them, which were gained by means of metaphorizing on the basis of the idea of *Tian Ren He Yi*.

The formation of the theory of *Zang Xiang* was a process of integrating knowledge on the man and Classical Chinese philosophy: first anatomical knowledge, then the attributes of the organs to the yin-yang and five phases in the way of *Qu Xiang Bi Lei* or metaphorizing guided by the idea of *Tian Ren He Yi*, then proving and modifying the theory in the clinical practice.

Huang Di's Inner Classic. Miraculous Pivot. Rivers and Vessels states that "Regard the body of an eight *chi* (feet) man; when alive, take his measurement, feel his pulses; when dead, dissect his body and regard the strength of his *zang* organs, the size of his *fu* organs, the volume of the trunk cavity and the organs within it, then the length of the vessels, the clarity of the blood and the state of the *qi* … All are shown to conform to a standard.", which shows that the ancient Chinese people had got a rough idea on the positions of the organs of the body. For example, the lungs were analogized as "canopy" for their uppermost position in the *Huang Di's Inner Classic*. The ancient drawings on the organs also show that the almost correct positions of the organs in the body such as the liver at the right side and the spleen at the left side.

Huang Di's Inner Classic. Basic Questions. On Contraindications in Acupuncture started with Huang Di's question "Can you tell me the areas that are contraindicated in acupuncture?" Qi Bo answered that "The five *zang* organs are the vital parts of the body, so you should be very careful in acupuncture treatment as so to avoid damaging them. The liver grows at the left, the lung stores at the right". It is clear that what they were discussing are the areas contraindicated in acupuncture, so the positions of the organs should be their real locations in the body. But why here is quoted as the liver at the left and the lung at the right?

There were two versions as regards to the attributes of the five *zang* organs to the five phases in the ancient times. One is recorded in *Lu Shi Chun Qiu* or *Lu's Spring Autumn Annals*[371], which attributes the spleen to wood (east, left), the lungs to fire (south, upper), the heart to soil (middle), the liver to metal (west, right), and the kidneys to water (north, lower). The other is the same as that stated in the *Huang Di's Inner Classic*, which attributes the spleen to soil (middle), the

---

370 See "**3.2.1.3 The *Xiang* Taken: Image**" of this part for the four concepts indicating the progressive process of *qu xiang*.

371 *Lü Shi Chun Qiu* or *Lu's Spring Autumn Annals*, is an encyclopedic Chinese classical text compiled around 239 B.C. under the patronage of the Qin Dynasty Chancellor Lü Buwei 吕不韦 (?-235B.C.).

lungs to metal (west, right), the heart to fire (south, upper), the liver to wood (east, left), and the kidneys to water (north, lower). In the two versions, only the attributes of the kidneys to water are identical with each other. Then some scholars believe that the positions of the five *zang* organs in the *Huang Di's Inner Classic* do not refer to their real positions but imagery positions instead. But *Huang Di's Inner Classic · Basic Questions · Discourse on Contraindications in Acupuncture* talks about which areas should be avoided in acupuncture, so the positions of the five *zang* organs in it should refer to their actual positions in the body.

Li Ding 李鼎 holds that the former version accords with their actual positions of the back view which was arranged according to the order of animals' internal organs in the offer sacrifices to the gods or ancestors; While the latter accords with their actual positions of the front view for the doctor sits face to face to the patient when diagnosing and treating him. Therefore the left and the right in the formulation "the liver grows at the left, the lung stores at the right" do not conform to the patient's left and right hand respectively, but refer to their opposites. The *He Tu* 河圖 and *Luo Shu* 洛書, the two mysterious patterns of numbers of the Bearings of the Eight Trigrams (*Li* 離-South, *Kan* 坎-North, *Zhen* 震-East, *Dui* 兌-West) also takes the East as the left and the West as right.[372] I agree with this explanation. That is to say, the theory of *Zang Xiang* established in the *Huang Di's Inner Classic* is first of all based on the ancient anatomical knowledge; then, on the attributes of the organs to the yin-yang and five phases in the way of *Qu Xiang Bi Lei* or metaphorizing guided by the idea of *Tian Ren He Yi*, and then has been proved and modified in the clinical practice.

To sum up, *The Book of Changes* and Chinese medicine are of the same origin: shamans' practice; *Qi* and *Xiang* are the fundamental metaphors to bridge *The Book of Changes* and Chinese medicine; *Tian Ren He Yi* is the cultural presupposition for metaphorizings of Chinese medicine; *Qu Xiang Bi Lei* is the metaphorizing process and the methodology to form metaphors of Chinese medicine; and metaphorizing is the way to bridge *The Book of Changes* (the philosophy of Chinese medicine) and medicine. Therefore, the metaphors of Chinese medicine are systematic, carrying unique Chinese cultural and philosophical characteristics, and embodying the core methodology of Chinese medicine.

372 Li Ding. 1998: 99-191.

Universe and Man are all composed by the movement and mutation of *Qi*, which makes up the underlying foundation for the cultural presupposition of Chinese medicine – *Tian Ren He Yi* or Universe and Man Uniting and Resembling Each Other, and metaphorizations of Chinese medicine.

- The Author

5 Metaphorizing: A Vital Way to Understand the Human Being

Metaphorizing is the major way of Chinese medicine to form its ontological concepts, fundamental theories, and to develop its clinical explorations. By analyzing metaphors in Chinese medicine, we become clear about implicit ontological convictions in Chinese medicine. And only by understanding the metaphors in Chinese medicine, we know that Chinese medicine is a different medical system from Western medicine which weaves natural and social phenomena together with rudimentary correct understanding of human beings as an integrity, thus revealing its methodology "*Qu Xiang Bi Lei* 取象比类 or Taking Image and Analogizing" under the guidance of "*Tian Ren He Yi* 天人合一 or Universe and Man Uniting and Resembling Each Other", the core idea of classical Chinese philosophy. By this way it becomes clear that Chinese medicine must not be taken as a natural science in the Western sense, but it goes closer to geisteswissenschaften.

Here I would like to clarify this viewpoint - what Chinese medicine is based on is Chinese understanding of the live human being, compared to what Western medicine is based on is Western understanding of the dead body. For example, you can not find *Qi* and *Jing-Luo* (the meridians or vessels) by dissecting dead bodies.

5.1 Essence, *Qi*, Shen: From Universe to Man

Essence, *Qi*, *Shen* are said to be the three treasures of Chinese medicine. First let us take a look at the Blood and *Qi*, two symbols of life. Confucius divided the life process into three stages: young, prime, and old. Confucius said that "There are three things against which a man with honour is on his guard. In his youth, when his blood and *qi* are not yet settled down, he is on guard against lust. Having reached his prime, when his blood and *qi* have become full and strong, he is on guard against strife. Having reached his old age, when his blood and *qi* is weakening, he is on guard against avarice." (*The Analects of Confucius*), which shows that blood and *qi* were regarded as symbols of life at Confucius's time.

The sinogram for blood is 血, written as "" in the oracle script and "" in the Lesser Seal Script. It is an ideograph, the lower part of which is a vessel, and the dot inside the vessel is a drop of the blood. Its original meaning shown by the sinogram is a blood drop from sacrificed animals dropping down into the vessel. It thus clear that the Chinese concept of blood is a kind of vivid, direct, and visible material.

As we have already known that the concept of *Qi* in Chinese philosophy was formed through a metaphorizing process by means of taking and analogizing the image of air current or vapor. That is to say, the concept of *Qi* in Chinese philosophy evolved from air current or vapor in the universe to the basic invisible constituent of the universe and man, and the movement, mutations and changes of *qi* result in the formation of everything in the universe. *Qi* has finally become invisible and abstract, and more relates to functional activities in Chinese medicine. *Lao Tzu* states that

"Tao begets one,
The one begets two,
The two begets three,
The three begets all things in the universe.

Everything in the universe bears **yin** and embraces **yang**, where the central and harmonious ***qi*** makes them in harmony." (Chapter 42)

Lao Tzu has more than 5,000 sinograms, but only here *Qi* is addressed.

Tao is unnamable and the way of the nature; Tao is Non-being which begets Being.

The One is the Great Ultimate or *Qi*.

The Two is Yin and Yang.

The Three is Yin, Yang and *Qi*.

Here I would like to propose that Tao in Chinese culture and philosophy can be interpreted as the methodology of *Qu Xiang Bi Lei* or Taking Image and Analogizing, or the metaphorizing process for the fundamental concepts and understanding of the universe and man in Chinese culture and philosophy are chiefly evolved by this way. That is to say, Tao in Chinese culture refers to *Qu Xiang Bi Lei*. Of course, it is my original new point of view which needs to be further studied and discussed.

The *Lei Jing* or *Classified Inner Classic* states that "All the human life depends upon *Qi*". Physiologically, *Qi* has the propelling, warming, protecting, retaining, and metabolizing functions, which keeps the life activities going in the normal process.

The correlation between *Qi* and blood is usually expressed by "*Qi* is the commander of blood, and blood is the mother of *qi*." That *Qi* is the commander of the blood implies that *Qi* is the dynamic force for producing and moving blood as well as keeping the blood flowing within the vessels; That blood is the mother of *qi* means that blood carries *qi* on one hand and constantly supplies *qi* with food energy on the other. Both of them are the symbols of life, a live human being.

The sinogram 精 *Jing*, a signific-phonetic, originally refers to the selected good rice, or polished rice, which is then extended to mean "the purest, the most refine part, the essence of things". In Chinese medicine Jing or essence bears three meanings: ① the essential part of *qi*; ② all the substances useful for the human being, e.g. food essence from diet; ③ the essential substance stored in the kidney, also called kidney essence.

Jing or Essence as the essential part of *Qi* is also known as Essential *Qi*. Essence, *Qi*, and blood function as the material basis for Man. Then what is *Shen*?

Actually, *Shen* is a half religious and half scientific concept in Chinese culture, and bears many meanings. For example, *Dictionary of Commonly Used Characters in Archaic Chinese* explains *Shen* as "god or supernatural being; the law in the nature; spirit; magic, superb, excellent".[373] So first, let's start understanding *Shen* based on its etymology.

The sinogram 神 *Shen*, an associative compound, is composed of two parts: "示" and "申". The ancient form of the right part "申" is the image of lightning in the sky, and is actually the ancient writing form of "電", whose upper is the rain radical 雨 and the lower is 电 indicating the meaning); the ancient Chinese people named lightning as "*Shen* 申" for they believed that the lightning was so changeable, unpredictable, invincible, knew no bounds, and therefore mysterious, and was governed by or the embodiment of "*Shen* or Gods". *The Origin of Chinese Characters* explains that "申 refers to 神". The left part "示" is also an associative compound, and is made up of "二" (the ancient form of "上", means "upper" or "heaven"), and the three falls ("111"), representing the sun, the moon and the stars. The ancient form of "示" was written as "T", representing the image of a sacrificial altar. The part "示" is a radical in Chinese characters, and the meanings of the sinograms with "示" are usually related to offering sacrifices to gods or ancestors, or to rites. *The Origin of Chinese Characters* explains "示" as "The heaven hangs down images to show man good or ill luck, following 二. The three falls stand for the sun, the moon and the stars. Observing the images in the sky[374] to detect the current changes. 示 indicates *SHEN*'s things. All with 示 part follow such a connotation." Thus, we can figure out the ancient Chinese people's mysterious feeling about the future world and their great reverence for the gods.

The bronze script of 神 *Shen* is written as . Its original meaning is "*Tian* (Heaven) *Shen* who induces all things of creation" as explained in *The Origin of Chinese Characters*. The *Shen* in the compound *Tian-Shen* 天神 of this quotation may imply both "lightening" and "god". *Shen*'s extended meanings include the following three aspects:

① The spirits of all things on the earth, including the heaven, the earth, the mountains, the rivers, etc., e.g.: The people are the governor of *Shen* (the spirits). (*Zuo's Spring Autumn Annals*)

② The spirits of dead famous men, e.g.: Yao killed Gun, and Gun's *Shen* (spirit) transformed into a yellow bear, which went into a deep pool of the mountain. (*Zuo's Spring Autumn Annals*)

373 Dictionary of Commonly Used Characters in Archaic Chinese [Z]. 1998: 254.

374 "天文 Tian Wen" is usually translated into "astronomy", but I think here it is better to be translated into "the images in the sky".

③ The mysterious and wonderful changes, e.g.: The unpredictable changes of Yin-Yang are named *Shen*. (*The Book of Changes*)

It thus clear that the concept *Shen* evolved from the lightening in the Universe to the spirit in Man – first "Lightening in the nature", then "Heaven God who created the world", then "Unpredictable, marvelous, wonderful changes in the nature", and then "Spirit in Man". As the Chapter of *Moving Essence and Changing Qi* of *Huang Di's Inner Classic • Basic Questions* states that "A patient with *Shen* is apt to recover from illnesses, while a patient losing *Shen* has a poor prognosis".

A Concise Dictionary of Chinese Medicine interprets *Shen* as "a collective term for life activities of man in a broad sense" and "thinking and awareness activities in a narrow sense";[375] *The Fundamental Theories of Chinese Medicine*, the national textbook of the fifth edition on fundamental theories for higher education of Chinese medicine in China, reads that "*Shen* bears 3 meanings in the Chinese medical theory: the first, the transformations, the changes, and the functions of the materials in the nature; the second, all of the activities of man's life; the third, thinking and awareness of man".[376]

To maintain a wellbeing of body and spirit" 形与神俱 is the very point to preserve, cultivate and promote health, which reads in the first chapter of *Basic Questions* that "The people of the remote antiquity practiced Tao by following the rules of yin-yang, harmonizing themselves with the universe by performing some exercises such as *Dao-Yin*,[377] having a balanced diet, arising and retiring at regular hours, avoiding overstressing their body and mind, therefore they maintained a wellbeing of body and spirit, and lived over one hundred years which was beyond their natural life span". Besides, *Shen*'s condition also affects man's healthy conditions, as the 62nd chapter of *Basic Questions* reads that "Spirit (*Shen*) in excess results in continuous laughing; while Spirit (*Shen*) in deficiency leads to being grief."

As regards to the relationship between the body and the spirit, there are two famous metaphors in classical philosophical texts. One is the metaphor of candle and its flame, in which candle metaphorizes the body and its flame the spirit.[378] The flame (the spirit) will immediately disappear as long as the candle (the body) burns out and does not exist, which shows that the spirit exists on the body. The other is the metaphor of a sword and its sharpness, which was put forward by Fan Zhen (范缜, ca. 450-515)[379]. He said, "The body is the substantial foundation of

375 Li Jingwei, Ou Yongxin, Yu Ying'ao, et al. 2001: 775.

376 Yin Huihe. 1984: 3.

377 *Dao-Yin* 导引 refers to an exercise combining stretching, massaging, and breathing to promote the flow of *qi*.

378 See *Xin Lun • Xing Shen* 新论•形神 by Huan Tan 桓谭 (23 B.C.- 50 A.D.), the first treatise on body and spirit in the history of Chinese philosophy.

379 Fan Zhen 范缜 (ca. 450-515) was a Chinese philosopher of the Southern Dynasty, remembered today for his treatise *Shén Miè Lùn* (神灭论, "On the Annihilation of the Spirit").

the spirit, and the spirit is the function of the body. … The relationship between the spirit and its substantial foundation is just like that between the sword and its sharpness; the relationship between the body and its function is just like that between the sword and its sharpness. However, there is neither sword without its sharpness nor sharpness without the sword. As there is no sharpness without a blade, it is impossible for a spirit to exist without its body. ”

To sum up, the concepts of Essence, *Qi*, and *Shen*, or rather *Qi*, Essence, and *Shen,* the three treasures of Chinese medicine, are all formed by the way of *Qu Xiang Bi Lei* or Taking Image and Analogizing or the metaphorizing process from the Universe to Man:

Qi: originally from the "cloud air or vapor" in the nature, then to "the invisible basic substance that forms the universe and man and produces everything in the world through movements, mutations and changes";

Essence: originally from "the selected good rice" in the nature, then to "the purest, the most refine part, essence of things", and then to "the essential part of *Qi*";

Shen: originally from "lightening" in the nature, then to "Heaven God who created the world", then to "unpredictable, marvelous, wonderful changes in the nature", and then to "Spirit in Man"; Shen can also be understood as the liveliness derived from Essence and *Qi*.

5.2 The Visceral Image: Weaving Yin-Yang, Five Phases, and Social Phenomena with Basic Understanding of Internal Organs Together

All of the knowledge related to *zang fu* organs was systematized as the visceral image theory. *Zang Fu* 藏府, now written as 脏腑 in Chinese, is a collective term for the internal organs and a pair of specific concepts in Chinese medicine, which are metaphors formed in the way of observing, taking images from and analogizing the social storing system of the remote antiquity.

5.2.1 *Zang Fu* 藏府: Metaphorizing the Social Storing System of the Remote Antiquity

5.2.1.1 *Zang* 藏: Storing but Not Discharging

The sinogram "脏 *Zang*" underwent such an evolution process "臧-藏-臟-脏". 脏 *Zang* was originally written as "臧" before the Han Dynasty (206B.C.-220A.D.), such as in *Han Shu·Yi Wen Zhi* or *Treatise on Literature* of *The History of the Former Han Dynasty* where all the sinograms of "藏" were written as "臧". Later on, "臟" was made to be used as a specific sinogram for man's *zang* organs by adding the flesh moon 月 part to "藏". "脏" is the simplified writing form of "臟".

As regards to the meaning of "藏", Chinese medical books usually interpret it as follows: "藏 zang4，藏 cang2 也", which means "藏 zang4 is used to store"[380]. "*The Origin of Chinese Characters* with Annotations from Duan Yucai" states that "藏 *Zang*" is the place to store valuable and precious things, i.e. "storehouse".

The sinogram "藏" bears two pronunciations, one is "cang2", mainly used as a verb，means to "hide 隐藏", "to collect and store up 收藏", "to save and preserve 储藏" or "to store 储藏"; the other is "zang4"，originally refers to "a place to store valuable and precious things", i.e. "precious deposits 宝藏", "treasure house 宝库", which is the original meaning of "脏 *zang*" in the compound words "内脏 the internal organs". *Shi Ji·Lao Zi Zhuan* or *The Historical Records·Biography of Lao Tzu* states that Lao Tzu was "the official to guard the treasure house of the Zhou Dynasty (ca.1100-256 B.C.)". One annotation interprets "the official to guard the treasure house" as "the official to guard the treasure house for storing valuable documents and files". Such a specialized establishment for storing imperial mandates, files, gold, jades and other precious things had been handed down to later generations. For example, *Zhong Zang Fu* 中藏府, also know as *Zhong Zang* 中藏, was set up in the Han Dynasty (206B.C.-220A.D) with officials known as *Ling* 令 and *Cheng* 丞 to be in charge of documents and precious things.

Therefore, we see that the prototype of *zang* 藏 is a kind of storehouse established by kings of the remote antiquity for storing precious documents, files, imperial mandates, imperial jade seal, and other valuable things. All the things inside the storehouse "藏" are extremely precious or invaluable, which are generally stored inside and not taken out. The five *zang* organs "五藏" in Chinese medicine function to store the essential *qi* and not discharge it, which resembles the function of zang "藏", therefore, "藏" is used to name man's five *zang* organs "五脏（藏）" and state their common physiological function by the way of *Qu Xiang Bi Lei*.

5.2.1.2 *Fu* 府: Discharging but Not Storing

Fu 腑 was originally written as "府" in the ancient times. The part "flesh moon 月" was supplemented to "府" afterwards to make a specific sinogram "腑" for expressing man's *fu* organs.

In the ancient literature, "府" at least bears the following meanings:

① the place to store money, goods, or documents. *The Origin of Chinese Characters* interprets the original meaning of *Fu* 府 as "the place to store documents".

② the official being in charge of money, goods, and documents. *The Rites of Zhou [Dynasty]* (*Zhou Li ·Tian Guan ·Zai Fu* 周礼•天官•宰夫) states that "the fifth is ***Fu***, who has official contract to administer the storehouse".

---

380 Note: The number after the pinyin indicates the tone of the pronunciation of the character.

③ the place of gathering something. *Zuo's Spring and Autumn Annals• The 27th Year of Xigong's Reign* states that "*The Book of Songs* and *The Book of Documents* are the ***Fu*** of Yi, the place of gathering meanings".

④ a general name for feudal official or local authorities. *The Rites of Zhou [Dynasty]* (*Zhou Li ·Tian Guan ·Da Zai* 周礼•天官•大宰) states that "Eight methods are used to govern the feudal officials". One annotation interprets ***Fu*** as "the places where all the officials reside".

⑤ high officials' or noble lords' residences.

Actually, the earliest meaning of "*fu* 府" is a storing system established by kings of the remote antiquity to govern six kinds of money and goods. *The Book of Documents* (*Shang Shu·Da Yu Mo* 尚书•大禹谟) states that "The earth is even, the heaven is ready-made, and the six ***Fu*** and three kinds of things are all in order, which will be relied on by all the later generations to live". Kong Yingda's[381] annotation reads that "***Fu*** is the place to store money". *Yu Pian· Guang Part* 玉篇•广部[382] reads that "***Fu*** is the place to store goods". What kinds of goods were stored in the ***Fu***? Six kinds of money or goods, i.e. water, fire, metal, soil, wood, and grain, were stored in the "*Fu*", which were often consumed in the daily life and indispensable to ancients' life. The six kinds of money or goods to consume were administered by six officials of six departments respectively, and the institutions where the officials reside are also known as six *Fu*.

The Rites of Zhou [Dynasty] (*Zhou Li·Qu Li* 周礼·曲礼) states that "The son of Heaven's six ***Fu*** are set up to administer soil, wood, water, grass, utensils, and goods". It can be seen that the specific names of the six ***Fu*** in the Zhou Dynasty (ca.1100-256B.C.) slightly changed, but their functions and official system remained the same.

Six kinds of money or goods were to be constantly consumed, which of course needed corresponding fresh supplies. How to supply them? They should be supplied by collecting and gathering them from the common people. As a matter of fact, "six ***Fu***" were also the tax bureau of the remote antiquity, the officials of the six ***Fu*** were a general name of "six tax officials" of the king's official system of that time, as what was recorded in the annotation on six ***Fu*** of the *The Rites of Zhou [Dynasty]* (*Zhou Li·Qu Li*) that "(six) ***Fu*** governs the storing of the tax of six kinds of things" in the remote antiquity. It is thus clear that the six ***Fu*** administered by the six corresponding officials stored six kinds of necessities for everyday life, which were consumed and supplied everyday, so coming in and out were their characteristics. While "藏 *Zang*" was characterized by only coming in without coming out.

---

381 Kong Yingda 孔颖达 (574-648), a famous Confucian scholar and an expert in Confucian classics of the Sui-Tang Dynasties.

382 *Yu Pian* 玉篇, a dictionary arranged according to forms and structures of sinograms compiled by Gu Yewang 顾野王 (519-581) in 543.

To sum up, "府 *Fu*" was a kind of storehouse established by kings of the remote antiquity to hold six necessities for everyday life, known as "six materials"; the institutions were also known as six "*Fu*", governing collecting or levying tax, therefore, the official names administering the six *Fu* also had the sinogram "府 *Fu*". The "六府 six *Fu*" were characterized by constantly coming in and out of the money or goods, resembling the function of man's "六腑(府) six *fu* organs" which receive, transform, move water and grain and discharge the waste out of the body but not to store, therefore, "府 *fu*" is used to name man's "六腑(府) six *fu* organs" and state their common physiological function by the way of *Qu Xiang Bi Lei*.

It can be seen that the establishment of "臧 *zang*" and "府 *fu*" started in the Xia Dynasty (ca.2100-ca.1600), was gradually perfected till Shang and Zhou Dynasties (ca.1600-256B.C.) according to the record in *The Book of Documents* (*Shang Shu Da Yu Mo* 尚书·大禹谟). It can be inferred that the origin and formation of the Chinese medical theory were really time-honored.

To Sum up, the sinogram 脏 *Zang* underwent such an evolution *Zang* process "臧—-藏—臟—脏". "Zang 藏" originally refers to "a place to store precious things or treasure house". *The Origin of Chinese Characters* reads that "藏 zang4 is used to store (藏 cang2)", which was annotated by Duan Yucai that "*Zang* 藏" is the place to store valuable and precious things, i.e. "storehouse." In the remote antiquity, *Zang* 藏 is a specialized establishment for storing imperial mandates, files, gold, jades and other precious things, and all the things inside the storehouse "*Zang* 藏" were extremely precious or invaluable, which were generally stored inside and not taken out. Such "*Zang* 藏" was taken and analogized the five organs in the body which are said to store the essential *qi* but not discharge it – Heart, Liver, Spleen, Lungs, and Kidneys.

Fu 腑 was originally written as "府". The earliest meaning of "*fu* 府" is a storing system established by kings of the remote antiquity to govern six kinds of money and goods, known as "Six Materials", i.e. water, fire, metal, soil, wood, and grain. What were stored in the "*Fu*" were often consumed and of course needed corresponding fresh supplies and indispensable to ancients' life. Therefore the Six *Fu* were taken and analogized the organs in the body which are said to receive, transform, move water and grain and discharge the waste out of the body but not to store.

5.2.1.3 *Zang* 藏 or *Fu* 府: Who Decided?

Who decided which organ was attributed to *Zang* or *Fu* is still unclear. *Huang Di Nei Jing Su Wen • Yin-Yang Ying Xiang Da Lun* or *Huang Di's Inner Classic ·Basic Questions• Great Discourse on Images Corresponding to Yin-Yang* states in the name of Huang Di that "I have heard that in the remote antiquity, the sages talked about and theorized the human body by differentiating *zang* from *fu*, understanding the distribution and function of the vessels, giving the names to the acupuncture points …" *Huang Di Nei Jing Su Wen • Wu Zang Bie Lun* or *Huang*

Di's Inner Classic ·Basic Questions• Further Discourse on the Five Zang Organs states also in the name of Huang Di that "I have heard from persons educated in medicine the different classifications of the *zang* and *fu* organs. Some regard the brain and marrow, the intestines and stomach as *zang* organs; others regard these organs as *fu*. People all disagree".

The two quotations indicate that the ancient Chinese had formulated the meanings of "藏府 *zang fu*", but developed into different schools as regards to the specific classification or differentiation of them.

5.2.2 The Visceral Image: Weaving Social Phenomena with Basic Understanding of Internal Organs Together

How did the Visceral Image theory in Chinese medicine evolve and form?

5.2.2.1 Anatomical Knowledge of the Body

First, the visceral image theory is based on a correct anatomical knowledge of the body. *Huang Di's Inner Classic · Miraculous Pivot ·Rivers and Vessels* reads that "Regard the body of an eight *chi* (feet) man, when alive, take his measurement, feel his pulses; when dead, dissect his body and regard the strength of his *zang* organs, the size of his *fu* organs, the volume of the trunk cavity and the organs within it, then the length of the vessels, the clarity of the blood and the state of the *qi* … All are shown to conform to a standard". I think that is the basic requirement for medical practitioners of that time. Actually there are some more accurate anatomical records in the *Huang Di's Inner Classic*. For example, the ratio of the esophagus and the intestinal canal of human beings was 1.6 *chi* : 55.8 *chi*, i.e. 1: 34.87, which is very close to 1:34 in the modern anatomy.[383]

Anatomical knowledge was the foundation to construct the theoretical system of Chinese medicine. The procedure of dissecting the body is just like to open a treasure house, from which the concepts of exterior-interior and *Zang-Fu* came out, and the physical structure level – skin, vessel, flesh, sinew, and bone was understood. Then the further anatomical practice showed shapes or structures of internal organs, helped build the concept of *San Jiao* or Triple Energizer[384] and its relative theory, learned relationship among internal organs, and discovered the partial physiological functions of internal organs.

---

383 Wang Hongtu. 2004: 25.

384 Energizer is a standard translation for "Jiao 焦", which is approved by World Health Organization, such as Triple Energizer for "San Jiao 三焦". Actually, Burner is more popular in the English literature on Chinese medicine published in the West. But actually both translations are misleading. Pinyin transliteration is the best but far away from well-known, so the standard translation "Energizer" is adopted here to avoid misunderstanding. See Lan Fengli. A Corpus-Based Study on Cultural Connotations and Translation of Fundamental Concepts in Classical Chinese Texts (Post-Doctoral Report). Shanghai: Shanghai Jiao Tong University, 2008.

For example, the sinogram for **heart** evolved from a direct vision of the organ, which underwent from  in the oracle script through  in the bronze script and  in the lesser seal script to 心 in the regular script; others like the sinogram  in the lesser seal script and 肺 in the regular script for the **lungs**, and the sinogram  in the bronze script,  in the lesser seal script, and 胃 in the regular script for the **stomach**, etc. all embody the direct vision of the internal organs.

San Jiao is well-known for it is "has just name but no form". Is that true? The sinogram 焦 *Jiao* is interchangeable with 膲, which carries the flesh moon radical, thus indicating a fleshy organ in the body like the diaphragm or the pleuroperitoneal membrane. The chapter 80 of *Huang Di's Inner Classic Miraculous Pivot* states that "The evil *qi* remains in the Upper *Jiao* 上膲, and thus the Upper *Jiao* 上膲 is blocked up". *Zhong Xi Yi Xue Hui Tong Wu Zhong* or *Five Kinds of Books on Merging Western medicine with Chinese Medicine* published in 1892 by Tang Rongchuan 唐荣川 holds that the original writing form of 焦 *Jiao* was composed of three parts: 采(米) - layers are differentiable and analyzable, 韦 – for its membrane resembles the cowhide, 焦 – with wrinkles just like burning the skin with fire. *The Origin of Chinese Characters* interprets this writing form as "something contracting or bring together", thus indicating that it is a kind of something like soft skin or hide which contracts from the all sides to the center, i.e. the pleuroperitoneal membrane to cover or wrap the organs.[385] Also based on anatomical knowledge about the pleuroperitoneal cavity, the *San Jiao* was divided into the three segments known as Upper *Jiao*, which contains organs in the thoracic cavity and above the diaphragm, i.e. Lungs and Heart; Middle *Jiao*, which contains organs locating inside the peritoneum, i.e. Spleen, Stomach, Small Intestine; and Lower *Jiao*, which contains organs locating outside of the peritoneum, i.e. Liver, Gallbladder, Kidney, Large Intestine, and Uterus. Based on such an understanding, medical experts developed the *San Jiao* Theory into a specific theory in Chinese medicine.

Physiological functions of the organs were also discovered partly by dissecting dead bodies, for example:

① The heart governs blood and vessels; The vessels are the residence of the blood;

② The lungs govern *qi*, perform respiration, open at the nose, relate to all the vessels, help the heart to move the blood;

③ The kidneys govern water metabolism;

④ The major physiological functions of the stomach, the small intestine, and the large intestine: The stomach governs food intake and decomposition, then

385 Wang Hongtu. 1997: 197.

sends the decomposed food down to the small intestine, where it is separated into the clear and the turbid; Then the clear is absorbed and distributed through the body, while the turbid is further passed down to the large intestine, through which it becomes the waste and is discharged from the body through the anus.

All of the above mentioned take the anatomical knowledge as their background and foundation. Bacause of the limitation of anatomical knowledge, *Huang Di's Inner Classic* interpretes the life phenomena and constructs its own system by integrating the philosophical theories of essential *qi*, yin-yang, and five phases with the accumulation of practical knowledge together with the limited anatomical knowledge.

5.2.2.2 The Attributes of the Organs To the Yin-Yang and Five Phases by the Way of Metaphorizing Guided by the idea of *Tian Ren He Yi*

The five *zang* organs were attributed to the five phases at least partly according to their colors in ancients' eyes, which gained from observing the organs after dissecting dead bodies:

Heart – red –fire,
Liver – brown (blue-green) - wood,
Spleen – yellow – soil,
Lungs – pink to grey (white) – metal[386],
Kidneys – dark red (black) – water.

Thereby, their physiological functions, pathological changes, and their relationships were inferred through analogizing the five phases' characteristics and the engendering and restricting relationship among them.

5.2.2.3 Long-term Observation on Physiological and Pathological Phenomena

For example, if people wear too less or the weather is too cold, people may catch a cold, and then may present with the following symptoms such as nasal obstruction, running nose, sneezing, and coughing. Long-term observation of this series of phenomena resulted in the understanding of the close relationship among the skin, nose and lungs – Lungs govern the skin and the hair of the body, and open at the nose.

5.2.2.4 The Theory Being Modified and Proved in the Long-term Clinical Practice

Repeated medical practice explained and proved some physiological functions from the aspects of pathological phenomena and therapeutic effects. For example, many eye diseases were cured by treating the liver, so "the liver opening into the eyes" was concluded as a theory; many kidney-supplementing agents promoted

386 Nowadays, many people's lungs tend to be black because of smoking and/or air pollution.

the healing of fractures, thereby that "the kidney essential *qi* has the function of promoting the growth of bone" was drawn out, which resulted in the theory that "the kidneys govern bones and engender marrow".[387]

5.2.2.5 Why Did Anatomy Decline in Chinese Medicine?[388]

Why does not Chinese medicine need anatomy anymore for a better understanding of *zang fu* organs? Actually, this question can be transformed into the question "why the concepts and theory of *Zang Fu* organs of Chinese medicine have evolved from anatomical organs to functional entities". Based on the genesis of the Visceral Image Theory, I would like to advance the following viewpoints:

① The main reason that medical practitioners lost motive force of dissecting dead bodies to know the structure of the human body was not the restriction from the Confucian or feudal ethical codes, but the influences of Chinese thinking ways – *Si Wai Zhuai Nei* or Inspecting the exterior to predict the interior, *Qu Xiang Bi Lei* or Taking image and analogizing, and *Yi Xiang Ce Zang* or Speculating the internal organs' pathological changes by observing the external manifestations of life guided by *Tian Ren He Yi* or Universe and man uniting and resembling each other;

② The ontology of Chinese culture decides the holistic, dynamic, functional, interacting and interrelating thinking to be the core thinking of Chinese medicine, which does not need reductionist ideology to understand the human being;

③ Chinese medicine is a practical, clinical, medical system, which pays much more attention to practical knowledge which aims to prevent and cure illnesses, not the basic anatomical knowledge which only aims to understand the human body;

④ The integration of *Qi*, Yin-Yang, and Five-Phase theories into Visceral Image Theory systematizes the open and complicated system of human being, successfully explains all of the physiological functions and pathological changes of the organs;

⑤ Repeated clinical observations and practices have proved that the transformation of the concepts and theory of *Zang Fu* organs of Chinese medicine from anatomical organs to functional entities is successful.

Take "Pi 脾" or the spleen for example.

Pi or spleen in Chinese medicine is located in the Middle *Jiao* and below the diaphragm; it is attributed to Soil in the five phases, which is sowing and reaping,

---

387 Yin Huihe. 1984: 28.

388 Lan Fengli. Why Anatomy Declined in Chinese Medicine: The Concepts and Theory of Zang Fu Organs. CMIR, London, 2009.

thus representing the features of receiving, generating, transforming, and supporting; by metaphorizing the soil's characteristics it governs movement and transformation of water and grain (food), i.e. transforms the water and grain into essence, then moves and sends the essence to the whole body, and thus is regarded as the source of the formation of *qi* and blood, and the foundation of postnatal existence; it controls blood, governs the flesh and the limbs, opens into the mouth, manifests its brilliance in the lips, is interrelated with anxiety in the emotions and saliva in the fluids, and stands in exterior-interior relationship with the stomach, etc.; in the nature, it is related to the late summer in the season, and dampness in the climate, etc.[389] It is thus clear that Pi or spleen in Chinese medicine is responsible for digesting food, and is extremely important and indispensable to a man. Abdominal pain or distension, poor appetite, loose stool, diarrhear, jaundice, fatigue or weakness of the limbs, edema, etc. are common symptoms of the spleen disease, which can be relieved or cured by treating the spleen.

While Western medicine understands the spleen as the largest lymphatic organ, which is located in the top part of the abdominal cavity behind the stomach and below the diaphragm; it appears to act to remove dead blood cells and fight infection, but its functions are not fully understood and an adult can live normally after his spleen has been removed; etc.[390]

You see Chinese understanding of the spleen is so different from Western understanding of the spleen. What's the underlying reason? The underlying reason is that they are based on different cultural presuppositions. Chinese understanding of the spleen is based on the specific cultural foundation of classical Chinese science, e.g. the philosophical theories of yin-yang and five phases, the methodology of *Qu Xiang Bi Lei* or Taking Image and Analogizing guided by the idea of *Tian Ren He Yi* or Universe and Man Uniting and Resembling Each Other, etc. and thus finally forming **a spleen complex system** which involves Universe and Man but centers the spleen; While Western understanding of the spleen is based on the cultural foundation of Western science, e.g. the analytic approach based on reductionist ideology, mechanism, dichotomy, the methodology of deduction and induction, the methods of anatomy and experiments, etc. Successful practice of Chinese medicine and Western medicine demonstrates that each of the both understandings about the spleen is true under its specific cultural presuppositions.

5.3 The Vessel Theory: From the Rivers in the Universe to the Vessels in Man

What is *Jing-Luo* system? Several translations are available for *Jing-Luo* system 經絡系統: "Meridian System" is the standard translation approved by WHO, but

389 Yin Huihe. 1984: 34-36.
390 Collin, P.H. 2001: 550.

the word "Meridian" only indicates a two-dimensional grid while *Jing-Luo* system is supposed to carry *qi* and blood, and thus must be a three-dimensional system; “Channel System” is the most popular translation in the English literature on Chinese medicine, but the word "Channel" is polysemous; I think "Vessel System", a translation shown in *Huang Di Nei Jing Su Wen* by Paul U. Unschuld in 2003 is the best if we take into account the origin and development of the concepts of *Mai* 脈 and *Jing-Luo* 經絡.

Based on some anatomical knowledge on *Mai* (脈, vessel) and medical practice esp. the application of acupuncture, moxibustion, *tuina*, and *qigong*, the concepts of *Jing-Luo* 經絡 are actually metaphors formed in the way of observing, taking images of and analogizing the water flow in the rivers under the earth and the longitudinal lines of the textiles, which are embodied in their writing forms. The chapter *Water & Earth* of *Guan Tzu* states that “Water is the *qi* and blood of the earth, running on (under) the earth just like *qi* and blood flowing in the vessels”.

The sinograms 脈 and 衇 are two common original complex forms of 脉. Its lesser seal script is . This sinogram is a signifc-phonetic compound: the left part is the signific component 月 (flesh moon) or 血 (blood), indicating that *mai* 脈 functions to carry and move blood and is a part of the body; and the right part is the phonetic, indicating both pronunciation and meaning at the same time. In the medical books unearthed from Mawangdui Han Tomb, most of *mai* 脈 were written as “温”. “氺” is the variant form of “氵”, “目” the variant form of “flesh 月”, “皿” the variant form of “blood 血”. The structure of the sinogram has clearly illustrated that the ancients analogized or metaphorized water flow with blood flow.[391] It is thus clear that “*mai*” of the early days referred to blood vessels, so “*mai* 脉” is also known as “blood vessel 血脈”, as stated in *Huang Di Nei Jing Su Wen · Mai Yao Jing Wei Lun* or *Huang Di's Inner Classic ·Basic Questions ·Discourse on Subtleties and Essentials of Vessels* that “the vessels 脈 are the residence of the blood” (Attention: *Qi* does not appear in this quotation).

The concepts “*jing*” and “*luo*” appeared later than “*mai* or vessel”. *Jing* and *luo* are further divisions of “*mai* or vessel”, i.e. “*jing*” vessel and “*luo*” vessel, which was first recorded in the *Huang Di Nei Jing Ling Shu Mai Du* or *Huang Di's Inner Classic·Miraculous Pivot · On Vessels*: “*Jing* vessels reside in the interior; their branches running transversely are known as *luo* vessels; the branches of *luo* vessels are known as grandchild vessels”.

The sinograms “經 *jing*” and “絡 *luo*” share the same silk part “糸”, which is originally used in the textiles. The concept “*jing-mai* 經脈” is a metaphor formed in the way of *Qu Xiang Bi Lei* or taking images and analogizing. The right part of “經” is “巠”, indicating both pronunciation and meaning, which is interpreted in

391 Li Ding. 1998: 2-3.

The Origin of Chinese Characters as "water vessels, following <<< (川), pictographic, indicating rivers, under the 一; 一, refers to the earth", that is to say, "巠" refers to the water vessels running under the earth. *Jing* 經 is explained in *The Origin of Chinese Characters* as "the longitudinal lines of the textiles". The reason that "*jing* 經" is used to name the main stems of the vessels is closely related to the origin of the sinogram "*jing* 經", which contains two images and reflects the similarities between the longitudinal lines of the textiles, the rivers running under the earth and the running routes of the main stems of the vessels. Another part of "*luo* 絡" is "各", indicating both pronunciation and meaning, which is interpreted in *The Origin of Chinese Characters* as "divergence of views being different". Another interpretation of "*luo* 絡" is that "It originally meant unreeled silk, hemp, or cotton fiber, and from its association with stringy fibers came to be used in Chinese medicine as a noun that means network and as a verb that means to net".[392] Anyway, *luo* 絡 is used to name divergent branches of the vessels.

Huang Di Nei Jing Ling Shu Ben Zang or *Huang Di's Inner Classic · Miraculous Pivot · On Viscera* states that "*Jing* vessels 經脈 function to move *qi* and blood, nourish yin and yang, moisten tendons and bones, and lubricate joints". Compared to the statement that "The vessels 脈 are the residence of the blood", quite a lot new contents were supplemented to *jing* vessels, among which the most remarkable point is that the function of moving **blood** was extended to moving ***qi*** **and blood**.

"*Xue mai* 血脈", "*jing* 經" and "*luo* 絡" appeared together in the *Han Shu·Yi Wen Zhi* or *Treatise on Literature* of *The History of The Former Han Dynasty*, "Medical classics explore the origins of **blood vessels** 血脈, ***jing-luo*** 經絡, bone marrow, yin-yang, exterior and interior in order to treat various diseases from the root", where seemingly differentiated blood vessels from *jing-luo.*

Jing-luo 經絡 functions to carry and move *qi* and blood in the body. *Guan Tzu · Water & Earth* states that "water is the qi and blood of the earth, running on the earth which is just like *qi* and blood flowing in the vessels". Judged from the cognizing order, the flow of *qi* and blood in man is analogized and inferred from the natural phenomenon of water flow in the rivers under the earth. The extensions from "vessel 脈" to "*jing-luo* 經絡" and from "blood" to "*qi* and blood" are also closely related to the application of acupuncture, moxibustion, *tuina*, *qigong*, etc, which explore the phenomenon of *qi* and blood flowing in the body, thus enriching the understanding on the "vessels".

To sum up, the concepts and theory of *jing-luo* were formed first on the basis of some anatomical knowledge on "vessels 脈"; then by the way of *Qu Xiang Bi Lei*, i.e. observing and taking images of the water flow in the rivers on/under the

---

392 Wiseman Nigel and Zhang Yuhuan. 2003: 174.

earth and the longitudinal lines of textiles, then analogizing, enlightened by the idea of *Tian Ren He Yi*; and then have been proved and modified in the medical practice esp. the application of acupuncture, moxibustion, *tuina*, and *qigong*. That is to say, *jing-luo* or the vessels are metaphors, referring to the circular or round pathways of the living system.

Therefore, we believe that it will take forever to find any three-dimensional structure of *jing-luo* 經絡 through dissecting dead human bodies. *Jing-luo* 經絡 system or the vessel system is more like a functional concept reflecting a certain image, which is embodied in their writing forms. As stated in the *Huang Di Nei Jing Su Wen·Li He Zhen Xie Lun* or *Huang Di's Inner Classic · Basic Questions · Discourse on Leaving and Uniting of True Qi and Evil Qi* that "The sages formulated principles, which must conform to the nature. Therefore, the heaven has 365 degrees and 28 constellations, the earth has 12 *jing* rivers, and man has 12 *jing* vessels".

Here we can conclude that metaphorizing or *Qu Xiang Bi Lei* is a vital way to understand the human being for the concepts of Essence, *Qi*, Shen, the Visceral Image theory, and the Vessel Theory were all formed by the way of *Qu Xiang Bi Lei* or Taking Image and Analogizing, the metaphorizing process, guided by the idea of *Tian Ren He Yi* or Universe and Man Uniting and Resembling Each Other.

"To truly modernize Chinese medicine, we must first demystify these theories."
(Wang Ming-wei)[393]

6 Metaphorizing: A Vital Way to Understand and Modernize Chinese Herbal Medicine

The formulation of most of the books on Chinese materia medica has been almost fixed in the writing pattern of "General Introduction" and "Classified Medicinals" arranged according to their chief actions with "Properties, Flavors, Meridians Entered, Actions, Cautions & Contraindications" since the era of *Shennong's Classic of Materia Medica*[394], but few explain or illustrate whys and hows. The Chinese herbal medicine, just like Chinese medicine, has evolved under the guidance of *Tian Ren He Yi* 天人合一 or Universe and Man Uniting and Resembling Each Other through *Qu Xiang Bi Lei* 取象比類 or Taking Image and Analogizing, which refers to the Metaphorizing Process in Chinese Herbal Medicine.

6.1 Differences between *Ben Cao* and *Yao*

It is well known that Chinese medicine uses mixtures of different medicinal substances formulated according to a certain strategy in a holistic approach to disease. Here first of all, I would like to discuss the differences between *Ben Cao* (Materia Medica，本草) and *Yao* (Medicine, 藥).

Ben Cao (Materia Medica，本草) and *Yao* (Medicine, 藥) have been taken as the same since the teaching mode of Chinese medicine has transformed into the modernized or Westernized or professional one at the early of the 20th century. That is to say, *Yao* is a modernized term of *Ben Cao.* Actually, they do not refer to the same thing.

Ben Cao, the materia medica, is a collective term for all of the individual substances with healing properties, i.e. the medicinal substances or the medicinals, including herbs, minerals and animal parts. *Ben Cao* is divided into three grades in the *Shennong's Classic of Materia Medica*:

- ➢ Top-grade medicinal is non-toxic, possesses a rejuvenating effect and can be taken frequently and for a long period of time without causing any harm;
- ➢ Medium-grade medicinal has no or only slight toxic effect and is effective in treating diseases or supplementing deficiencies;
- ➢ Low-grade medicinal is effective in expelling pathogens, but is toxic and should not be taken for a long period of time.

Yao 药, with its original sinogram as 藥, is explained to be "harmony of different medicinal substances", and is used to "treat illnesses" (the sinogram is 疒 with 樂 inside it, a variant form of *liao* 療, the simplified writing form is 疗),

393 Qiu, Jane. China Plans to Modernize Traditional Medicine [J]. Nature, April 2007: 590-591.
394 Ling Yikui. Textbook for Medical Higher Education (5th Edition): Chinese Herbal Medicine [M]. Shanghai: Shanghai Scientific and Technical Publishers, 1984: 1.

i.e. restoring the harmonious state to the individual. The two sinograms of the original forms share the same part 樂 (the simplified form is 乐, means music, and is explained to be "harmony of different tones" in *The Origin of Chinese Characters*). Thus, it is clear that *Yao* 藥 refers to the medicine ready to be taken for treating illnesses, which is usually composed of more than one medicinal substance formulated according to the strategies of *Jun Chen Zuo Shi* or Chief, Associate, Assistant and Guide medicinals, i.e. formula. I think the Chinese Herbal Medicine is composed of the two parts: *Ben Cao* (Materia Medica, 本草) – discussion of individual medicinals and *Yao* (Medicine made from a Formula, 藥) – Formulas and Strategies.

6.2 Properties, Flavors, and Meridian Entry

Theory of Chinese materia medica comes from metaphorizing *qi*, yin-yang and five phases. Everything in the universe, including Man and Chinese Materia Medica, comes into being by the movement and mutation of *Qi*, which begets Yin-Yang, and the five phases (two pairs of yin and yang, i.e. water and fire & wood and metal, plus one middle soil).

The Four Properties (*si qi*, 四气 result from metaphorizing the Yin-Yang of the Heaven, varying according to the four seasons – Warm and Hot, the Yang of the Heaven; Cool and Cold, the Yin of the Heaven. In specific, properties of a medicinal come from metaphorizing its living environment, growing seasons and rules, collecting time, and/or medicinal part (including its shape, color, etc.), etc.

The Five Flavors (*wu wei*, 五味) result from metaphorizing the Yin-Yang of the Earth, varying according to the five phases – Acrid, Sweet, and Bland, the Yang of the Earth; Sour, Bitter, and Salty, the Yin of the Earth. It is well know that flavors of many medicinals are far away from their real tastes.

The Meridian Entry (*gui jing*, 歸經) results from attributing the medicinal's properties and flavors to Man's *zang-fu* organs according to the theories of Yin-Yang, Five Phases and Meridians.

6.3 Metaphorizing: A Vital Way for Genesis of Actions of Materia Medica

Tian Ren He Yi or Universe and Man Uniting and Resembling Each Other is the cultural presupposition for metaphorizings of Chinese materia medica, and metaphorizing is the way to understand actionns of Chinese medicinals, which of course have been confirmed and proved in the clinical practice.

Actions of a Chinese medicinal are from metaphorizing its property, or its flavor, or its color, or its shape, or its quality, or its disposition, or its growing time, or its growing place, or its pronunciation, etc. which is used to harmonize the *zang-fu* organs and restore Yin-Yang balance to the individual with its predominating actions. Briefly speaking, actions of Chinese medicinals are chiefly based on the principle of "**Like attracts like**".

Metaphorizing Its Property: Cool or cold medicinals have the actions of clearing heat, draining fire, cooling blood and reducing toxicity, etc; while warm or hot medicinals have the actions of warming the interior, dispersing cold, supplementing fire, reinforcing yang, warming the meridians and freeing the network vessels, restoring yang from collapse, etc.

Metaphorizing Its Flavour: Generally speaking, acrid medicinals can disperse and promote the flow of *qi* and blood; sweet can tonify, moderate, and harmonize; sour can astringe; bitter can drain fire and dry dampness; salty can soften the hardness and free the bowels; bland can promote urination, etc.

Metaphorizing Its Colour: Such a viewpoint has been systematized and theorized by the aid of the five-phase theory since the Han dynasty (206B.C.-220A.D.). *Essentials of Materia Medica*[395] (Ben Cao Bei Yao. Yao Xing Zong Yi) states that medicinals of green-blue with sour taste pertains to wood, all enter the Liver and Gallbladder Meridians (The liver stands interior-exterior relationship with the gallbladder, the gallbladder is *Jia* wood, the liver is *Yi* wood); medicinals of red with bitter taste pertains to fire, all enter the Heart and Small Intestine Meridians (The heart stands interior-exterior relationship with the small intestine, the small intestine is *Bing* fire, the heart is *Ding* fire) ; medicinals of yellow with sweet taste pertains to earth, all enter the Spleen and Stomach Meridians (The spleen stands interior-exterior relationship with the stomach, the stomach is *Wu* earth, the spleen is *Ji* earth); medicinals of white with acrid taste pertains to metal, all enter the Lung and Large Intestine Meridians (The lung stands interior-exterior relationship with the large intestine, the large intestine is *Geng* metal, the lung is *Xin* metal); and that medicinals of black with salty taste pertains to water, all enter the Kidney and the Bladder Meridians (the kidney stands interior-exterior relationship with the bladder, the bladder is *Ren* water, the kidney is *Gui* water.).[396]

For example: There are five colours of beans to enter the five zang organs respectively. Black bean, black in color, its shape is like that of the kidney, the grain of the kidney, so can tonify the kidney; Red bean, red in color, the grain of the heart, with downbearing property, can free the small intestine and has the function of diuresis; the white hyacinth bean, white and yellowish, the grain of the spleen, can regulate the spleen and warm the stomach. The following are some other examples illustrated with pictures.

395 *Ben Cao Bei Yao* 本草备要, or *Essentials of Materia Medica*： a clinical manual of materia medica and a door to Chinese medicine with 8 volumes and published in 1694 by Wang Ang 汪昂 (1615-1695).

396 *Jia, Yi, Bing, Ding, Wu, Ji, Geng, Xin, Ren, Gui*: the ten heavenly stems.

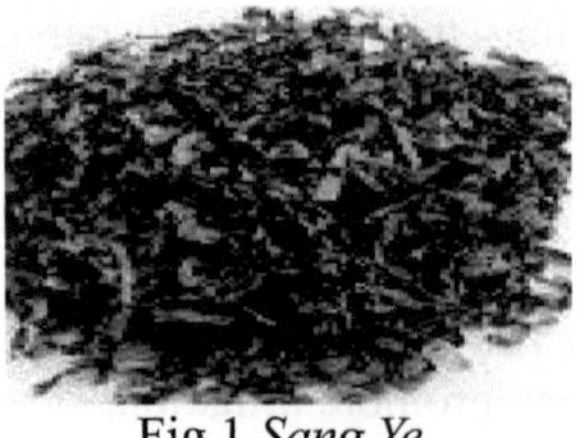

Fig.1 *Sang Ye*

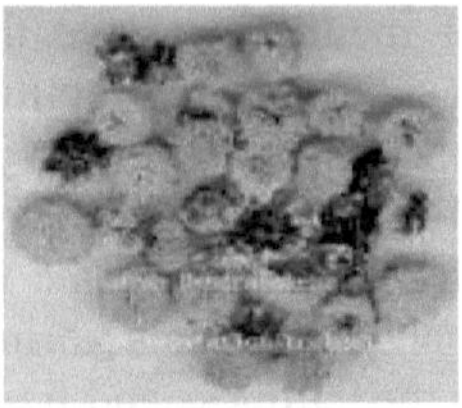

Fig.2 *Ju Hua*

The greenish, whitish, yellowish medicinals are usually said to enter the phase of *qi*, used to treat exterior pattern, such as mulberry leaf (Folium Mori, *Sang Ye*; Fig.1) and chrysanthemum (Flos Chrysanthemi, *Ju Hua*; Fig.2)

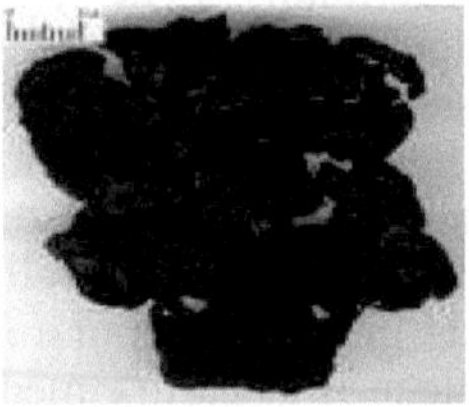

Fig.3 *Di Huang*

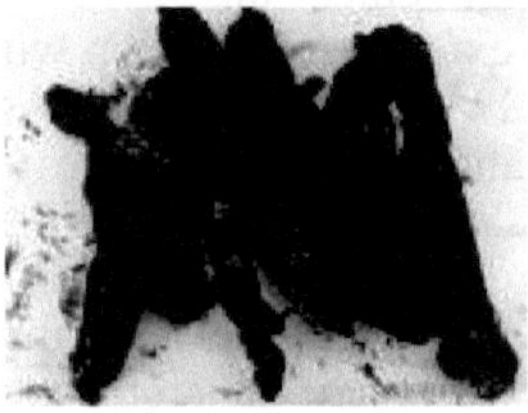

Fig.4 *Xuan Shen*

The reddish, blackish, dark yellow medicinals are usually said to enter the phase of blood, used to treat interior pattern, such as rehmannia (Radix Rehmanniae, *Di Huang*; Fig.3) and scrophularia (Radix Scrophulariae, *Xuan Shen*; Fig.4).

Besides, green-blue, red, yellow, white and black medicinals are attributed to different zang-fu organs according to the five-phase theory. For example:

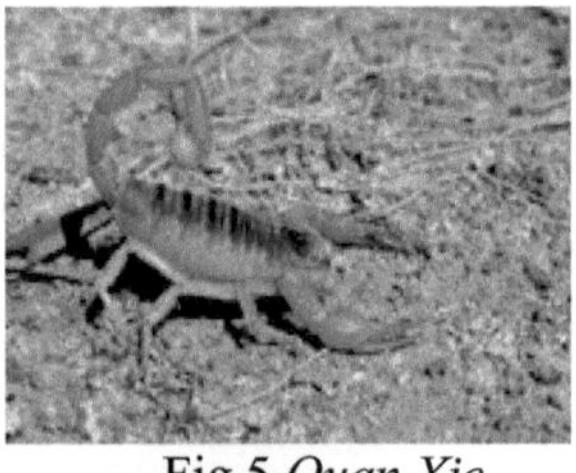

Fig.5 *Quan Xie*

Scorpion (Buthus, *Quan Xie*, Fig 5), whose body colour is *green-blue*, is said to enter the *Liver* Meridian, and is therefore used to treat *wind disease*, such as convulsion, spasm, stubborn *bi* syndrome, e.g. arthritis, etc.

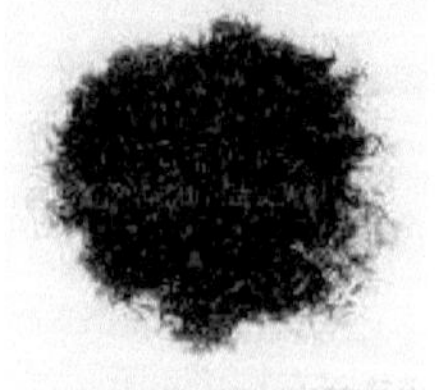

Fig.6 *Hong Hua*

Carthamus (Flos Carthami, *Hong Hua*, Fig.6), whose colour is *red*, is said to enter the *Heart and Liver* Meridians, and therefore is used to promote the flow of blood, remove blood stasis, and free menstruation for the *blood* is from the heart and is stored in the liver.

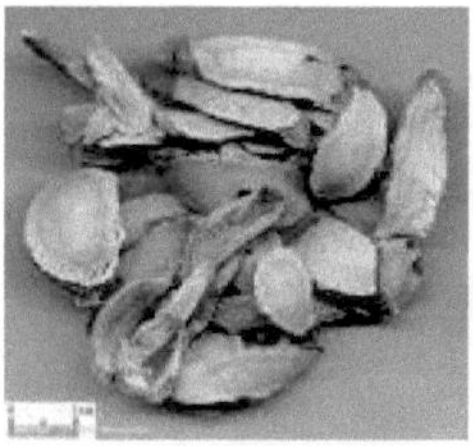

Fig.7 *Huang Qi*

Astragalus (Radix Astragali, *Huang Qi*, Fig.7), whose colour is *yellow* and whose flavour is *sweet*, is said to enter the *Spleen* Meridian, and is therefore very effective in *tonifying the Spleen and benefiting Qi*.

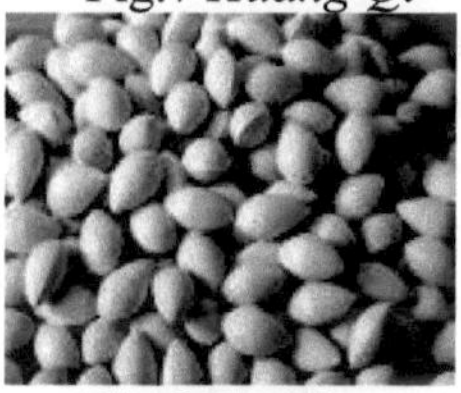

Fig.8 *Yin Xing*

Gingko (*Yin Xing*, Fig.8), whose colour is *white*, is said to enter the *Lung* Meridian, and is therefore used to supplement the Lung *Qi* and arrest coughing.

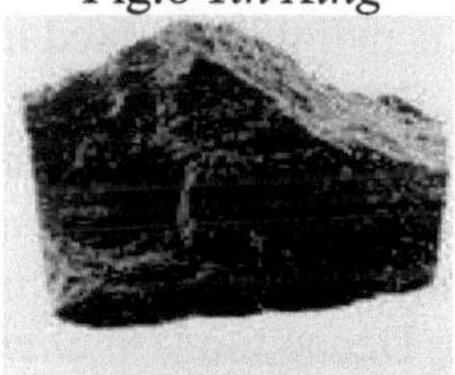

Fig.9 *Ci Shi*

Magnetite (*Ci Shi*, Fig.9), whose colour is *black* and *heavy* in quality, is said to enter the *Kidney* Meridian, and is therefore used to tonify the Kidney and subdue yang, arrest panting, deafness and tinnitus caused by Kidney deficiency, downbear the reverse upward flow of *Qi*.

Some medicinals with more than one colour or even five colours can be used to treat various diseases. For example, Jujube is formed from small white flower to fruit of first green, then white and yellow, then red after being ripe, then blackish after being picked up and dried under the sun, bearing the colours and qualities of the five phases, and therefore can nourish the Spleen and Stomach, free and open the nine orifices, benefit the twelve meridians, supplement *qi*, engender fluid, tonify the blood, supplement deficiencies of all kinds, harmonize all of the other medicinals, etc. (Zhang Zhicong, *Ben Cao Chong Yuan* or *The Origin of Materia Medica*[397]. *Ben Jing Shang Pin* or Top Grade Medicinals of *Shennong's Classic of Materia Medica*)

397 *Ben Cao Chong Yuan* 本草崇原 or *The Origin of Materia Medica:* a monograph on materia medica, which annotates *Shennong's Classic of Materia Medica,* by Zhang Zhicong 张志聪 (1616-1674). Based on the five circuit phases, six climatic factors, and waxing and waning between yin and yang, Zhang Zhicong founded the *Yao Qi* 药气 theory to expound actions of medicinals in details, which starts from the formation of properties and flavors, attributes of yin-yang and five-phases as well as shapes and colors of medicinals, and correlates the machanism of curing an illness. His approach deeply influenced such medical experts as Xu Dachun 徐大椿 (1693-1771) and Chen Xiuyuan 陈修园 (1753-1823).

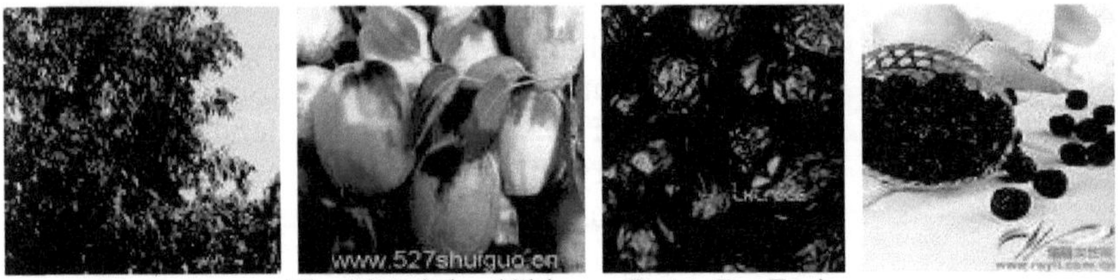

Fig.10 Jujube (Chinese Date, *Da Zao*)

Metaphorizing Its Shape: The typical example is ginseng. The Chinese name is *Ren Shen* 人参, of which *Ren* 人 means human being. *The Origin of Materia Medica.* Top Grade Medicinals of *Shennong's Classic of Materia Medica* (Ben Cao Chong Yuan. Ben Jing Shang Pin) by Zhang Zhicong states that the root of ginseng is like the shape of the human being with head, face, and the four limbs. It receives the brilliance of the Heaven and the vastness and richness of the Earth, and forms into the shape of the human being after a long time, thus having the quality of the Heaven, Earth, and human being. Therefore, it is mainly indicated in supplementing or tonifying the human being.

Besides, Ginseng mainly grows in the damp shadow places of forests in the North-East of China, can survive in one of the world coldest places, and is therefore very effective in restoring yang from collapse and contraindicated in excessive and heat patterns, such as the famous Pure Ginseng Decoction (*Du Shen Tang*).

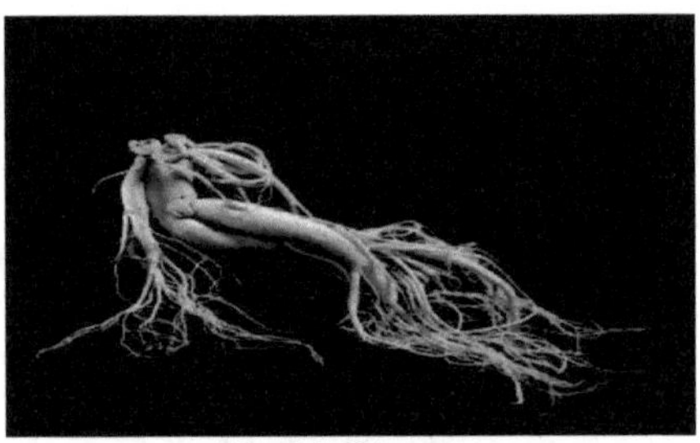
Fig.11 Ginseng

Metaphorizing Its Disposition: Generally speaking, flower is usually on the tip of a branch, and therefore can expel the pathogenic factors on the head and eyes; the leaves distribute around a plant in different directions, and therefore can disperse; stem and branch can treat diseases of the limbs; seed conceives a new life, and therefore can tonify the Kidney, strengthen sexuality, help conceiving a fetus, and treat sterility (male) and/or infertility (female); hollow medicinals or with holes can free the flow of *qi* and free the network vessels; medicinals rich in fluid can increase humour; vine can free the network vessels; and so and so forth. Take krait for example.

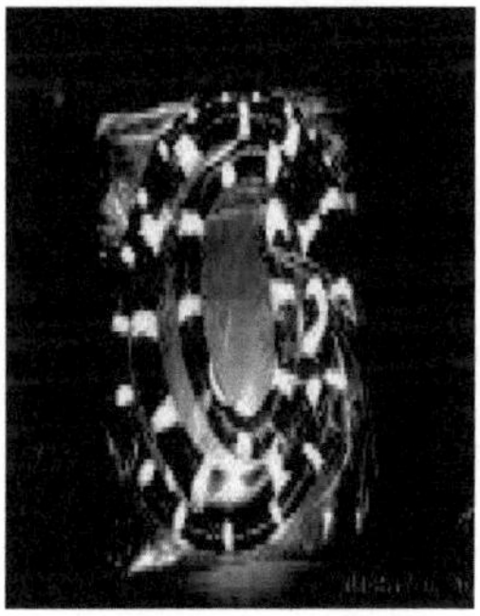

Fig.12 Krait

"The snake can treat all kinds of wind diseases. … The wind moves swiftly and is changeable. The snake also moves swiftly and exuviates (casts off or sheds) many times in its life. Therefore, it can track wind deep into the bone, stabilize convulsions (caused by wind), and is an important medicinal for wind blockage disease, convulsions, leprosy, tinea, serious sores and ulcers for it can move through the bowels and viscera inside, run through the skin outside, can reach nowhere in the body". (Li Shizhen, *Ben Cao Gang Mu* or *The Compendium of Materia Medica*)

Metaphorizing its pronunciation[398]*:* Take seeds as another example. "*The seed* (籽) *can produce semen* （子）". Seed conceives a new life. *Shen Nong's Classic of Materia Medica* read that *Wu Wei Zi* (schisandra, Schisandrae Fructus) can benefit or supplement the male's semen; *Ben Cao Jing Ji Zhu* or *A Collection of Annotations on Classic of Materia Medica* states that *Gou Qi Zi* (lycium berry, Lycii Fructus) can tonify essential *qi*, strengthen sexuality; *Yao Xing Lun* or *On Properties of Medicinals* records that *Tu Si Zi* (cuscuta, Cuscutae Semen) can benefit essence or semen and supplement marrow, and that *Fu Pen Zi* (rubus, Rubi Fructus) is indicated in deficiency or depletion of kidney essence for the male and infertility for the female; *Ben Cao Hui Yan* or *A Collection of Words on Materia Medica* states that *Che Qian Zi* (plantago seed, Plantaginis Semen) can strengthen sexuality and help conceiving a fetus; and so and so forth. A version of textbook "*Chinese Herbal Medicine*" published in the 1950's states that "most of the medicinals rich in seed are said to enter the kidney", and we know that kidney is responsible for growth, development and reproduction (maturation) in Chinese medicine. There are some formulae which are mainly composed of different seeds, such as Seven-Seed Powder recorded in the *Bei Ji Qian Jin Yao Fang* or *Invaluable Prescriptions for Emergencies* mainly for male's sterility due to

398 There are three important methods to explain a sinogram in ancient Chinese texts: "discerning meaning by interpreting and analyzing its structure", "discerning meaning in the light of pronunciation", and "discerning meaning in its contexts". It is worth to note that "structure" here refers to that of sinograms in Oracle, Bronze, or Lesser Seal Script such as the approach in *Shuo Wen Jie Zi* or *The Origin of Chinese Characters,* not that in Simplied Lesser Seal or Regular Script; that "pronunciation" refers to that of sinograms of the Zhou, Qin, and Han Dynasties (ca. 11th Century B.C. – A.D. 220), which are generally known as pronunciation of the ancient times; All of the three methods should be used in a rigorous way, esp. the second one "discerning meaning in the light of pronunciation", and observe the principle that "Single evidence is untenable". Actually "discerning meaning in the light of pronunciation" is also a specific Chinese cultural phenomenon. Take *Hu Lu* 葫芦 or the bottle gourd as an example. Its pronunciation sounds like *Fu Lu* 福禄 or blessing and emolument, so it has long been regarded as a traditional symbol for blessing and emolument among Chinese people.

deficiency of essential *qi*, Five-Seed Progeny Pill recorded in *Yi Xue Ru Men* or *Introduction to Medicine* as "the No.1 prescription for conceiving a fetus of all times", and Pill of Five-Seed and Whole Deer recorded in *Chi Shui Xuan Zhu* or *The Black Bead in the Red Water* for sterility and infertility due to yang deficiency.

To sum up, all of the Chinese medicinals come into being and shape from the *Qi* of the Heaven and Earth, have different actions, and therefore can treat different illnesses, which can be inferred from metaphorizing their *qi* (property), flavour, colour, shape, quality, etc. through *Qu Xiang Bi Lei* outlined in the framework of *Tian Ren He Yi*.

6.4 Metaphorizing: A Vital Way to Understand Medicine made from a Formula/Prescription[399] (*Yao*)

It is a great qualitative leap of the development of Chinese herbal medicine from the use of a single medicinal to a compound formula, in which therapeutic interactions among different medicinals are strengthened, and toxicity or side effect is reduced through coordinating actions of different medicinals. To identify the pattern and establish a treating principle is the premise of formulating a formula/prescription, which is generally composed of Chief, Associate, Assistant and Guide medicinals, a holistic approach to disease treatment of harmonizing different aspects of the patient:

- *Sovereign [Chief]:* provides the principal therapeutic action;
- *Minister [Associate]*: helps strengthen the principal action;
- *Adjuvant [Assistant]*: relieves secondary symptoms or tempers the action of the Chief when the latter is too potent;
- *Courier [Guide]*: directs action to the affected Meridian or site.

6.5 Metaphorizing: A Vital Way to Modernize Chinese Herbal Medicine

Previous attempts to modernize Chinese herbal medicine have focused on isolating active ingredients from herbal remedies and screening them one at a time, which accords with the Western way of thinking, i.e. analytical or abstract thinking. And such an approach has led to a handful of new treatments, such as artemisinin for treating malaria and the decongestant ephedrine, "but there has been no goldrush of approved drugs." The Western way of thinking can be an ideal complement to the Chinese way of thinking, and the corresponding research outcome provides valuable references for both researchers and practitioners. But I think the Chinese way of thinking should be of more significance in guiding the studies on modernizing Chinese herbal medicine.

399 I use "formula" for one with a fixed name and a fixed group of component medicinals with fixed dosages, and "prescription" for one prescribed by a practitioner aimed at a specific patient in his/her specific condition.

The 1st Example – Tripterygium Wilfrodis (*Lei Gong Teng*, 雷公藤)[400]: Li Leishi 黎磊石 discovered for the first time the therapeutic effect of Tripterygium Wilfrodis in treating various chronic nephritis, lupus nephritis, and purpuric nephritis, and spread it to the whole country through metaphorizing Tripterygium Wilfrodis's immunosuppressive action in taking effect in treating nephritis and allergic dermatological diseases. Later on he proved the effect of an ingredient isolated from this herb in acute rejection after renal transplantation, and clarified Tripterygium Wilfrodis's immunosuppressive action in an all round way.

The 2nd Example – Realgar-Indigo Naturalis Formula (RIF, *Fu Fang Qing Dai Wan*, 复方青黛丸)[401]: The main components of RIF are realgar (*xiong huang*, 雄黄), *Indigo naturalis* (*qing dai*, 青黛) and *Salvia miltiorrhiza* (*dan shen*, 丹参) with tetraarsenic tetrasulfide (A), indirubin (I), and tanshinone IIA (T) as their major active ingredients respectively. The research group took the active ingredients as the representatives of the three medicinals (a kind of metaphorizing) to study the synergy in the treatment of a murine APL model *in vivo* and in the induction of APL cell differentiation *in vitro*. Their data also indicate A as the principal component of the formula, whereas T and I serve as adjuvant ingredients. They therefore suggest that dissecting the mode of action of clinically effective formulae at the molecular, cellular, and organism levels may be a good strategy in exploring the value of traditional medicine. This case has been regarded as a successful case of researching compound formulas of Chinese medicine. Therefore, the strategy of composing a formula (Chief, Associate, Assistant and Guide medicinals) will be a valuable strategy in discovering or synthesizing new drugs. [402]

To sum up, I think metaphorizing is a vital way to understand, to research, to and modernize Chinese herbal medicine, and will be also a valuable strategy in discovering or synthesizing new drugs.

---

400 Li Leishi. Personal Experiences in Integrating Chinese Medicine with Western Medicine [J]. Chinese Journal of Integrated Traditional and Western Medicine, 1998, 18 (12):707.

401 Wang Lan, Zhou Guangbiao, Liu Ping, et al.. Dissection of Mechanisms of Chinese Medicinal Formula Realgar-Indigo Naturalis as An Effective Treatment for Promyelocytic Leukemia [J]. PNAS (Proceedings of the National Academy of Sciences of the United States of America), 2008, Vol. 125 (12): 4826-4831.

402 Qiu, Jane. 'Back to the future' for Chinese herbal medicines [J]. Nature, 2007 (6): 506-507.

The numbers start at one, end with ten, and complete with three.

- *Shi Ji. Lu Shu* or *Historical Records. Calendar*

7 Number Metaphors for Constructing the Theoretical System of Chinese Medicine

The numbers in Chinese medicine embody philosophy of numbers in Chinese culture.

7.1 Numbers in Chinese Medicine

Numbers are everywhere in Chinese medicine, for example:

- ❖ One: *Tian Ren He Yi* 天人合一: Literally means "Universe and Man Uniting into One", while my translation is "Universe and Man Uniting and Resembling Each Other"; and One pillow for pulse taking;
- ❖ Two *Qi*: Yin and Yang;
- ❖ Three Materials: three resources of Chinese materia medica - herbs, minerals, and animal parts;
- ❖ Three Grades: three grades of Chinese material medica – Top, Medium, and Low Grade Medicinals;
- ❖ Three treasures: Essence, *Qi*, and Spirit - man as one unity with three dimensions;
- ❖ Three *Jiao*: also known as "triple energizer" or "triple burner", a collective term for the three portions of the body cavity, i.e. Upper, Middle and Lower *Jiao*, through which *qi* and fluids are transmitted;
- ❖ Three pathogenic categorizations: All of the disease-causing factors can be classified into three - internal, external, non-external & non-internal pathogens;
- ❖ Four *Qi*: four properties of Chinese medicinal substances – cold, hot, warm and cool;
- ❖ Four examinations: inspection, listening & smelling, inquiry (history-taking), and palpation (including pulse taking) - four diagnostic methods of examining a patient and collecting information for making a diagnosis;
- ❖ Five flavors: five flavors of Chinese medicinal substances – sour, bitter, sweet, acrid, and salty;
- ❖ Five *zang* organs: heart, liver, spleen, lungs, and kidneys;
- ❖ Six *fu* organs: gallbladder, stomach, large intestine, small intestine, bladder, Triple energizer;
- ❖ Six *Qi*: six climatic influences, i.e. wind, cold, summer-heat, dampness, dryness and fire, the normal climatic conditions in the nature;
- ❖ Six excesses: the six pathogenic excessive or untimely climatic influences as exopathogenic factors – pathogenic wind, cold, summer-heat, dampness, dryness and fire; `

- ❖ Six meridians: Taiyang, Yangming, Shaoyang, Taiyin, Shaoyin, and Jueyin;
- ❖ Seven emotions: also known as "seven affects" - Joy, anger, melancholy, anxiety, grief, fear, and fright;
- ❖ Eight therapeutic methods: sweating, vomiting, precipitating (mainly refers to "purgation"), warming, clearing, harmonizing, supplementing, dispersing;
- ❖ Eight principal patterns: yin and yang, exterior and interior, cold and heat, deficiency and excess patterns;
- ❖ Eight extraordinary vessels: governing, controlling, girdling, thoroughfare, yin heel, yang heel, yin link, yang link vessels;
- ❖ Twelve regular meridian-vessels: the main passages for *qi* and blood, namely Lung Meridian of Hand-Taiyin (LU), Large Intestine Meridian of Hand-Yangming (LI), Stomach Meridian of Foot-Yangming (ST), Spleen Meridian of Foot-Taiyin (SP), Heart Meridian of Hand-Shaoyin (HT), Small Intestine Meridian of Hand-Taiyang (SI), Bladder Meridian of Foot-Taiyang (BL), Kidney Meridian of Foot-Shaoyin (KI), Pericardium Meridian of Hand-Jueyin (PC), Triple *Jiao* Meridian of Hand-Shaoyang (TJ), Gallbladder Meridian of Foot-Shaoyang (GB), and Liver Meridian of Foot-Jueyin (LR);

...

Shi Ji. Lu Shu or *Historical Records. Calendar* reads that "The numbers start at one, end with ten, and complete with three". Now let us take a look at some commonly emcountered important numbers - one, three, five, six, and twelve.

7.2 One (一 and 壹): The Origin of All things

"One (*yi* 一) is the original great beginning. Tao is based on one (*yi* 一), and then is to separate the heaven from the earth and to create all the things".

- *The Origin of Chinese Characters*

"The movements under the heaven start from one (*yi* 一)."

- *The Book of Changes*

"At the great beginning there was Non-being, [but] no Being nor Name. That was where one (*yi* 一) started, but still no physical appearance."

- *Chuang Tzu. Chapter of Heaven and Earth*

"Where do the rules start to be established? They start to be established at the great oneness. The great oneness is the root of all the beings and the bottom of all the phenomena."

- *Arts of Painting. The Great Oneness of Visual Arts*[403]

403 The author is Shi Tao 石涛 (1630-1724), a great artist in Chinese painting. As Kaptchuk said that "The arts in China were nourished by the same natualist and Taoist sensibility that fed Chinese philosophy and medicine". See Kaptchuk, Ted J. 2000: 17.

One is far beyond the number one. In philosophers' eyes, one is the origin of all the things. *The Origin of Chinese Characters* starts from "*yi* 一", ends with "hai 亥", the last of the twelve earthly branches. The interpretation of "*yi* 一" in *The Origin of Chinese Characters* completely carries on the concepts in the myth of creating the world, thus conceiving the system of the concepts of the genesis of the universe in Chinese philosophy. "*Yi* 一" is far beyond the number one, and is the opposite of the multiple as the myriad of things in the universe, and is the exact mysterious being or state before the beginning of the world.[404]

In Chinese, both 一 and 壹 means one. Actually, 壹 is derived from 一. *Yi* 壹, written as  in lesser seal script, resembles the image of a pot with a lid. *The Origin of Chinese Characters* interprets it as "undivided. Following 壺 (Pot)". *The Book of Songs · July* reads that "To pick up bottle gourds in August"(八月断壶), where Mao's interpretation reads that "*Hu* 壶 refers to the bottle gourd". The bottle gourd stands for the creation myth of the world: the upper became the heaven and the lower became the earth. See the Illus. 10.

In Chinese legends, the bottle gourd had functioned as a vessel to save people from flooding like Noah's ark. There are unearthed bottle gourds and bottle gourd-shaped potteries from some early ruins of 7,000 years ago in China. You see, in ancient Chinese people's eyes, the bottle gourd was a symbol for uterus, and so for the female as well. The bottle gourd can be divided into two, which has been an essential utensil for a family, functioning as a spoon or a container. It has long been an original mascot for Chinese people, a symbol of good fortune, happiness, and official salary.

Giradort, Norman J., an American sinologist, believed that the bottle gourd was the sub-type of cosmological egg. He said that bottle gourd and egg, chaos and nothing, hermaphroditic giant, and incestuous primordial couple can all be understood as the mythological symbol of "the fullness of being", which stresses the primordial unity of the sexes.[405]

The Fu Xi & Nü Wa Coupling Figure has many different versions, from stone figures of the Han Dynasty (206B.C.-220A.D.) to paintings on silk, or paper of later dynasties, esp. until the Northern Dynasties (386-581). Paintings on silk or paper tend to be easily destroyed and decomposed, so are difficult to be found. But a large number of them are available in Turpan[406], Xinjiang. The Illus. 11 is one of those paintings. Fu Xi and Nü Wa in this painting have high noses and deep

404 Ye Shuxian, Tian Daxian. 1998:3.

405 Translated from Chinese. See the original reference *Myth and Meaning in Early Taoism*. Berkeley and Los Angeles: University of California Press, 1983.

406 Turpan has long been the centre of a fertile oasis and an important trade centre. It was historically located along the Silk Road's northern route, thus being international and intercultural. It was originally one kingdom called Gushi 故師 which the Chinese conquered in 107 B.C.. During the Han era the city changed hands several times between the Xiongnu, an ancient nationality in China, and the Han, interspersed with short periods of independence.

eyes, just like persons of mixed blood. Wen Yiduo 闻一多 (1899-1946), a Chinese poet and scholar, did a textual research on Fu Xi. He believed that Fu Xi and Nü Wa, two names but one person, were personified bottle gourds, among which the only difference was the gender.[407]

Pan Gu separated the heaven from the earth. "The chaotic universe is just like an egg". And one was the chaotic universe, and the egg. *The Book of Changes* reads that "Therefore there is in the Changes the Great Primal Beginning. This generates the two primary forces (Yin and Yang). The two primary forces generate the four images (the four seasons). The four images generate the eight trigrams". Here in this quotation one is the *Tai Ji,* or the Great Primal Beginning.

Actually, Tao and One can be mutually interpretive. In fact, Tao bears two qualities, i.e., nothing and being. Nothing means without shape or image, i.e., the chaotic universe; Being means with shape and image, i.e. the one. So *Lao Tzu* reads that "Tao gives birth to one", which means that which has physical appearance is generated by that which has no physical appearance.

Qian Zuo Du of *The Book of Changes* 易.乾凿度 reads that "Confucius states that 'Changes start from *Tai Ji*. *Tai Ji* gives birth to two, i.e. yin and yang, so to generate the heaven and the earth. In between the heaven and the earth there are the seasons of Spring, Summer, Autumn, and Winter, i.e. the four seasons. Each of the four seasons has the qualities of yin and yang, hardness and softness; therefore, the eight trigrams are generated. The eight trigrams establish the Tao of the heaven and Earth, so the images of thunder, wind, water, fire, mountain and swamp are determined'".

To sum up, "*yi* 一" is the first beginning of the numbers; "*yi* 壹" represents the image of the bottle gourd, means "undivided". One is far beyond the number one. Philosophers' interpretation of One is the origin of all things. All in all, One is *Tai Ji* or the Great Primal Beginning, the foundation of Tao, and the mystical state before the Genesis of the world.

The reasons that *The Origin of Chinese Characters* starts with "*yi* 一" and ends with "*hai* 亥" lie in that "*yi* 一" refers to *Tai Ji* or the Great Primal Beginning, the foundation of Tao, and the mystical state before the Genesis of the world; while "hai 亥" is interpreted as "the image of a pregnant woman, delivering a baby, then starting again from *yi* 一", then transforming again into everything in the universe. Such an arrangement also suggests the circular reasoning of Chinese philosophy.

7.3 Three Gives Birth to All Things

Lao Tzu reads that

"Tao begets the one,

---

407 See the first volume of *The Complete Works of Wen Yiduo*.

The one begets the two,
The two begets the three,
and the three gives birth to all things (in the universe)".

Tao and One can be mutually interpretive. In fact, Tao bears two qualities, i.e., nothing and being. Nothing means without shape or image, i.e., the chaotic universe; Being means with shape and image, i.e. the one. So "Tao gives birth to one" means that which has physical appearance is generated by that which has no physical appearance. Two refers to the heaven and the earth, and yin and yang; "The two begets the three" can be understood as the union of the heaven *qi* and the earth *qi* makes man. And then three, i.e. the heaven, the earth and the man, is the first complete unit of the creation of the world. Therefore three is the foundation for the birth, growth and development of all things in the universe.

Here I would like to suggest you to read Stephen Hawking's works such as *Stephen Hawking's Universe* (1997) and *A Brief History of Time* (1988). You will learn more by reading them together with *Lao Tzu*.

Zuo Zhuan or *Zuo's Spring Autumn Annals* states that "Three is the number of the heaven, the earth and the man". *The Origin of Chinese Characters* explains "three" as "the Tao (way) of Heaven, Earth and Man". *The Historical Records* reads that "The numbers start at one, end with ten, and complete with three". *The Book of Changes* names the heaven, the earth, and man as "Three *Cai*". *Cai* 才, written as  in the oracle script, is a pictographic, in which the upper horizontal line stands for the soil, the part below it resembles the image of the tender shoot just sprouting from the seed but not coming up out of the ground, and so its original meaning is "(of trees and grasses, or plant) newborn".

Let's now go back to *Lao Tzu. the 42nd Chapter.*

"Tao begets the one,
The one begets the two,
The two begets the three,
and the three gives birth to all things (in the universe).
All things in the universe bear yin and embrace yang,
where the central and harmonious *qi* makes them in harmony."

The relationship of "the central and harmonious *qi*" and "the Three Newborns" is just like that of "the soil" and "the five phases", where the soil is in the Center of the other four phases, i.e. Wood-East, Fire-South, Metal-West, and Water-North. If without the middle there would be no Left Wing nor Right Wing; if without the central and harmonious *qi* there would be no Yin *qi* nor Yang *qi*. Take the structure of an atom as an example. Its outer is the electrons (-), while its inner is composed of the protons (+) and neutrons. If without the neutrons, an atom could not be kept as a stable entity. It is clear that the central and harmonious *qi* bears the same importance as the neutrons. And Heaven – Earth - Man make up a holistic system, among which they are independent and closely related to each other and Man is the dominator.

Five Phases are actually the foundation for constructing the visceral image theory, meridian theory, and herbal theory, etc. in Chinese medicine.

7.4 Five *Zang* Organs and Six *Fu* Organs

The Book of Changes states that "Heaven is one, earth is two; heaven is three, earth is four; heaven is five, earth is six; heaven is seven, earth is eight; heaven is nine, earth is ten. There are five heavenly numbers, and there are also five earthly numbers. When they are distributed among the five places, each finds its complement. The sum of the heavenly numbers is twenty-five, and that of the earthly numbers is thirty. The sum total of heavenly numbers and earthly numbers is fifty-five. It is this which results in the changes and transformations and moves demons and gods."

That is to say, in the numbers from one to ten, the odd are heavenly numbers, while the even are earthly numbers. Six is a heavenly number, while five is an earthly number. Therefore, the heaven has six climatic influences, i.e. wind, cold, summer-heat, dampness, dryness, and fire, and man has six *fu* organs, which pertain to Yang; The earth has five phases, i.e. wood, fire, soil, metal, and water, and man has five *zang* organs, which pertain to Yin.

Six to five, why? I have consulted ancient Chinese classics and have got some related quotations for your information.

Guo Yu. Zhou Yu or *Records of States. Records of Zhou* reads that "The heaven is six and the earth is five, which are the rules of the numbers".

Zuo Zhuan. Zhao Gong Yuan Nian or *Zuo's Spring and Autumn Annals. The 1st Year of Zhao Gong's Reign* reads that "The heaven has six climatic influences, which go down to give birth to five flavors, to present with five colors, and to manifest in five tones".

Han Shu. Lu Li Zhi or *History of the Former Han Dynasty. Treatise on Calendar* reads that "The heaven is six and the earth is five, which are the rules of the numbers. The heaven has six climatic influences, which go down to give birth to five flavors. The five plus the six is the number in between the heaven and the earth. … The eleven terminates the way of the heaven and the earth".

In ancient Chinese people's eyes, the evolution of the *zang fu* organs was a kind of group development following the rule of the nature. *Nan Jing Ji Zhu* or *A Collection of Annotations on The Classic of Difficult Issues*[408] reads that "The reason that the *zang* organs are five and *fu* organs are six is that the five *zang* organs respond to the five phases on the earth, and the six *fu* organs echo the six

408 *Nan Jing Ji Zhu* 难经集注 or *A Collection of Annotations on The Classic of Difficult Issues*: a collection of annotations on *The Classic of Difficult Issues* from Lu Guang 吕广 of the Three Kingdoms (220-265), Yang Xuancao 杨玄操 of the Tang Dynasty (618-907), and Ding Deyong 丁德用, et al of the Song Dynasty (960-1279) by Wang Jiusi 王九思 in 1505 of the Ming Dynasty (1384-1644), the extant earliest collection of annotations on *The Classic of Difficult Issues*. It has 5 volumes and 13 chapters.

climatic influences upon the heaven, among which the triple *jiao* is the premier fire and is attributed to hand lesser yang. Therefore, only *fu* organs are six".

All of the knowledge related to *zang fu* organs was systematized as the visceral image theory. *Zang Fu* 藏府, now written as 脏腑 in Chinese, are metaphors formed in the way of observing, taking images from and analogizing the social storing system of the remote antiquity. Five *zang* organs 五藏 store the essential *qi* but not drain, like *zang* 藏 or depots which stored the invaluable treasures and were not allowed to take out; Six *fu* organs 六府 transform the water and grain (food) but not store, like *fu* 府 or six palaces which stored six kinds of goods and were daily consumed and supplemented with.

Zuo Zhuan. Wen Gong Qi Nian or *Zuo's Spring & Autumn Annals. The 7th Year of Wen Gong's Reign* reads that "Water, fire, metal, wood, soil, and grain are termed six *Fu*". An annotation reads that "Six is the number of man's *fu* organs".

Why is that - the heaven six and the earth five? The answer would be that culture depends on natural and social environments, and that science depends on culture. This point of view has been developed through

① Thomas Samuel Kuhn (1922-1996), one of the most influential philosophers of science of the twentieth century, see *The Structure of Scientific Revolutions,* Chicago: University Of Chicago Press, 1996;

② Paul Feyerabend (1924-1994), a critic of Karl Popper's "critical rationalism" and one of the twentieth century's most famous philosophers of science, see *Against Method*, London: New Left Books, 1975; and *Realism, Rationalism and Scientific Methods: Philosophical Papers,* Volume 1, Cambridge: Cambridge University Press, 1981;

③ Friedrich G. Wallner (1945-), the founding father of Constructive Realism, an intercultural and interdisciplinary philosophy of science with the aim of making the manifold scientific approaches depending on different cultures understandable, see *Constructive Realism: Aspects of A New Epistemological Movement*, Wien: W. Braumueller, 1994.

7.5 Regular Meridians: From Eleven to Twelve

There were only 11 vessels recorded in *The Moxibustion Classic of 11 Vessels of Arms & Feet* and *The Moxibustion Classic of 11 Vessels of Yin & Yang,* two monographs on moxibustion unearthed from Mawangdui Han Tomb. But as we know, there have been 12 regular meridians since the time of *Ling Shu* or *Miraculous Pivot.* Then which one is missing? In the above mentioned two monographs on moxibustion unearthed from Mawangdui Han Tomb, there were only two hand yin meridian-vessels, and one was missing for the heart in Chinese medicine is said to be "the governor of the five *zang* and six *fu* organs ... Evils are not permitted to invade the heart"; and then that "the pericardium protects the heart by taking the invading evils instead" (*Ling Shu. Xie Ke* or *Miraculous Pivot. Evils Visited*). Later on, one heart meridian-vessel became divided into two, i.e.

Heart Meridian of Hand-Shaoyin (HT) and Pericardium Meridian of Hand-Jueyin (PC). And then the six pairs of meridian vessels - one *zang* and one *fu*, one yin and one yang; three yin and three yang, six hand medians and six foot meridians, were recorded in the *Ling Shu. Jing Mai* or *Miraculous Pivot. Meridian Vessels,* thus forming the so-called the Twelve Regular Meridians.

In Chinese culture, the number twelve was a specific and the greatest number of the heaven as well. For example, the Ten Heavenly Stems have been used as serial numbers and also in combination with the Twelve Earthly Branches to designate years, months, days, and hours since oracle scripts of the Yin-Shang Dynasty (ca. 17th - 11th Century B.C.).

Shi Ji. Lu Shu or *Historical Records. Calendar* reads that "The numbers start at one, end with ten, and complete with three". *Shuo Wen Jie Zi* or *The Origin of Chinese Characters* reads that "*Shi* 十 or Ten completes the numbers. The horizontal stroke '一' indicates East-West; the vertical '丨' indicates South-North, and then the sinogram 十 possesses the four directions and the center". Kong Yingda 孔颖达 (574-648) annotated that "Ten is the extreme of the numbers". Such understanding may result from that the counting of man's fingers ends with ten. In ancient Greece, Pythagoras (580? – 500? B.C.) school also attached great importance to the number Ten. As we know from *The Book of Changes* that from one to ten, the odd numbers "one, three, five, seven, and nine" are heavenly numbers, while the even numbers "two, four, six, eight, and ten" are earthly numbers, so the number Ten is the largest earthly number. In classical Chinese culture, the number "ten" represent the mysterious perfect, and many, numerous. For example, "*Shi Quan Shi Mei* 十全十美", an Chinese idiom, literally means "ten completenesses and ten beauties", actually means "be perfect in every aspect", "flawless and perfection", "be done to perfection"; "*Shi Mu Suo Shi, Shi Shou Suo Zhi* 十目所视，十手所指", another Chinese idiom originally from *Li Ji. Da Xue* or *The Book of Rites. The Great Learning*, literally means "ten eyes watching, and fingers of ten hands pointing", actually means "with many eyes watching and many fngers pointing – One cannot do wrong without being seen; Nothing could be done without public supervision".

The Twelve Earthly Branches are usually used to echo the twelve months. *Shi Ji. Lu Shu* or *The Historical Records. Calendar* names the Ten Heavenly Stems and the Twelve Earthly Branches as "Ten mothers and twelve sons". *Huai Nai Tzu. Tian Wen Xun* reads that "The numbers start from *Jia* 甲 and Zi 子, in which mother and son are matching to each other". *Bai Hu Tong* 白虎通[409] reads that

409 *Bai Hu Tong* 白虎通 was compiled during the reign of Han Zhang Di 漢章帝 (58－88 A.D.). The work started in the year 79 A.D. when he summoned his officers to hold a conference. The results were recorded and compiled by Ban Gu 班固 (32-92), a famous scholar. This becomes standard answers to questions about the study of *Jing Xue* 經學 or study of Confucian classics. It is interesting that this book even includes a section on sex education.

"The heavenly stems such as *Jia* 甲 and *Yi* 乙 are the trunk (stem), while the earthly branches such as *Zi* 子 and *Chou* 丑 are the branches". Actually the number twelve reflects the classical Chinese thinking of *Tian Ren He Yi* 天人合一 or Universe and Man Uniting and Resembling Each Other, such as the twelve months in a year, the twleve two-hour periods in a day – Midnight (PM23:00 – AM1:00), Rooster Crowing (AM1:00 -3:00), Daybreak (AM3:00-5:00), Sunrise (AM5:00-7:00), Eating Time (AM7:00-9:00), Midmorning (AM9:00-11:00), Midday (AM11:00-PM1:00), Sun Westing (PM1:00-3:00), Late Afternoon (PM3:00-5:00), Sunset (PM5:00-7:00), Dusk (PM7:00-9:00), Man Sleep (PM 9:00-11:00), which takes the movement of the sun to show the time order, and the twelve animals used to symbolize the year in which a person is born, etc.

Huai Nan Tzu. Patterns of Heave reads that "The heaven has the four seasons to regulate the twelve months; the man has the four limbs to make the twelve joints". And *Ling Shu. Wu Luan* reads that "The twelve vessels are supposed to respond to the twelve months".

Therefore we see that numbers in Chinese culture are far beyond the numbers. Numbers reflect the world view of ancient Chinese people. Numbers in Chinese medicine show that understanding of Man is based on the understanding of the universe, that Man and Universe unit and resemble each other, and that man mirrors the universe.

Chinese medicine needs to be developed and modernized in the way it was formed rather than to be westernized in accordance with Western scientific methods and criteria.

- The Author

8. Metaphorizing: A Vital Way to Develop and Modernize Chinese Medicine

As we know now that the theories of *qi*, yin-yang, the five phases, visceral image (*zang xiang*), the vessels (*jing luo*) and Chinese herbal medicine, the fundamental theories of Chinese medicine, were mainly formed by means of metaphorizing in the way of *Qu Xiang Bi Lei,* and Chinese medicine has been mainly developed also in this way, and thus sharing the same unique Chinese cultural and philosophical background. They are not discovered or detected by the modern Western scientific technology or methods, so their origin and essence cannot be revealed by Western scientific way, either. They can be only understood by means of interpreting metaphors.

In the recent last years, a famous research on acupuncture was done in Germany. Assurance companies in Germany wanted to know if acupuncture is really effective in treating some diseases, such as the low back pain, migraine, and headache in the sense of science, of course, the Western science, and so they sponsored a series of studies on the effect of acupuncture. This was a huge research project which had lasted some years and used many millions of Euros.[410, 411, 412, 413] They grouped patients into 3. The first group was treated by conventional therapy, pills of Western Medicine or put into the waiting list control; the second group was treated by real acupuncture given by German acupuncture experts; and the third group was treated by sham acupuncture, superficial needling at non-acupuncture points. The results were in every aspect funny. Firstly, Western medicine or conventional therapy or waiting list control was worse than acupuncture treatment group for the low back pain, tension-type headache and migraine; secondly, the sham acupuncture group had really near the same effect as the real acupuncture. Can we draw a conclusion that acupuncture theories are all

---

410 Klaus Linde, Andrea Streng, Susanne Jurgens, et al. Acupuncture for Patients With Migraine: A Randomized Controlled Trial [J]. The Journal of the Amerian Medical Association (*JAMA).* 2005; 293: 2118-2125.

411 Dieter Melchart, Andrea Streng, Andrea Hoppe, et al. Acupuncture in patients with tension-type headache: randomised controlled trial [J]. British Medical Journal, 2005, 331 (8): 376-382.

412 Michael Haake, Hans-Helge Muller, Carmen Schade-Brittinger, et al. German Acupuncture Trials (GERAC) for Chronic Low Back Pain: Randomized, Multicenter, Blinded, Parallel-Group Trial With 3 Groups [J].*Arch Intern Med.* 2007;167(17):1892-1898.

413 Klaus Linde, Claudia M. Witt, Andrea Streng, et al. The impact of patient expectations on outcomes in four randomized controlled trials of acupuncture in patients with chronic pain [J]. Journal of the International Association for the Study of Pain. 2007, 128 (3): 264-271.

nonsense? Can acupuncture and Chinese herbal medicine be treated and researched in the same as Western drugs? Of course not. The pure objective therapeutic effects have never been possible in the acupuncture treatment because mind-regulating has been attached great significance for both the patient and practitioner from the very beginning of acupuncture treatment.

An important aspect of creativity is the ability to create something new by relating it to something already done, known or understood. Clearly metaphorizing fits in well here because this is also its task. Metaphorizing has been a chief means by which famous physicians of the past generations created new thoughts, and thus developing Chinese medicine in both theoretical and clinical explorations.

"In the beginning, metaphors in scientific discourse may be not a kind of standardized scientific language, but can produce important scientific findings or even lead to the occurrence of scientific revolutions. Metaphorization stands for an approach which frees from the shackles of a kind of literal meaning, and being divergent and being creative constitute its intrinsic essence. In the scientific activities, scientists use metaphors mainly for the purpose of theoretical innovation not out of their interest of appreciation of the beauty".[414] In Chinese medicine, *Qu Xiang Bi Lei* or Taking Image and Analogizing, the metaphorizing process, not only states, constructs its theoretical system, guides its clinical practice, but is also a vital way to develop the system. Chinese medical experts are good at taking image and analogizing, and applying metaphorizing to make new explorations so as to develop Chinese medicine. Here I give you some examples:

8.1 Metaphorizing: A Vital Way to Develop Clinical Explorations of Chinese Medicine

8.1.1 *Ti Hu Jie Ga*: Carrying a Kettle and Uncovering Its Lid to Treat Dysuria

Ti Hu Jie Ga or Carrying a Kettle and Uncovering Its Lid to Treat Dysuria is a treating method created by Zhu Danxi 朱丹溪 (1281-1358), a famous physician and the founder of Yin-Nourishing School of the Jin-Yuan Dynasties (1115-1368). He was enlightened from a phenomena in daily life that uncovering the upper lid of a kettle filled with boiling water can make the water be poured out, and then inferred a treating method of "*Ti Hu Jie Gai*", which literally means "carrying a kettle and uncovering its lid (in order to pour out water)". What does this mean? The story reads that:

One day, a male patient with dysuria visited him, who was formerly treated by other physicians with diuretics of Chinese medicine which in fact aggravated his condition. Zhu Danxi felt that his right *cun* pulse (indicating the condition of

414 Guo Guichun. 2007: 36.

the lungs) was quite wiry and slippery, and then treated the patient with the method of dispersing the lung *qi*, then diuresis was successfully induced, and finally the patient was cured of the disease.

Zhu Danxi pointed out that the disease was caused by accumulation of phlegm in the lungs, and that the lungs are located in the upper *jiao* and the urinary bladder in the lower *jiao*, and that when the upper *jiao* is blocked the lower *jiao* will surely be obstructed, just like a kettle, only after the lid is uncovered, can water be poured out. This therapeutic method is known as *Ti Hu Jie Gai*, which literally means "carrying a kettle and uncovering its lid (in order to pour out water)", and actually refers to the method of dispersing the lung *qi* to induce diuresis, which is usually used to treat edema, dysuria, or anuria when the patient does not respond to the routine methods.

8.1.2 *Ni Liu Wan Zhou*: Saving the Boat in an Adverse Current to Treat Dysentery

Yu Jiayan 喻嘉言 (1585-1664), a famous physician in the early Qing Dynasty (1644-1911), created a therapeutic method named *Ni Liu Wan Zhou*, or saving the boat in an adverse (swift) current to treat enduring dysentery. He believed that dysentery was caused by external pathogen sinking into the interior, should be treated by lifting the external pathogen out of the exterior from the interior, just like saving a boat in an adverse and swift current to make the boat move upward. Accordingly, he formulated a formula named Ginseng Toxin-Vanquishing Powder to treat the disease. Afterwards, physicians of Chinese medicine usually apply this method and the formula to treat the dysentery with external pattern complicated with dampness.

8.1.3 *Zeng Shui Xing Zhou*: Increasing Water to Move the Boat to Treat Constipation

The term *Zeng Shui Xing Zhou* or Increasing Water to Move the Boat implies that: When the river flow cuts off for the lack of water, then boat will surely run aground. When the water is supplied and rises, then the boat will move in it easily.

Wu Jutong 吴鞠通 (1758-1836), a distinguished expert in warm disease of the Qing Dynasty (1644-1911), created the treating method termed as *Zeng Shui Xing Zhou,* or Increasing Water to Move the Boat to treat constipation caused by humor insufficiency or heat drying the humor, which is just like the boat running aground for the lack of water. Accordingly, he also formulated a formula named Humor-Increasing Decoction to treat the disease, which has become a famous and effective formula to treat constipation of this kind.

Besides, many other effective treating methods created by the way of *Qu Xiang Bi Lei* or Taking Image and Analogizing, the metaphorizing process, have been still in use in the clinical practice, such as:

Yin Huo Gui Yuan or Conducting Fire Back to Its Origin: a therapeutic method of leading the rising fire to the kidney, used in the treatment of declining fire of the life gate with floating of deficient yang;

Fu Di Chou Xin or Taking Away firewood from under the Cauldron: a therapeutic method of clearing heat or fire by purgation;

Zi Shui Han Mu or Enriching Water to Moisten Wood, a therapeutic method of nourishing kidney yin to subdue liver yang for hyperactivity of liver yang due to liver-kidney yin deficiency, which presents with such symptoms as dizziness, red complexion due to rising fire, and hypertension in some cases.

There are still many other methods or theories in Chinese medicine created by the way of *Qu Xiang Bi Lei*. We can see that the process of constructing and understanding metaphors is a typical example for creativity. The creative nature of metaphor is to find new relationships in two or more existing concepts or phenomena so as to explore new mental spaces and to advance new theories, thus developing Chinese medicine in both theoretical and clinical explorations.

8.2 Metaphorizing: A Vital Way to Develop and Modernize Chinese Medicine

Modernization of Chinese medicine has been a hot issue for dozens of years. The problem now is how to modernize but not westernize Chinese medicine. Therefore first it is essential to regard the differences between Chinese medicine and Western medicine, and the advantages of Chinese medicine as well. I advocate that there are no ranking but just different cultures, and that all cultures and sciences should be treated on an equal footing.

Based on what we have discussed before - metaphorizing is the process of *Qu Xiang Bi Lei* or Taking Image and Analogizing and the way of forming of metaphors; metaphorizing is the major way to form the ontological concepts, the fundamental theories, and to develop clinical explorations of Chinese medicine as well; and metaphorizing reveals the cultural presupposition of Chinese medicine - "*Tian Ren He Yi* 天人合一" or Universe and Man Uniting and Resembling Each Other, and the core methodology of Chinese medicine - "*Qu Xiang Bi Lei* 取象比类" or Taking Image and Analogizing; metaphorizing is also a vital approach to modernize Chinese medicine – to develop and modernize in the way how it was formed and has developed in the past thousands of years. Here again I give you some examples.

8.2.1 Metaphorizing: Pattern Identification based on Microcosmic Findings

Identifying pattern and instituting treatment is a major feature of Chinese clinical medicine. "Pattern Identification based on Microcosmic Findings" refers to a method of identifying pattern by using microcosmic findings gained through modern science and technology such as gastroscopy and ultrasound techniques but guided by Chinese medical theories.[415] For example, the color and state of the gastric mucusa can be seen through gastroscopy, so the light color usually indicates deficiency of *Qi* and blood; congestion and edema indicate the pattern being heat; the gastric mucusa in red and white check with submucous blood vessels visible indicates *qi* deficiency and blood stasis.

8.2.2 Metaphorizing: Discovery and Application of Effects of Tripterygium Wilfrodis

Li Leishi[416] discovered for the first time the therapeutic effect of Tripterygium Wilfrodis (*Lei Gong Ten,* 雷公藤) in treating various chronic nephritis, lupus nephritis, and purpuric nephritis, and spread it to the whole country through metaphorizing its immunosuppressive action in taking effect in treating nephritis and allergic dermatological diseases.

8.2.3 Metaphorizing: A Vital Way to Reveal Essence of Patterns

Zheng 证 or Pattern is a specific and significant concept in Chinese medicine. Actually, both acupuncture and herbal treatments are based on pattern understanding and identifying. That is to say, prescriptions of both acupoints and medicinal agents should be formulated according to the same procedure: *Li* or Theory – *Fa* or Method – *Fang* or Prescription – *Yao* or Agents (acupoints or herbs), a thinking way of the comprehensive application of Chinese medical theories, diagnosing and treating methods in the clinical practice. Therefore revealing the essence of the common patterns of acupuncture and herbal treatments bears both theoretical and practical significance.

Studies on essence of patterns of Chinese medicine are usually performed by the reductionist and analytic approach with Western scientific methods, i.e. interpreting patterns of Chinese medicine with modern science. This approach has been very fruitful in these years, and is also very important. For example, the pattern of Yin Deficiency can be interpreted by lab indexes of endocrine system, blood system, energy metabolism, cyclic nucleotide, trace elements, blood lipid, etc., and the research outcome can provide a foundation for further studies on its possible causes and pathogenesis as well as prevention and treatment of related diseases in Western medicine.

But how do we deal with these data and go one step further? My answer is to trace back to the source of a pattern, to investigate how this pattern was formed in Chinese medicine, and analyze the data in the way of metaphorizing, and then try to take metaphorizing as the philosophical approach to do the research. For

415 See Xue Feifei. The Emergence and Development of Pattern Identification based on Microcosmic Findings [D]. Beijing University of Chinese Medicine, 2006.

416 Li Leishi. Personal Experiences in Integrating Chinese Medicine with Western Medicine [J]. Chinese Journal of Integrated Traditional and Western Medicine, 1998, 18 (12):707.

example, inflammation is a pathological condition in Western medicine, manifesting in local redness, swelling, pain, ulcer and dysfunction as well as fever of different degrees, leukocytosis, fatigue, poor appetite, and so on, which is usually treated by antibiotics; While inflammation in Chinese medicine can be generally identified as fire - excessive fire which connects with heat, damp, phlegm, *qi* stagnation, or blood stasis, and deficient fire which connects with yin deficiency, and thus accordingly the fire can be relieved or reduced by different methods – clearing heat, eliminating dampness, resolving phlegm, freeing *qi*, promoting the flow of blood, or supplementing yin, which can be achieved with acupuncture or herbal prescriptions. In this case fire is the key metaphor, which runs through the aspects from the theoretical understanding of inflammation to its clinical treatment. The modern research can also take this point of view into consideration – fire as the central metaphor, and try to reveal the essence of fire of different kinds and their relationship to different inflammations in Western medicine. To sum up, metaphorizing is a vital way to reveal essence of patterns of Chinese medicine.

8.2.4 Metaphorizing: Philosophical Examinations of Treatments of Cancer

Of all major diseases that afflict us today, perhaps the most feared, and in many ways the most mysterious, is cancer. Cancer has become an increasingly prominent and feared cause of death. In modern Western medicine, the treatments of cancer can be generally classified into three forms, surgery, radiotherapy, and chemotherapy. Surgery is effective when the primary tumor has not begun to invade the tissue around it; Radiotherapy and chemotherapy are supposed to inhibit, kill the malignant cells, and/or increase the body resistance to the tumor cells. Such approaches achieve success in some cases, but at the same time produce serious side effects. Some patients did not die of cancer but died of radiotherapy or/and chemotherapy.

Based on the principle of comprehensive treatments and the care of the well-being of the cancer patient, Chinese medicine cannot be ignored when concerning the treatment of cancer, esp. for patients who have just undergone a surgical operation, or whose cancer is in the late stage or where metastasis happens. A lot of successful cases reported in China have shown that Chinese medicine can make the active malignant cells rest, thus making a tumor patient live with the tumor, or we could say, live in harmony with the tumor. Chinese medicine takes the being as a whole, cares the relationship among the phonomena and events that happen to the being at the same time, and activates the self-healing and self-organizing power of the being.

Here I propose this topic - How to Deal with Tumor: Killing, Inhibiting, or Living in Harmony with it? Killing and inhibiting are approaches of allopathic medicine, i.e. Western medicine. Then how can a human being live in harmony with tumor? Chinese herbal medicine and acupuncture can work as coordinators to coordinate, harmonize the relationship between the normal cells and the malignant cells. Whether coordinators are efficient or not hinges on the qualification of the practitioner, the patient's condition, and the relationship between the doctor and the patient, etc.. The therapeutic effects reflect in several aspects, such as the life quality of tumor patients being improved, the survival rate being raised, and the survival time being lengthened, etc..

Please don't misunderstand me! I do not let you give up the Western approaches to tumor treatments; I just propose to combine (or integrate if possible) the available treating methods, such as surgical operation, radiotherapy, chemotherapy, acupuncture, moxibustion, and Chinese herbal medicine, in a proper way so as to benefit tumor patients as much as possible. It is your job to probe into the scienticity or rationality of treatments of cancer for you are majoring in philosophy, philosophy of science in particular. When doing so, keep metaphorizing in your mind!

I would like to finish this course with this quotation from the Chapter 25 of *Lao Tzu*:

"Therefore, Tao is great.
Heaven is great.
Earth is great.
Man is great.
In the universe, there are four great things, and man is one of them.
Man abides by the earth.
Earth abides by the heaven.
Heaven abides by Tao.
Tao abides by the nature".

Metaphorizing bridges Tao (The Way) of the Nature and Medicine. "Heaven", "Earth", and "Man" compose a whole system; In *Lao Tzu*, Tao abides by the nature; In the *Huang Di's Inner Classic*, medicine abides by the Tao; In essence, medicine abides by the nature. That is the way of seeing, thinking and working of Chinese medicine.

We should not content ourselves to the present state of language. We have to trace back to the origins of words if we want to discover the ties which link the words and their references. ... Etymology has thus become not only the heart of linguistics, but also the foundation stone of philosophy of language.

- Ernst Cassirer[417]

Epilogue

Etymology-Based Literal Translation Approach and Strangification: Efficient Methods for Successful Intercultural Communications

Dissemination of foreign cultures in large scales occurred twice in the history of China. One is the dissemination of Buddhism since Han Dynasty (206 B.C. – A.D. 220) of about 2,000 years ago, and the other is the dissemination of Catholicism since Ming Dynasty (1368-1644) of about 400 years ago, plus later the dissemination of Christian religion. Both disseminations seem to be the dissemination of different religions on the surface, but in essence, what have been actually introduced into China are Indian and Western cultures, including philosophy, arts, sciences, technologies, and so and so forth. If without these two disseminations, the development of science, technology, and culture of the present days in China would have had been definitely not the case. That is an indisputable fact, leaving no leeway for further debate.[418]

Of course, translation and intercultural activities are essential for the success of these two disseminations, during which conflicts transformed into mutual understanding, and then even to integration of different cultures. Chinese culture is a typical inclusive culture with manifoldness – modern Western culture, classical Chinese culture, Indian Buddhism culture, and culture of national minorities coexist in China today.

Here I would like to take the dissemination of Chinese medicine in the West as the example to illustrate how significant the proper translation approach and intercultural methodology are in the process from conflicts to mutual understanding to coexistence in a complementary way between medicine East and West.

417 Translated into English from Chinese. Gan Yang, Translator; Ernst Cassirer, Author. 2004: 158. Its Original Version is: An Essay on Man: An Introduction to a Philosophy of Human Culture [M]. New Heaven: Yale University Press, 1944.

418 This quotation is from Ji Xianlin's *Preface to Figures of Disseminating Western Studies to the East Series* published by Beijing: Science Press in 2000. Ji Xianlin 季羡林 (1911-2009), a famous writer, linguist, philologist, educator, translator, essayist, and social activist, acquired proficiency in 12 languages, and had been a deputy president of Peking University.

1 Etymology-Based Translation Approach: Key to Eliminate Confusions and Ambiguities

Actually, "Translations of Chinese Medical Concepts Being Confusing" is the major problem in translating Chinese medical texts. Hereafter the table 15 shows translations of "六節藏象論" and "藏象何如" of *Huang Di Nei Jing Su Wen* by different translators.

Translators	六節藏象論	藏象何如
K. CHIMIN WONG & WU LIEN-TEH	Numerical Categories of the Five Viscera	/
VEITH, ILZA	Treatise on the Six Regulations Governing the Manifestations of the Viscera	How can you explain the outer appearances of the viscera
NI, MAOSHING	The Energetic Cycles of the Universe and Their Effects on Human Beings	How do the functional aspects of the zang organs manifest outwardly?
WU LIANSHENG & WU QI	The Close Relation between the Viscera in Human Body with the Environment of the Outside World	What are the outer appearances like when the viscera corresponding to heaven, earth, Yin and Yang?
UNSCHULD, PAUL U.	Discourse on the Six Terms [of a Year] and on Phenomena [associated with the Condition of] the Depots	What are the phenomena [associated with the condition] of the depots?

Table 15 Translations of "六節藏象論" &"藏象何如" by Different Translators

It is well known that the *Zang Xiang* Theory is of vital significance in Chinese medicine. *Zang Xiang* 藏象 is generally considered as a compound term. But the translations of *Zang Xiang* 藏象 in the Table15 given by different tranlators are so different from each other.

1.1 Translations of Chinese Medical Concepts Being Confusing

At least 33 different versions of "Chinese-English Dictionary of Chinese Medicine" have got published in the years between 1980 and 2011 in mainland China, in which English translations of the same concept are very far away from each other; English terminology of Chinese medicine by Dr. Nigel Wiseman has been adopted by two of the three major Chinese medical publishers in the United States (Paradigm Publications and Blue Poppy Press) as the standard terminology for their publications; In Europe, Prof. Paul U. Unschuld and Dr. Giovanni

Maciocia have adopted different terminology systems. Obviously, English translations of the same original text from different translators are very different from each other, which undoubtedly hinders translation, transmission, and exchange of Chinese medicine and the culture it is loaded to the West.

Chinese and international experts have been making unremitting efforts in order to standardize English translation of Chinese medical terminology: WHO issued two English standard acupuncture nomenclatures -- *A Proposed Standard International Acupuncture Nomenclature* (Geneva, 1989) and *Standard Acupuncture Nomenclature* (Revised ed., Manila, 1991) as the outcome of an international cooperation since 1982; Prof. Xie Zhufan was assigned by the State Administration of Traditional Chinese Medicine a research project on the standardization of English translation of Chinese medical terminology in 2000, the research outcome of which was published by Foreign Languages Press in Beijing; Academician Wang Yongyan took the lead of a research project approved by Ministry of Science and Technology on "Standardization of Basic Chinese Medical Terminology", the research outcome of which was published by Science Press in Beijing after being examined and approved by "China National Committee for Terms in Sciences and Technologies"; and WHO approved and issued the *WHO International Standard Terminologies on Traditional Medicine in the Western Pacific Region* in 2007 as the outcome of an international cooperation since 2004; and so and so forth.

So many different versions of "Chinese-English Dictionary of Chinese Medicine" and so many different authoritative standardization proposals will unavoidably make people lost and confused as to which to follow: Which proposal on earth is the real "standard" one? Each has been sticking to his own version and argument for so many years.

Several translations available for one term are very common in the English translation of Chinese medical terminology, which may result from different understanding of the same concept or from different translation strategies. The following table shows translations of some basic concepts of Chinese medicine.

	Translation1	Translation2	Translation 3	Translation 4
五行	five elements	five phases	five agents	five elemental phases
經脈	meridian	channel	vessel	meridian vessel
五藏	five *zang* organs	five viscera	five depots	the yin organs
六府	six *fu* organs	six bowels	six palaces	the yang organs
正气	healthy *qi*	upright *qi*	normal *qi*	Body resistance
邪气	pathogenic *qi*	evil *qi*	pathogenic agent	pathogen; pathogenic factor
證	syndrome	pattern	configuration	conformation
虛	vacuity	deficiency	asthenia	emptiness
實	repletion	excess	sthenia	fullness
疝	hernia	genital disease	lower abdominal colic	mounting
消渴	diabetes	dispersion-thirst	wasting-thirst	melting-thirst
奔豚	gastroenteroneuro-sis	running-piglet	"running-pig" syndrome	/

Table 16 Translations of Some Basic Concepts of Chinese Medicine

Even the *Standard Acupuncture Nomenclature* approved and issued by WHO has not been well implemented and widely used in the reality, see the Table 16. A standard terminology system is of no value and significance no matter how good and authoritative it is if it cannot be carried out and adopted by translators in English publications.

ORIGINAL TERMS	STANDARD TRANSLATION (WHO)	POPULAR TRANSLATIONS IN THE WEST
經脈	Meridian	Channel
三焦	Triple Energizer	Triple Burner
督脈	Governor Vessel	Governing Vessel
任脈	Conception Vessel	Directing (or Controlling) Vessel
沖脈	Thoroughfare Vessel	Penetrating Vessel
帶脈	Belt Vessel	Girdle (or Girdling) Vessel
太陽、陽明、少陽	Taiyang, Yangming, Shaoyang	Greater Yang, Bright Yang, Lesser Yang
太陰、少陰、厥陰	Taiyin, Shaoyin, Jueyin	Greater Yin, Lesser Yin, Terminal (or Absolute) Yin

Table 17 A Comparison between Standardized Translation Approved by WHO and Popular Translations in the West

It is well known that Chinese medicine is the product of systematizing the knowledge contained in the ancient Chinese medical classics, esp. "the Four Great Medical Classics". The academic and cultural exchanges between different medical systems are first embodied in their terminologies, and terminology is the sole means by which we understand concepts. English Translation of concepts of classical Chinese medical texts not only deals with the historical texts but rather the present practice and research for Chinese medicine has still claimed to follow and observe the system established by ancient Chinese medical classics, and "the Four Great Medical Classics" in particular. The concepts of classical Chinese medical texts embody the cultural presupposition *Tian Ren He Yi* 天人合一 or Universe and Man Uniting and Resembling Each Other and the core methodology of *Qu Xiang Bi Lei* 取象比類 or Taking Image and Analogizing of Chinese medicine. Therefore I propose to clarify the confusing translations by referring to etymologies of the original. Then what is the value of *Qu Xiang Bi Lei* 取象比類 or Taking Image and Analogizing for Chinese medicine?

1.2 Chinese Medical Concepts: Embodying Methodology of *Qu Xiang Bi Lei*

Chinese medical concepts embody the methodology of *Qu Xiang Bi Lei or* Taking Image and Analogizing, 取象比类, which weaves natural and social phenomena together with rudimentary understanding of the human being[419] into the knowledge system of Chinese medicine.

419The paper prefers being instead of body for Chinese medicine actually studies the being (the live system being composed of body and mind) while Western medicine mainly cares the body.

1.2.1 Understanding *Qu Xiang Bi Lei*

Shuo Wen Jie Zi or *The Origin of Chinese Characters* states that "*xiang*, with long nose and teeth, a big mammal in the Southern Yue area, will be pregnant every three years", so the original meaning of "*xiang*" is elephant. In the remote antiquity, the elephant had lived in the Central Plains of China. Later on, the elephant had to migrate south because of the changes in climate, so the people in the Central Plains had few opportunities to see the live elephant again. Han Fei, a famous philosopher and the representative of the Legalists of the late Warring States Period (475-221B.C.), said in his *Jie Lao Pian* 解老篇 that "people seldom see the live elephant, but has gained the skeleton of a dead one, so they can imagine what it is like after investigating the picture or image of its skeleton. Therefore, all in people's imagination is known as *'xiang*'". This quotation also reveals the mystery of the origin of the Chinese compound "*xiang xiang*" (想象，literally means "thinking or imagining elephant", and actually means "imaging" or "imagination"), and thus setting off *xiang*'s "imagining" cultural connotations.

In the meanwhile, we can see that "*xiang*" originally evolved from "seeking similarities" between things from the angle of genetics, as stated in *The Book of Changes* "*xiang* refers to something being like or resembling this thing". Transforming *xiang* into a cultural symbol is related to divining activities – *Bu* 卜 with tortoise shell and *shi* 筮 with stalk of *shi* grass – the two main ways to hunt for information of the cosmos in the Yin and Zhou dynasties (16th century -256 B.C.). *Zuo's Spring Autumn Annals · The Fifteenth Year of Xi Gong's Reign* states that "tortoise is *xiang*"; *The Book of Changes* states that "change is *xiang*". That is to say, the omens on the tortoise shell and the trigrams were called *xiang* for they were regarded as being capable of communicating the Heaven with the Man and ruling all the cultural information. Thereafter, *xiang* has become a symbol which carries all the cultural information.

Xiang has a very strong adhesive power, and is a vital part of a series of compounds such as *jing* (scenery) *xiang* 景象, *xing* (star) *xiang* 星象, *mai* (pulse) *xiang* 脉象, *she* (tongue) *xiang* 舌象 and *zang* (visceral) *xiang* 藏象, including everything from the concrete *xiang* of objects which can be felt to the metaphysical subtle *xiang* such as the big *xiang* (大象) - Tao 道, the primitive motive force of the origin of everything in the universe, which is difficult to grasp, thus possessing both perceptual and rational ingredients, and also indicating relationships.

Qu Xiang Bi Lei can be summarized into four steps as stated in *The Book of Changes*: ① Observing object or phenomenon (*guan wu,* 观物): directly observing an object or a phenomenon; ② Taking image (*qu xiang,* 取象): summarizing and refining the image of the object or phenomenon after repeatedly observing and feeling it; ③ Analogizing (*bi lei,* 比类): comparing the things which need to know with the known "image (*xiang* 象)"; ④ Understanding the Way or Rule (*ti dao,* 体道): finding the rules, which can be achieved by applying metaphors.

Qu Xiang Bi Lei, the core methodology of Chinese medicine, plays a vital role in stating, constructing and developing the theoretical system and clinical practice of Chinese medicine mainly in the following three aspects: ① Forming systematic metaphors (Theory): naming basic concepts, stating and constructing the theoretical system; ② Gaining knowledge through metaphorizing (Practice): Grasping the hidden essence or telling the interior through observing the external image or manifestation such as in the processes of making diagnosis and identifying pattern in the practice; and ③ Understanding rules through metaphorizing (Development and Modernization): inferring the unknown through the known image such as developing new theories and therapeutic methods.

1.2.2 Enlightenments of Philosophy of Language

Modernization of Chinese medicine must be directed by scientific methodology, and scientific methodology is in the field of philosophy, esp. the field of philosophy of science. The key tone of the modern Western philosophy focuses on language analysis and understanding. Today, language is redefined as "the means and process of man cognizing, understanding and stating the world".[420] The characteristics of the definition of language manifest in the following three aspects: first, "cognizing" and "stating" instead of being "communicative" and "systematic" ; second, "means", a kind of subjective behavior and manifestation of subjectivities, instead of "tool", an object; third, emphasizing "process". It is well known that language is dynamic, constantly changing, generating new words to meet the needs of the developments and changes of the world.

The founding of philosophy of language at the beginning of the last century is another "Copernican revolution" in the history of philosophy, which has deeply influenced philosophy of science, highlighting the vital role of linguistic analysis in the scientific methodology, thus promoting the development of modern logic.

Modern logic stresses the role of language, regards a scientific theory as a language system, being composed of word items, sentences, and their logic relationships. When analyzing Chinese medical system, how the ontological Chinese medical concepts and theories were formed, stated and constructed, and how Chinese medicine has been developed should be clarified in the first place for the purpose of understanding the system itself, bridging classical Chinese medicine and modern Western medicine in deep level and making them complement each other, thus laying foundation for modernization of Chinese medicine.

"Languages are metaphoric in its essence and nature. …"; "We should not content ourselves to the present state of language. We have to trace back to the

420 Pan Wenguo. Redefining Language: Means and Process of Man Cognizing and Stating the Genuine World [J]. (Hongkong) Chinese Philology Correspondence. 2002, 2: 33-36.

origins of words if we want to discover the ties which link the words and their references".[421]

Metaphors in Chinese medicine reveal relationships, and metaphor thinking is an exact thinking. The metaphor system of Chinese medicine is the deep structure of Chinese medicine, and the key to understand Chinese medicine.

1.2.3 Example: Translation of *Jing Luo*

Several translations are available for "經絡系統": "Meridian System" is the standard translation approved by WHO, but the word "Meridian" only indicates a two-dimensional grid while *Jing Luo* system is supposed to carry *qi* and blood, and thus must be a three-dimensional system; "Channel System" is the most popular translation in the English literature on Chinese medicine, but the word "Channel" is polysemous; I think "Vessel System", a translation in *Huang Di Nei Jing Su Wen* by Paul U. Unschuld in 2003 is the best translation if we take into account the origin and development of the concepts of *Mai* (脈, vessel) and *Jing-Luo* (經絡).

Based on some anatomical knowledge on *Mai* (脈, vessel) and medical practice esp. the application of acupuncture, moxibustion, *tuina*, and *qigong*, the concepts of *Jing-Luo* (經絡) are actually metaphors formed in the way of observing, taking images of and analogizing the water flow in the rivers under the earth and the longitudinal lines of the textiles, which are embodied in their writing forms. The chapter *Water & Earth* of *Guan Tzu* states that "Water is the *qi* and blood of the earth, running on/under the earth just like *qi* and blood flowing in the vessels".

The sinograms 脈 and 衇 are two common original complex forms of *mai* 脉. Its lesser seal script is . This sinogram is a signifc-phonetic compound: the left part is the signific component 月 (flesh moon) or 血 (blood), indicating that *mai* (脈) functions to carry and move blood and is a part of the body; and the right part is the phonetic, indicating both pronunciation and meaning at the same time. In the medical books unearthed from Mawangdui Han Tomb, most of *mai* 脈 were written as "温". "水" is the variant form of "氵", "目" the variant form of "flesh moon 月", "皿" the variant form of "blood 血". The structure of the sinogram has clearly illustrated that the ancient Chinese analogized and metaphorized water flow with blood flow.[422] It is thus clear that "*mai*" of the early days referred to "blood vessels", so "*mai* 脉" is also known as "blood vessel 血脈", as stated in *Huang Di's Inner Classic ·Basic Questions ·Discourse on Subtleties and Essentials of Vessels* "The vessels 脈 are the residence of the blood"(Attention: *Qi* does not appear in this quotation).

---

421 Ernst Cassirer, From *Essays on Man*, Translated into English from Chinese.
422 Li Ding. 1998: 2-3.

The concepts "*jing*" and "*luo*" appeared later than "*mai* or vessel". *Jing* and *luo* are further divisions of "*mai* or vessel", i.e. "*jing*" vessel and "*luo*" vessel, which was first recorded in the *Huang Di's Inner Classic·Miraculous Pivot · On Vessels* "*Jing* vessels reside in the interior; their branches running transversely are known as *luo* vessels; the branches of *luo* vessels are known as grandchild vessels".

The sinograms "經 *jing*" and "絡 *luo*" share the same silk part "糸", which is originally used in the textiles. The concept "*jing-mai* 經脈" is a metaphor formed in the way of *Qu Xiang Bi Lei* or taking images and analogizing. The right part of "經" is "巠", indicating both pronunciation and meaning, which is interpreted in *The Origin of Chinese Characters* as "water vessels, following <<< （川, pictographic, indicating rivers）, under the 一; 一, refers to the earth", that is to say, "巠" refers to the water vessels running under the earth. *Jing* 經 is explained in *The Origin of Chinese Characters* as "the longitudinal lines of the textiles". The reason that "*jing* 經" is used to name the main stems of the vessels is closely related to the origin of the sinogram "*jing* 經", which contains two images and reflects the similarities between the longitudinal lines of the textiles, the rivers running under the earth and the running routes of the main stems of the vessels. Another part of "*luo* 絡" is "各", indicating both pronunciation and meaning, which is interpreted in *The Origin of Chinese Characters* as "divergence of views being different". Another interpretation of *luo* 絡 is that "It originally meant unreeled silk, hemp, or cotton fiber, and from its association with stringy fibers came to be used in Chinese medicine as a noun that means network and as a verb that means to net".[423] Anyway, *luo* 絡 is used to name divergent branches of the vessels.

Huang Di's Inner Classic · Miraculous Pivot · On Viscera states that "*Jing* vessels 經脈 function to move *qi* and blood, nourish yin and yang, moisten tendons and bones, and lubricate joints". Compared to the statement that "The vessels 脈 are the residence of the blood", quite a lot new contents were supplemented to *jing* vessels, among which the most remarkable point is that the function of *jing* vessels in moving **blood** was extended to moving ***qi* and blood**.

"*Xue mai* 血脈", "*jing* 經" and "*luo* 絡" appeared together in the *Treatise on Literature* of *The History of The Former Han Dynasty* that "Medical classics explore the origins of **blood vessels 血脈, *jing-luo*** 經絡, bone marrow, yin-yang, exterior and interior in order to treat various diseases from the root", where seemingly differentiated blood vessels from *jing-luo*.

Jing-luo 經絡 functions to carry and move *qi* and blood in the body. *Guan Tzu · Water & Earth* states that "water is the *qi* and blood of the earth, running on the earth which is just like *qi* and blood flowing in the vessels". Judged from the

423 Wiseman Nigel and Zhang Yuhuan. 2003: 174.

cognizing order, the flow of *qi* and blood in man is analogized and inferred from the natural phenomenon of water flow in the rivers under the earth. The extensions from "vessel 脈" to "*jing-luo* 經絡" and from "blood" to "*qi* and blood" are also closely related to the application of acupuncture, moxibustion, *tuina*, *qigong*, etc, which explore the phenomenon of *qi* and blood flowing in the body, thus enriching the understanding on the "vessels".

To sum up, the concepts and theory of *jing-luo* were formed first on the basis of some anatomical knowledge on "vessels 脈"; then by the way of *Qu Xiang Bi Lei*, i.e. observing and taking images of the water flow in the rivers on/under the earth and the longitudinal lines of textiles, then analogizing, enlightened by the idea of *Tian Ren He Yi*; and then have been proved and modified in the medical practice esp. the application of acupuncture, moxibustion, *tuina*, and *qigong*. That is to say, *jing-luo* or the vessels are metaphors, referring to the circular or round pathways of the living system.

Therefore, I believe that it will take forever to find any three-dimensional structure of *jing-luo* 經絡 through dissecting dead human bodies. *Jing-luo* 經絡 system or the vessel system is more like a functional concept reflecting a certain image, which is embodied in their writing forms. As stated in the *Huang Di's Inner Classic · Basic Questions · Discourse on Leaving and Uniting of True Qi and Evil Qi* "The sages formulated principles, which must conform to the nature. Therefore, the heaven has 365 degrees and 28 constellations, the earth has 12 *jing* rivers, and man has 12 *jing* vessels".

Seeing that *jing* and *luo* are further divisions of *mai* or vessels, i.e., *jing* vessel and *luo* vessel, the proper translation for *jing-luo* 經絡 system would be "the vessel system".

1.3 Standard and Methods for Translating Chinese Medical Concepts

1.3.1 English Translation of Chinese Medical Terminology: One Standard or Multiple Standards?

It is well known that even up till today, Chinese medicine still claims to follow the system established by such Chinese medical classics as *Huang Di's Inner Classic*, *The Classic of Difficult Issues*, *Treatise on Cold-induced and Miscellaneous Diseases*, which were systematized and classified into *On Cold-induced Diseases* and *Synopsis of the Golden Chamber* by later generations. Chinese medicine comes into being by systematizing the knowledge contained in ancient Chinese medical classics; Most of the specialized Chinese medical concepts formed for the first time in ancient Chinese medical classics by means of metaphorization and analogization, thus embodying the specific core Chinese methodology *Qu Xiang Bi Lei* or taking image and analogizing, thus bearing historical, cultural and medical values at the same time. But when translating a Chinese medical concept, most of translators no matter of China or other countries lay stress only on its medical value and ignoring its cultural and historical values, and thus making the English translation lose the central methodology of Chinese medicine - *Qu Xiang Bi Lei* or taking image and analogizing.

I hold that specialized terms of both Chinese and Western medicine reflect that they are based on specific and different cultural traditions and thinking ways; and that Chinese medicine is a systematic, complete, and unique medical system incompatible with Western medicine; and therefore, English translation of concepts of Chinese medical classics, esp. those formed by means of metaphorization and analogization, should apply the translation strategy which can reflect their metaphorical connotations and the specific Chinese methodology of *Qu Xiang Bi Lei*, thus observing the only one standard.

1.3.2 Method: Literal Translation Approach Based on Etymology Investigation

"However, in communicative as in semantic translation, provided that equivalent-effect is secured, the literal word-for-word translation is not only the best, it is the only valid method of translation. There is no excuse for unnecessary 'synonyms', let alone paraphrase, in any type of translation".[424]

Actually, English Chinese medical terminology formed through literal translation approach bears the following merits: ① accuracy in content, form, and logic, i.e. the translation gives the ideas, words, and logic of the original; ② conciseness and pithiness in style, i.e. the translation reproduces the conciseness and pithiness of the original compared to the lengthy paraphrase for the original is usually concise in form but profound in meaning; ③ systematicness, i.e. the literal translation approach makes the English Chinese medical terminology being systematic, and thus faithfully reflecting the integrity and inter-relationship in its concept system for Chinese medical terminology comes from the way of *Qu Xiang Bi Lei* based on the ancient Chinese people's daily life experiences; ④ back-translation, i.e. literal translation improves or realizes translation of English Chinese medical terminology back into original Chinese terminology, thus keeping distinguishing features of Chinese medical culture and being beneficial for the double direction information interchange.

Compared to Western medicine, an applied science based on achievements of Western science and technology, Chinese medicine is a typical linguistic medical knowledge system in essence for it is formed in the way of linguistication and is recorded in self-interpreting sinograms. Therefore Chinese medicine can be regarded as a linguistic medical system being composed of its logographic language writing forms, concepts, terminology, formulations, sentences, and their logic relationships.

424 Newmark, Peter. 1981: 39.

The core knowledge of Chinese medicine is from classical Chinese medical texts, which are written in self-interpreting characters, or more exact, sinograms. Compared to phonetic writing forms, Chinese language (logographic writing) is more stable and accumulative. In Chinese language, giving the original sinogram new meanings by the way of metaphorizing instead of creating new sinograms is the major way to reflect the changes and developments of the world and the means and process of Chinese people cognizing, understanding and stating the world. After tracing back to the original meanings of sinograms, concepts and statements are not difficult to understand in their contexts in a broad sense, which also provide us extensive but close links among different disciplines of Chinese culture and science. Therefore, etymology investigation is of vital significance for etymology of a sinogram can unify all the migrating meanings of concepts based on the one sinogram with the same etymology. The theoretical system of Chinese medicine is stated and expressed in a natural language with the two major characteristics: being polysemous and ambiguous, which can also be clarified and unified by etymology investigation and metaphor understanding.

2 Strangification: Intercultural Approach to Successful Intercultural Communication

After reviewing the successful disseminations of Indian and Western cultures in China (with disseminating Buddhism and Catholism as the original purposes) in the past centuries, I have found that intercultural approach is an essential approach to successful intercultural communication. The general features of the successful intercultural communication methods coincide with "Strangification", the methodology of Constructive Realism developed by Prof. Dr. Friedrich Wallner in the 1980s. Constructive Realism connects a hermeneutical philosophy of science with a constructive philosophy of science, which connects interpretation with construction. Thus it is an interdisciplinary and intercultural hermeneutical philosophy of science, and its methodology "strangification" aims to make the implicit presuppositions explicit.

Constructive Realism aims at making the manifold scientific approaches depending on different cultures understandable. In fact, studies on the manifold scientific approaches are intimately related to another proposition that modern science results from European culture under specific conditions. Prof. Wallner holds that European science is not the only rational way of constructing the world and there are still some other reasonable ways of constructing different aspects of the world in different approaches and based on different cultures, such as classical Chinese science.

Constructive Realism stresses the importance of understanding and interpreting science, and so Prof. Wallner introduced "Strangification" as its methodology for the sake of a valid and effective interpretation of a scientific system. "Strangification" is a coined word, a translation of the German word

"Verfremdung". This methodology comes from the field of hermeneutics, a way of interpreting and understanding. Strangification is able to show the presuppositions of a scientific system, and represents one of the core ideas of Constructive Realism. How does the procedure of Strangification go? It follows a simple strategy: Take a proposition system or a concept out of its original context and put it into another different context, then observe what happens with the proposition system. The more different the other context is the better it is for the use of this methodology.

Strangification is advanced on that a scientific system is a proposition system based on certain presuppositions. That is to say, a certain scientific proposition system is not always true but only true under certain conditions. Strangification aims to improve scientific understanding by revealing and expressing the implicit theoretical presuppositions, which are actually the foundation of the scientific theories, arguments, approaches, conclusions and results. The equality and no ranking of different cultures and sciences is an essential prerequisite to the application of this methodology. "Mutual Strangification", i.e. strangification in double directions, can promote and realize self-understanding and mutual understanding between different cultures and different sciences.

For instance, transfer a proposition system from the context of Chinese medicine to the context of Western medicine but not in the aim of direct comparison. Then observe what will happen with the proposition system of Chinese medicine.[425] Take *Pi* 脾 or Spleen as an example.[426]

In Western medicine, the spleen refers to the organ in the top part of the abdominal cavity behind the stomach and below the diaphragm; it is the largest lymphatic organ, appears to act to remove dead blood cells and fight infection; and an adult can live normally after his spleen has been removed. But the spleen in Chinese medicine is radically different from that in Western medicine except its location: The spleen is located in the middle *jiao* (the center) and below the diaphragm. According to its central position and its yellow color, Chinese medicine attributes the spleen to the soil in the five phases. Soil is sowing and reaping, corresponding to the late summer in the seasons and dampness in the climate, representing the features of receiving, generating, transforming, and supporting. Therefore, the spleen's function in Chinese medicine is metaphorized as transforming the water and grain into essence, then moving and sending the essence to the whole body; thereby, the spleen is regarded as the foundation of postnatal existence, the source of the formation of *qi* and blood, is interrelated with the flesh, governs the limbs, opens into the mouth, manifests its brilliance in the lips, and so on. Finally a spleen complex system is formed. The common symptoms of the spleen diseases such as abdominal pain or distension, poor appetite, loose stool, diarrhea, jaundice, fatigue or weakness of the limbs, edema

---

425 Wallner Fritz G.How to Deal with Science If You Care for Other Cultures: Constructive Realism in the Intercultural World [M]. Wien: Wilhelm Braumuller, 1997.

426 Lan Fengli. Metaphorizing: The Way to Bridge *The Book of Changes* and Chinese Medicine. In Wallner F.G, Schmisberger F., Wimmer F.M. (eds). 2010: 177-192.

can be successfully relieved by treating the spleen in Chinese medicine. It is clear that the spleen in Chinese medicine does not refer to any concrete organ, maybe not the organ spleen at all (according to its central position and the yellow color, this organ may be the pancreas, which was not perceived by Chinese medicine in the ancient time), but to a functional system by applying the five-phase theory in the way of *Qu Xiang Bi Lei,* the methodological principle which demonstrates the circular reasoning and phenomena as reality guided by the idea of *Tian Ren He Yi,* the ontological principle and the presupposition of Chinese medicine. The spleen in Chinese medicine suggests a complex system, which is understood based on a holistic approach and emphasis of relations and functions.

Strangification has been always a way of mutual learning and understanding. Therefore, meanwhile it is also clear that understanding of the spleen in Western medicine is based on Reductionist Ideology with deduction and induction as its methodologies by taking an analytic approach, emphasizing morphological structure based on experimental studies.

Strangification is really pretty precious under the background of the current prevalence of "West-Centralism" or "Europe-Centralism" in the world, just as Prof. Vincent Shen comments, "Strangification is a miraculous cure to resolve human dilemmas and philosophical difficulties, and a driving force that suggests the willingness to go unceasingly out of oneself, to head for others and the society, for other disciplines, for other cultures, for the nature, for the ideals and the holiness. It implies the primary noble generous spirit that is willing to go out of oneself and perfect oneself by mutual enriching each other"[427].

Based on the standpoint of Constructive Realism, Prof. Wallner advocates that Chinese medicine is a scientific system with its own specific methodology, and thus is completely incompatible with Western medicine for the ways they construct their microworlds are totally different from each other; that compared to science in general sense, Chinese medicine comes closer to humanities; and that "Chinese medicine has its claims for truth".

Science depends on culture. There are different cultures in the world, such as Islamic, Indian, Chinese, and Western cultures. Hence different scientific approaches based on different cultures are possible to reveal the manifoldness of the world to the mankind. I think that Chinese culture and Western culture are two major and influential different types of cultures originated and developed in incompatible but complementary approaches, from which classical Chinese science and modern Western science have evolved and developed. Strangification is a vital method for us to learn from and understand each other, on the basis of which a harmonious sustainable world will be set up.

I would like to reformulate Confucius's statement "Man with honor can be harmonious but different" in this way: Culture, Philosophy and Medicine of East and West are different but together can make a harmonious world.

---

427 Shen Qingsong (known as Vincent Shen in the West). 2005: the Cover.

Chief References

1 Collin, P.H. Dictionary of Medicine [Z]. Beijing: Foreign Language Teaching and Research Press, 2001.
2 Cassirer, Ernst. An Essay on Man: An Introduction to a Philosophy of Human Culture [M]. New Heaven: Yale University Press, 1944.
3 Dong Hongle. Metaphorization in Scientific Discourse [M]. Shanghai: Fudan University Press, 2005.
4 Fu Weikang. The Earliest National Medical universities. Essays on Medicine and Culture[C]. Shanghai: Shanghai Ancient Books Press, 2001.
5 Gan Yang, Translator; Author: Cassirer Ernest. An Essay on Man [M]. Shanghai: Shanghai Translation Publishing House, 2004.
6 Guo Guichun. Metaphor, Rhetoric, and Scientific Interpretation [M]. Beijing: Science Press, 2007.
7 Hou Weirui. English Styles of Writing [M]. Shanghai: Shanghai Foreign Language Education Press, 1988.
8 Hsu, Elisabeth. The Transmission of Chinese Medicine [M]. Cambridge: Cambridge University Press, 1999.
9 Lakoff, George; Johnson, Mark. Metaphors We Live By [M]. Chicago: The University of Chicago Press, 1980.
9 Lan Fengli. The Influence of *Huang Di's Inner Classic* on *The Origin of Chinese Characters*[J], Chinese Journal of Medical History, 2006, 36(4): 201-205.
10 Lan Fengli. A Corpus-Based Study on Cultural Connotations and Translation of Fundamental Concepts in Classical Chinese Texts [D]. Shanghai: Shanghai Jiao Tong University, 2008.
11 Lan Fengli. Philosophical Reflections on Standard English Terminology of Chinese Medicine [J]. Medicine and Philosophy, 2010, 31 (7): 72-73.
12 Lan Fengli, Wallner Friedrich G, Wobovnik Claudia (eds). Shen, Psychotherapy and Acupuncture: Theory, Methodology and Structure of Chinese Medicine [C]. 2011.
13 Li Ding. Interpretation of Difficult Issues in Acupuncture [M]. Shanghai: Shanghai Uiversity of TCM Press, 1998.
14 Li Jingwei, Ou Yongxin, Yu Ying'ao, et al. A Concise Dictionary of Chinese Medicine [Z]. Beijing: China Press of Traditional Chinese Medicine, 2001.
15 Michel Foucault. The Birth of the Clinic [M]. New York: Vintage Books, 1973.
16 Needham, Joseph. Science and Civilization in China [M] (Volume 1). Translation. Beijing: Science Press & Shanghai: Shanghai Ancient Books Press, 1990.
17 Newmark, Peter. Approaches to Translation [M].Shanghai: Shanghai Foreign Language Education Press, 1981.
18 Pang Pu. Observing One in Three: Textual Criticisms and Explanations of Chinese Traditional Thoughts [M]. Shenzhen: Haitian Press, 1995.

19 Shen Qingsong (known as Vincent Shen in the West). Shen Qingsong's Self Selections from [M]. Jinan: Shandong Education Press, 1995.
20 Unschuld, Paul U. Huang Di Nei Jing Su Wen: Nature, Knowledge, Imagery in an Ancient Chinese Medical Text [M]. Berkeley: University of California Press, 2003.
21 Unschuld, Paul U. & Tessenow, Hermann. Huang Di Nei Jing Su Wen: An Annotated Translation of Huang Di's Inner Classic Basic Questions. Berkeley: University of California Press, 2011.
22 Wallner Fritz G..How to Deal with Science If You Care for Other Cultures: Constructive Realism in the Intercultural World [M]. Wien: Wilhelm Braumuller, 1997.
23 Wallner Friedrich G. Five Lectures on the Foundations of Chinese Medicine [M]. Frankurt am Main: Peter Lang, 2009.
24 Wallner Friedrich G, Kubiena Gertrude, Jandl Martin J. (eds). Understanding Traditional Chinese Medicine [C]. Frankfurt am Main: Peter Lang, 2009.
25 Wallner Friedrich G., Schmisberger Florian, Wimmer Franz Martin (eds). Intercultural Philosophy: New Aspects and Methods [C]. Frankurt am Mein: Peter Lang, 2010.
26 Wallner Friedrich G, Lan Fengli, Jandl Martin (eds). The Way of Thinking in Chinese Medicine: Theory, Methodology and Structure of Chinese Medicine [C]. Frankfurt am Main: Peter Lang, 2010.
27 Wallner Friedrich G, Lan Fengli, Jandl Martin (eds). Chinese Medicine and Intercultural Philosophy: Theory, Methodology and Structure of Chinese Medicine [C]. Frankfurt am Main: Peter Lang, 2011.
28 Wallner Friedrich G. The Philosophical Foundation of A Comparison between Western Medicine and Chinese Medicine (English-Chinese) [M]. Beijing: Higher Education Press, 2011.
29 Wang Hongtu. The Study of *Nei Jing* [M]. Beijing: China Press of Traditional Chinese Medicine, 2004.
30 Wang Jimin, Fu Weikang. Catalogue of Publications on Medicine in China in Foreign Countries (1656-1962). Shanghai: Shanghai Academy of Chinese Medicine. Medical History Museum, 1963.
31 Wang Yuxiong. Investigation into Origins of Image [M]. Hefei: Anhui Education Press, 1996.
32 Wiseman, Nigel. English-Chinese & Chinese-English Dictionary of Chinese Medicine [Z]. Changsha: Hunan Science and Technology Press, 1996.
33 Wiseman Nigel, Zhang Yuhuan. Chinese Medical Characters Volume One: Basic Vocabulary. Brookline, Massachusetts: Paradigm Publications, 2003.
34 Xia Zhengnong. Sea of Words [Z]. Shanghai: Shanghai Dictionary Press, 2002.
35 Xing Yurui. The Theories and Methodology in the *Huang Di's Inner Classic* [M]. Xi'an: Shaanxi Science and Technology Press, 2004.
36 Zhang Boyu. Chinese Internal Medicine [M]. Shanghai: Shanghai Scientific and Technical Publishers. 1989.

Bilingual Glossary
(Chinese-English)

A

埃及圣书体	Egyptian hieroglyphic

B

八卦	Eight Trigrams
本草	Materia Medica
本体论	Ontology
本义	Original meaning
比	Analogy; Analogizing
笔划	Stroke
表意文字	Ideographic writing
表音文字	Phonetic writing
辨证论治	Pattern Identification and Treatment
兵家	School of Militarists
补充与替代医学	Complementary and Alternative Medicine (CAM)
部首	Radical; Signific

C

草书	Cursive Script
传统医学	Traditional Medicine
传统中医学	Traditional Chinese Medicine
春秋时期	the Spring and Autumn Period (770-476 B.C.)

D

大陆文化	Continental Culture
大篆	Larger Seal Script
道	Tao; Dao; Way
道家	School of Taoists; Taoist School; Philosophical Taoism; Taoist
道教	Taoist religion; Religious Taoism
德治	Rule with Virtue
对抗医学	Allopathic Medicine
对联	Antithetical Couplet
对仗	Antithesis

E

二分法，二元论	dichotomy

F

法家	School of Legalists; Legalist School
法治	Rule with Law
方法论	Methodology
方块字	Squared Shaped Sinogram
风寒暑湿燥火	wind, cold, summer-heat, damp, dryness, and fire

G

古（经）典中医学	Classical Chinese Medicine
故宫	The Imperial Palace
观象授时	Observing Phenomena and Issuing an Official Calendar
观象制器	Observing Phenomena and Making Instruments

H

海洋文化	Maritime Culture
汉语语言哲学	Philosophy of Chinese Language
汉字	Sinogram; Chinese character
合理性	Rationality
葫芦	Bottle gourd
会意	Associative compound, one of the six categories of Chinese graphs
活字印刷	Movable-type printing
混沌	Chaos

I

J

甲骨文	Oracle-Bone Inscription; Oracle Script
假借	Loan sinograms, one of the six categories of Chinese graphs
兼爱	All-Embracing Love; Universal Love
金文	Bronze Inscription ; Bronze Script
经脉	meridian-vessel; meridian
经络学说	The vessel theory; The meridian theory; The meridian-collateral theory
经史子集	Classics, history, philosophy, and belle-letters
君子	man with honor; Man of noble characters

K

楷书	Regular Script
科学性	Scienticity

L

礼	Propriety; Rite
理法方药	Theories, methods, formulas and medicinal agents
隶书	*Li Shu*; Simplified from Lesser Seal Script
六十四卦	Sixty-Four Hexagrams
六书	Six categories of Chinese graphs
络脉	network vessel; collateral

M

脉	vessel
名家	School of Names
墨家	School of Mohists; Mohism
木火土金水	wood, fire, soil, metal, and water

N

农家	School of Agriculturalists

O

P

拼音文字	Phonetic writing

Q

齐万物	Equaling all the beings
取 象 比 类	*Qu Xiang Bi Lei;* Taking Image and Analogizing; Metaphorizing

R

人副天数	Man Mirroring Heaven
儒	Literati; Scholars
儒家	School of Literati; Confucianism
儒医	Scholar Physicians

S

三才——天地人	Three Newborns: Heaven, Earth, Man
三位一体	Unity with three dimensions
伤寒	Cold-induced diseases
生克，相生相克	Engendering and Restraining
术	Skill
司外揣内	*Si Wai Chuai Nei;* Inspecting the exterior to predict the interior
苏美尔楔形文字	Sumerian cuneiform

T

太极	*Tai Ji*; the Great Ultimate; the Supreme Ultimate; the Great Primal Beginning
太极图	Yin-Yang Diagram
天人感应	Interactions between Heaven and Man
天人合一	*Tian Ren He Yi*; Universe and Man Uniting and Resembling Each Other; Heaven and Man Uniting and Resembling Each Other
天下	The Land under the Heaven; All Beneath the Sky; the World

U

V

W

温病	warm disease
文化际哲学	Intercultural Philosophy
无	Non-Being
无为	Having Effortless Action
五材	Five Materials
五德	Five Virtues
五方	Five Directions
五行	Five Phases; Five Agents; Five Elemental Phases
五运	Five Periods; Five Circuit Phases

X

希腊四元素系统	Greek System of Four Elements
侠	Knight
先秦	Pre-Qin Days （before 221 B.C.）

线性推理	Linear Reasoning
象	Elephant; Image; Imaging
象思维	Imaging Thinking
象形	Pictograph, one of the six categories of Chinese graphs
象形文字	Logographic writing
小说家	School of Story Tellers
小篆	Lesser Seal Script
孝	Filial Piety
信	Sincerity
形声	Pictophonetic, or Signific-Phonetic, one of the six categories of Chinese graphs
行书	Running Hand
循环推理	Circular Reasoning
玄学	Metaphysics

Y

言，象，意	Word, Image, Idea
养生	Health Cultivation
医家	School of Medical Practitioners
以象测藏	*Yi Xiang Ce Zang;* Speculating the internal organs' pathological changes by observing the external manifestations of life
义	Righteousness
阴阳家	School of Yin-Yang
引申义	Extended meaning
有	Being
有为	Having Action
语言化	Linguistication
喻	Metaphor; Metaphorizing
元气	Primordial *Qi*

Z

杂病	Miscellaneous diseases
杂家	The Eclectics
藏府	Depots and Palaces
藏象学说	Visceral Image Theory
战国时期	the Warring States Period (475-221 B.C.)
指事	Ideograph; or Indicator, one of the six categories of Chinese graphs
知，智	Knowledge
諸子百家	The Master Philosophers and Hundred Schools

紫禁城	The Forbidden City
字	Character
字体演变	Evolution of the Scripts
整体观念	Holism; Holistic Concept
忠	Loyalty
中草药	Chinese medicinal herbs
中药	Chinese medicinals
中药学	Chinese Herbal Medicine; Chinese Pharmacology
中医学	Chinese Medicine
中医药学	Chinese Medicine; Chinese Medicine and Pharmacology
轴心时代	The Axial Age (800 - 200 B.C.)
转注	Mutually interpretive, one of the six categories of Chinese graphs
纵横家	School of Political Strategists
尊经崇古	Venerating Classics and Worshiping History

Historical Bibliography

(Before 1911)

Historical bibliography quoted in the book is listed here. The titles are arranged in chronological order by dynasty. Each entry includes the original Chinese, Pinyin transliteration, and an English translation or rendering of the Chinese title, as well as a brief introduction.

Pre-Qin Days (Before 221 B.C.)

Confucian Classics

四书

The Four Books: *Lun Yu* or *The Analects of Confucius, Meng Zi* or *Mencius, Da Xue* or *The Great Learning,* and *Zhong Yong* or *The Doctrine of Mean,* collectively known as "The Four Books", are the Confucian fundamental texts to expound its philosophical viewpoints, political ideal, ethics, and educational principles so as to propagte its doctrines and instructing one's studies. "The Four Books" were selected by the founder of the Neo-Confucianism Zhu Xi 朱熹 (1130-1200) during the Song Dynasty as a foundational introduction to Confucianism and examinations for the state civil service in China.

论语

Lun Yu, or ***The Analects of Confucius:*** the first Confucian classic in book form appearing in the early Warring States Period (475-221 B.C.), comprising 20 chapters. It is a record of the words and deeds of Confucius (551-479 B.C.) and his disciples. The core idea of *The Analects* is *Ren* or Benevolence, which means "to love people". According to *The Analects*, to realize benevolence one has to use "*Li* or Rite or Propriety" as a norm for "To Restrain One's Selfishness and Restore Propriety is Benevolence". Besides, *The Analects* still embodies Confucius's political advocation of rule with virtue and opposition to harsh government, and his educational thought of "making no social distinctions in teaching" and of "teaching disciples in accordance with their aptitude".

孟子

Meng Zi, or ***Mencius,* or *The Book of Mencius:*** a record of conversations betweem Mencius and feudal lords of his time, and between him and his disciples. It dates from the second half of the 4th century B.C.. Mencius 孟子 (372 – 289 B.C.) spread Confucianism throughout China and developed it as the idealistic wing of Confucianism. He was arguably the most famous Confucianist after Confucius, and his ideas in *Mencius* were regarded as orthodox interpretation of Confucian thoughts.

大学

Da Xue, or ***The Great Learning***: The *Great Learning* had come from a chapter in *The Classic of Rites*, which forms one of "the Five Classics". It consists of a short main text attributed to the teachings of Confucius and then ten commentary chapters accredited to one of Confucius's disciples, Zeng Zi 曾子 (505-432 B.C.). The ideals of the book were supposedly Confucius's; however the text was written after his death.

中庸

Zhong Yong, or ***The Doctrine of Mean:*** *The Doctrine of Mean* had come from a chapter in *The Classic of Rites*, which forms one of the Five Classics. The composition of the text is attributed to Zi Si 子思, Kong Ji 孔伋 (481?-402 B.C.), the only grandson of Confucius. The term is originally derived from a verse of *The Analects of Confucius*, which reads that "The Master [Confucius] said, The virtue embodied in the doctrine of the Mean is of the highest order. But it has long been rare among people."

五经

The Five Classics: *Shi Jing* or *The Classic of Poetry, Shu Jing* or *The Classic of Documents, Li Ji* or *The Classic of Rites, The I Ching* or *The Classic of Changes,* and *Chun Qiu* or *The Spring and Autumn Annals*, collectively known as "The Five Classics", are five ancient Chinese books used in Confucianism as the basis of its studies. These books, or parts of them, were recorded to be either commented, compiled, or edited by Confucius himself. In 136 B.C., Han Wu Di Liu Che 刘彻 (156-87 B.C.), or Emperor Wu of Han Dynasty, set up official positions of Doctors for "the Five Classics", thus laying a solid foundation for the honourable position of the Confucian Classics in Chinese culture. The *Yue Jing* or *The Classic of Music* was considered as the sixth classic before. Since most parts of it were destroyed or lost, the remaining sections are said to be collected as two chapters in *The Classic of Rites*.

詩經

Shi Jing, or ***The Classic of Poetry:*** translated variously as *The Book of Songs* and *The Book of Odes*, the earliest existing collection of Chinese poems and songs. It comprises 305 poems and songs, with the earliest range from the 10th to the 7th centuries B.C.. The collection is classified into three parts according to their genre, namely *feng* 风, *ya* 雅 and *song* 颂: *Feng* 风, 160 folk songs of different localities; *Ya* 雅, 105 festal songs or odes; and *Song* 颂, 40 hymns and eulogies. *The Analects of Confucius* reads that "In *The Classic of Poetry* there are [around] 300 poems. But the essence of them can be covered in one sentence: 'Have no depraved thoughts'."

書經，尚書

Shu Jing, or ***The Classic of Documents; Shang Shu,*** literally ***Esteemed Documents:*** translated variously as *"The Classic of History"*, *"The Classic of Documents"*, *"The Book of History"*, *"The Book of Documents"*. It is the earliest compilation of documentary records related to events from the Yu Shun through Xia, Shang to Zhou Dynasties until the reign of Duke Mu of Qin (Qin Mu Gong), i.e. from ca. 22th Century to 621 B.C., in ancient history of China.

禮記

Li Ji, or ***The Classic of Rites***: also known as *The Book of Rites, The Book of Customs, The Record of Rites*, described the social forms, governmental system, and ancient ceremonial rites of the Zhou Dynasty (ca.1050–256 B.C.). The work is not to be confused with the two other classical texts on rites: *Zhou Li* or *The Rites of Zhou [Dynasty]* 周禮, which is a collection of bureaucratic establishment with characteristics of archives; and *Yi Li* or *The Book of Etiquette and Ceremonies* 儀禮, which records complicated ceremonial procedures of Zhou rulers, something like a schedule of a professional master of ceremonies.

易经

Yi Jing, or ***The I Ching***, or ***The Classic of Changes:*** also commonly known as *The Book of Changes* and *Zhou Yi*. It is one of the oldest classical Chinese texts, which "was completed by three sages, namely Fu Xi 伏羲, Wen Wang 文王 and Confucius, through three eras". Fu Xi made the Eight Trigrams by observing the Heaven and the Earth; King Wen of Zhou Dynasty (Zhou Wen Wang) doubled the Eight Trigrams into Sixty-Four Hexagrams and gave text comments on them; Confucius composed *Shi Yi* or *Ten Wings* 十翼 to interpret the sixty-four hexagrams, and thus transforming *The I Ching* from a divination book to a philosophical masterpiece, and finally to a classic of Confucianism. Actually, being composed of symbols (trigrams & hexagrams) and interpreting words, it is also a remarkable piece of writing on metaphor, and occupies an immeasurable place in the metaphor studies of China.

春秋

Chun Qiu, or ***The Spring and Autumn Annals***: the official chronicle of the State of Lu covering the period from 722 to 481 B.C.. It is the earliest surviving Chinese historical text to be arranged on annalistic principles. Its contents involve various aspects such as politics, military affairs, economics, culture, astronomy, meteorological phenomena, material production, and social life, which are original records with correct time, place and figure of that time. The text is extremely concise and, if all the commentaries are excluded, about 16,000 sinograms long. Because of this its meaning can only be appreciated with the aid of ancient commentaries, especially the traditional *Zuo Zhuan* or *Commentary of Zuo [Qiuming]*.

Well-Known Works of Other Thoughts of School

左传，左氏春秋

Zuo Zhuan, ***Zuo Shi Chun Qiu***, or ***Zuo's Spring Autumn Annals:*** a historical record from 722 to 453 B.C. which forms the three records or elucidations relative to events coverd in *Confucius's Spring and Autumn Annals*, and an important Confucian classic. Its authorship is generally attributed to Zuo Qiuming 左丘明 (502?-422?B.C.) of the Spring and Autumn Period.

老子，道德经

Lao Zi, or ***Lao Tzu; Dao De Jing,*** **or** ***Tao Te Ching:*** the most important Taoist text, also known as *Tao Te Ching,* as the Chapter 51 reads that "All things respect Tao and value Te". Its authorship is attributed to Lao Tzu 老子 (580?-500 B.C.). Dating back to the 3rd century B.C., it has 81 short chapters, contains altogether 5,635 sinograms, which is composed by 815 different ones. It contains many paradoxes and profound teachings on living in harmony with the nature.

墨子

Mo Zi, or ***Mo Tzu:*** the representative work of Mohism bearing Mo Tzu's name 墨子 (470?-391 B.C.?). It is a collection of writings by himself and his followers. It is rich in content and well-knit in structure in general, and some topics are closely elaborated with an incisive, penetrating analysis and sound argument. It not only deals with humanities such as epistemology, logics, economics, sociology, and social history etc., but also contains knowledge of natural sciences such as time and space, material structure, mechanics, optics, and geometry, thus having important scientific values.

荀子

Xun Zi, or ***Xun Tzu,*** or ***The Book of Xun Tzu:*** an important Confucian classic involving such aspects as philosophy, politics, ways of conducting oneself in society and doing scholarly research as well as academic augumentation. It is a collection of essays chiefly by Xun Tzu 荀子 (300?-230?B.C.), who spread Confucianism throughout China and developed it as the realistic wing of Confucianism. Unlike the aphoristic style of *The Analects of Confucius* and *Mencius*, Xun Tzu was a more rigorous thinker and wrote elaborately argued essays with well-knit syntax, plenty of metaphors and parallel constructions in form.

庄子

Zhuang Zi, or ***Chuang Tzu****:* a famous Taoist book named after its purported author Chuang Tzu 庄子 (369? – 286?B.C.), also known as *Nan Hua Zhen Jing* or T*rue Classic of Southern Florescence* since 742 A.D. alluding to the tradition that Chuang Tzu came from South China. According to *Han Shu Yi Wen Zhi* or *Treatise on Literature* of *History of the Former Han Dynasty*, it had 52 chapters, but only 33 has transmitted down until today, among which 7 are inner chapters, 15 outer chapters, and 11 miscellaneous chapters. The authorship of the inner chapters is generally attributed to Chuang Tzu himself, and the others to his followers and other Taoists afterwards. The popular version of *Chuang Tzu* with 33 chapters nowadays was compiled by Guo Xiang 郭象 (252-312) of the Western Jin Dynasty (265-316).

Chuang Tzu bears very high values in both literature and philosophy. Its achievements in the literature are mainly embodied in the aspects of romantic writing, realistic description, fables in different poses and with different expressions as well as forceful, boundless, free and natural language. Prose in *Chuang Tzu* can be regarded as the beginning of the romantic writings in China.

周礼

Zhou Li, or ***The Rites of Zhou [Dynasty]***: a collection of bureaucratic establishment of the Zhou Dynasty (ca.1050–256 B.C.) with characteristics of archives. It has six essays on respectively Heaven, Earth, Spring, Summer, Autumn, and Winter Officials. *Zhou Li* has become one of the Confucian classics, and one of the "Three Rites" with the other two *Li Ji* or *The Classic of Rites* and *Yi Li* or *The Book of Etiquette and Ceremonies* since the Tang Dynasty (618-907).

国语

Guo Yu, or ***Records of States:*** the earliest monograph of the history of different states from around 990 to 453 B.C. extant in China.

商君书，商子

Shang Ju Shu, or ***The Book of Shang Yang's Ideas***: also known as *Shang Zi* or *Shang Tzu*, consisting of 24 chapters, a collection of writings by Shang Yang 商鞅(395?-338 B.C.) and his followers, a representative work of the Legalist School.

韩非子

Han Fei Zi, or Han Fei Tzu: a collection of essays by Han Fei 韩非 (281?-233B.C.), a famous philosopher, thinker, and political commentator, who epitomized the thought of the Legalist School. His essays are well-knit with strict precise reasoning, penetrating, incisive analysis, and a trenchant humurous pen.

吕氏春秋

Lu Shi Chun Qiu, or ***Lu's Spring and Autumn Annals***: an encyclopedic classical Chinese text compiled around 239 B.C. under the patronage of the Chancellor of Qin Dynasty Lu Buwei 吕不韦 (?-235 B.C.), and a typical representative work of the Eclectics. Several chapters of it such as *Shang Nong* or *Valuing Farming*, *Bian Tu* or *Differentiating Soils*, *Shen Shi* or *Observing Seasons*, etc. are regarded as important materials to study the thought of the School of Agriculturalists.

管子

Guan Zi*, or *Guan Tzu: a collection of viewpoints of different thoughts of school including Schools of Legalists, Literati, Yin-Yang, Names, Militarists, and Agricultualists. The authorship is said to be Guan Zhong 管仲 (ca. 723? or 716? – 645 B.C.), a famous politician, militalist, and Prime Minsiter of the State of Qi, of the Spring and Autumn Period. The current version, originally 86 articles and 76 remaining until now, was edited and finalized by Liu Xiang 刘向 (77?-6 B.C.) of the Western Han Dynasty.

山海经

Shan Hai Jing*, or *The Classic of the Mountains and Seas, a classical Chinese text of the Pre-Qin Days, and largely a fabled geographical and cultural account of Pre-Qin China as well as a collection of mythology.

黄帝内经，内经

Huang Di Nei Jing*, or *Huang Di's Inner Classic: also known as *The Nei Jing*, comprising *Su Wen* 素问 or *Basic Questions*, and *Ling Shu* 灵枢, or *Miracullous Pivot*, the earliest systematic, complete and greatest medical classic extant in China. The authorship was attributed to an ancient legendary ruler Huang Di or Yellow Emperor (2698?-2589? B.C.). But actually the work was a product of various unknown authors in the Warring States Period (475-221 B.C.), and it is comparable in importance to the *Hippocratic Corpus* in Greek medicine. It is not only the breeding ground of the ontological concepts and the fundamental theories of Chinese medicine, but also an important component part of excellent cultural heritage of China. It has been guiding the development of Chinese medicine for over 2,000 years. As Donald Harper said, it is "the essential reference for ancient Chinese medicine and a valuable to research on early Chinese civilization".

Qin and Han Dynasties（221 B.C. – 220 A.D.）

尔雅

Er Ya*, or *Approaching to the Standard: one of "the Thirteen Classics" on Confucianism, and the earliest dictionary to explain meanings of *Ci* or significant single or compound sinograms arranged according to meanings. It was finished in between the Waing States Period and the early Han Dynasty, and was first recorded in the *Treatise on Literature* of *The History of the Former Han Dynast.* It is regarded as the first book on explaining words in ancient books in China, and has exerted important influences on exegetic studies, phonology, etymology, dialects, and philology.

论六家要旨

Lun Liu Jia Yao Zhi, or ***On the Essentials of Six Schools***: by Sima Tan 司马谈(?-110 B.C.), who was the first scholar to classify the "Hundred Schools" into the following six: "The Schools of Yin-Yang, Literati (or Confucianism), Mohists, Names, Legalists, and Tao Te (i.e. Taoist School) to strive on government's behalf, i.e. to take governing as their task".

淮南子

Huai Nan Zi, or ***Huai Nan Tzu:*** a collection of essays of the Western Han Dynasty (206B.C.-A.D.24), also known as *Huai Nan Hong Lie* or *Liu An Zi* for its compilation was directed by a royal family member, Duke of Huainan Liu An 刘安(179-122 B.C.). Based on thoughts of Taoist School before 221 B.C., it synthesizes essence of other thoughts of school like Schools of Yin-Yang, Mohists, Legalists, and Literati, and is listed as a work of the Eclectics by *Treatise on Literature* of *History of the Former Han Dynasty*.

史记

Shi Ji, or ***The Historical Records,*** or ***The Records of Grand Historian:*** China's first dynastic history, completed ca. 86 B.C. by Sima Qian 司马迁 (145 or 135 ? - ca. 86 B.C.), who is regarded as the father of Chinese historiography because of his highly praised work. It is a general history of China covering more than two thousand years from a legendary ruler Huang Di 黄帝 (2698?-2589? B.C.), known as the Yellow Emperor in the West, to Emperor Han Wu Di Liu Che (156-87 B.C.), and thus laying a solid foundation for later Chinese historiography.

难经，黄帝八十一难经

Nan Jing, or ***The Classic of Questioning***, or ***The Classic of Difficult Issues***: also known as *Huang Di's Eighty One Difficult Issues*, originally compiled during the first century A.D. by an unknown author though its authorship is often ascribed to Qin Yueren 秦越人 (407-310 B.C.). It deals with fundamental theories in the form of questions and answers. Acupoints, needling method, physiological and pathological conditions to *Jing Luo* or the vessels, and pulse-taking method are all discussed. "It marked the apex and the conclusion of the initial development phase of a conceptual system of health care based on the doctrines of the Five Phases and yinyang. As the classic of the medicine of systematic correspondence, the *Nan-Ching* covers all aspects of theoretical and practical health care within these doctrines in an unusually systematic fashion. Most important is its innovative discussion of pulse diagnosis and needle treatment". (From the Inside Front Cover of the *Nan-Ching*, translated and annotated by Paul U. Unschuld, published by The University of California Press, 1986.)

春秋繁露

Chun Qiu Fan Lu, or ***The Luxuriant Dew of the Spring and Autumn Annals:*** an important Confucian classic, and one of the works that was attributed to Dong Zhongshu 董仲舒 (179-104 B.C.), a famous thinker and politician, who proposed "To proscribe all non-Confucian schools of thoughts and to espouse Confucianism as the orthodox state ideology", which was taken by Han Wu Di Liu Che 刘彻 (156-87 B.C.). And thereafter Confucianism was established as an official religion of China and the leading philosophical thought in China until 1905. The book deified Confucius by propogating the doctrine of *Tian Ren Gan Ying* or Interactions between Heaven and Man and integrating yin-yang and five phases into an ethical and political framework, which lays down rules for deciding the legitimacy of a monarch as well as providing a set of checks and balances for reigning a monarch. Such a proposal legitimated the emperors' autocratic government for thousands of years since Han Wu Di in China.

神农本草经

Shen Nong Ben Cao Jing, or ***Shennong's Classic of Materia Medica:*** the earliest monograph on materia medica in China and one of "The Four Great Classics" on Chinese medicine, believed to be a work of the first century B.C. with its authorship attributed to Shennong, a god in charge of agriculture and medicine. The original ancient work has been lost. Its contents have been preserved in quotations in the books on materia medica of the past ages. It records properties, flavors, actions and indications of 365 medicinals in three grades: top, medium, and lower in details. Scholars restored it by collecting quotations from the books on materia medica of its later ages.

新论•形神

Xin Lun • Xing Shen, or ***Body and Spirit*** of ***New Argumentation*****:** the first treatise on body and spirit in the history of Chinese philosophy by Huan Tan 桓谭 (23 B.C.- 50 A.D.), which advances a famous metaphor – the relationship between body and spirit is just like that between the candle and its flame, in which candle metaphorizes the body and flame the spirit.

周礼郑司农解诂

Zhou Li Zheng Sinong Jie Gu, or **Zheng Zhong's Annotations of *The Rites of Zhou [Dynasty]:*** 6 volumes, collected by Ma Guohan 马国翰 (1794—1857). Zheng Zhong 郑众 (?～83), an expert in Confucian classics of Eastern Han Dynasty, whose works had been lost long before.

郑众春秋牒例章句

Zheng Zhong Chun Qiu Tie Li Zhang Ju, or **Zheng Zhong's Syntactic and Semantic Analysis of Examples of *The Spring and Autumn Annals:*** 1 volume, collected by Ma Guohan 马国翰 (1794—1857) . Zheng Zhong 郑众 (?～83), an expert in Confucian classics of Eastern Han Dynasty, whose works had been lost long before.

汉书•艺文志

Han Shu Yi Wen Zhi, or ***Treatise on Literature*** of ***The History of the Former Han Dynasty:*** the earliest literature on bibliography and the earliest systematic title catalogue extant in China, compiled by Ban Gu 班固 (A.D. 32-92), who took the *Qi Lue* 七略 by Liu Xiang 刘向 (78-8 B.C.) and his son Liu Xin 刘歆 (50 B.C.? - 23 A.D.) as the primary source. Liu Xiang and Liu Xin were the first two persons in the history of China to systematize the available books, which were presented to the Han Imperial Court from the whole country after the event of burning books (of poetics, master philosophers and their school thoughts) in 213 B.C. in Qin Shi Huang's reign. They were put in charge of writing a catalogue of the books that were stored in the imperial library in the late first century B.C. Their survey began in 26 B.C. Their catalogue, called *Qi Lue*, was later lost, but not before it was used by Ban Gu to compile the bibliographical monograph - *Treatise on Literature*, a part of *Han Shu* or *The History of the Former Han Dynasty*.

论衡

Lun Heng, or ***Critical Essays:*** an important work finished around 86 A.D. by Wang Chong 王充 (27-100 A.D), a famous thinker, philosopher, and educator. It contains 85 essays with one missing and over 200,000 sinograms. It has been listed in the category of the Eclectics in the bibliographies since *Sui Shu Jing Ji Zhi* or *Treatise on Classics and Documents* of *The History of Sui Dynasty* by Wei Zheng 魏征 (580-643), the second oldest historical bibliography after *Treatise on Literature* of *The History of the Former Han Dynasty*. The author discussed significant issues on philosophy, politics, religion, and culture, augued against the viewpoint of Interaction between Universe and Man proposed by Dong Zhongshu, held that all things in the universe, including man and universe, are all natural existant beings resulting from a natural process known as the movement and mutation of *qi*, and Universe is not a deified God; denied the existance of *Gui* or Ghost; and opposed the ideology of "Esteeming the Universe and Following the Old".

说文解字

Shuo Wen Jie Zi, or ***The Origin of Chinese Characters:*** *Shuo Wen Jie Zi* literally means "explaining pictographs and analyzing composite sinograms". I prefer to translate the title into *The Origin of Chinese Characters*. It is the first comprehensive systematic dictionary of sinograms arranged by sections with shared components, called radicals (*bùshǒu*, lit. "section headers") and finished in 100 A.D. by Xu Shen 许慎 (A.D.58? – 147?) of the Eastern Han Dynasty. It is also the first dictionary which interprets the original meaning of a sinogram by analyzing its structure and gives the rationale behind it, sometimes the etymology of the sinogram as well. Actually, it is far beyond a dictionary, and moreover it can be interpreted from cultural and philosophical perspectives. It is indeed the case that no monograph on philosophy of Chinese language has ever been available up till today except this book.

伤寒杂病论

Shang Han Za Bing Lun*,* or ***Treatise on Cold-induced and Miscellaneous Diseases****:* a famous work by a world famous medical expert Zhang Zhongjing 张仲景(150-219), systematized and rearranged into "*Shang Han Lun* or *On Cold-induced Diseases*" and "*Jin Gui Yao Lue* or *Synopsis of the Prescriptions from the Golden Chamber*", which are regarded as the two of the "Four Great Classics on Chinese Medicine" (the other two are *Huang Di's Inner Classic* and *Shennong's Classic of Materia Medica*), and have been the required readings and courses for majors of Chinese medicine even up till today.

伤寒论

Shang Han Lun, or ***On Cold-induced Diseases****:* one of the most influential works in the history of Chinese medicine, the part on "cold-induced diseases" of *Treatise on Cold-induced and Miscellaneous Diseases,* rearranged by Wang Shuhe in 10 volumes.

金匮要略

Jin Gui Yao Lue, or ***Synopsis of the Golden Chamber:*** one of the most influential works in the history of Chinese medicine, the part on "miscellaneous diseases" of *Treatise on Cold-induced and Miscellaneous Diseases,* dealing with miscellaneous diseases of internal medicine, and some external and women's diseases, rearranged by Wang Shuhe in 3 volumes and 25 chapters, including 262 prescriprions.

The Three Kingdoms (220-265)

广雅

Guang Ya*, or *Supplement to Er Ya*:* an encyclopediac dictionary to explain meanings of *Ci* or significant single or compound sinograms in literature before Wei (220-265), one of the Three Kingdoms by Zhang Yi 张揖, Doctor of Wei Kingdom (220-265). As an supplement to *Er Ya* 尔雅, it includes 18,150 sinograms.

脉经

Mai Jing, or ***The Classic of Pulse Diagnosis*****:** written by Wang Shuhe 王叔和(201-280), which records 24 pulses and is generally acknowledged as the standard work and the earliest comprehensive monograph on sphygmology extant.

The Northern and Southern Dynasties (420-589)

神灭论

Shén Miè Lùn, or ***On the Annihilation of the Spirit*****:** a famous work on annihilation of the Spirit by Fan Zhen 范缜 (ca. 450-515), a Chinese philosopher and thinker of the Southern Dynasty. It insists on the primary importance of the materials, systematically expounds the viewpoints of atheism, points out that man is the unity of body and spirit, and metaphorizes the relationship between the body and the spirit as that between the sword and its sharpness.

全元起注素问

Quan Yuaqi Zhu Su Wen, or ***Quan Yuanqi's Annotated Version of Su Wen:*** the earliest annotated version of *Su Wen* or *Basic Questions* in China by Quan Yuanqi 全元起 (?-?), a famous medical expert living in the Northern and Southern Dynasties. It lost in between Norther Song (960-1127) and Southern Song (1127-1279) Dynasty . A famous modern Chinese scholar Duan Yishan 段逸山 (1940-) tried to restore it based on his research, and published the outcome entitled "Su Wen Quan Yuanqi Ben Yan Jiu Yu Ji Fu" or "Research and Restoration of *Quan Yuanqi's Annotated Version of Su Wen*" 素问全元起本研究与辑复 in 2001.

玉篇

Yu Pian, or ***Jade Writings*****:** a dictionary arranged according to forms and structures of sinograms compiled by Gu Yewang 顾野王 (519-581) in 543.

Sui-Tang Dynasties (581-907)

五行大义

Wu Xing Da Yi, or ***The Great Connotations of the Five Phases:*** the most important work on five phases of the middle ancient times written by Xiao Ji 箫吉 in 594 for his emperor, a comment from Joseph Needham (1900-1995) , which not only epitomised the thoughts on five phases theory before its time, but is also a must for studying the entire developing course of five phases theory in China as well as the theory of Images and Numbers of *The Book of Changes*.

诸病源候论

Zhu Bing Yuan Hou Lun, or ***Treatise on Causes and Symptoms of Diseases:*** the earliest monograph on causes and symptoms of diseases in China compiled by

Chao Yuanfang 巢元方 (?-?), et al. in 610 with 30 volumes of detailed discussions on causes and symptoms of various diseases, including diseases of internal medicine, external medicine, gynecology, pediatrics, ENT, mouth and teeth, orthopedics and traumatology, and some infectious diseases, parasitic diseases, and surgery. It summarizes medical achievements before 610, and consists of 67 categories with 1,720 entries and many brilliant expositions frequently cited by authors of later generations.

备急千金要方

Bei Ji Qian Jin Yao Fang, or ***Invaluable Prescriptions for Emergencies:*** also known as *Qian Jin Yao Fang,* or *Invaluable Prescriptions* for short, a famous work compiled by Sun Simiao 孙思邈 (581-682), in 30 volumes with a general introduction, prescriptions of various clinical branches, diets, pulse-taking, acupuncture, etc. *Da Yi Jing Cheng* or *A Great Doctor Should Be Expert in Medical Skills and Sincere to His Patients* 大医精诚, an important essay on medical ethics, is from the first volume of the book.

Song Dynasty (960-1279)
太平御览

Tai Ping Yu Lan: a large-sized *Lei Shu* or reference book with materials taken from various sources and arranged according to subjects compiled by Li Fang 李昉 (925-996), et al. from 977 to 983. It has 1,000 volumes and 5 millions of sinograms. It quotes altogether 2,579 kinds of books including 1,690 historical and classical ones, most of which have lost, therefore it has preserved plenty of valuable materials for us.

嘉佑本草

Jia You Ben Cao, or ***Jiayou Materia Medica:*** a monograph on materia medica including 1,082 medicinals compiled by Zhang Yuxi 掌禹锡 (992-1068) and other Confucian officials, who followed an imperial decree to do so. It preserves many lost materials on materia medica.

图经本草

Tu Jing Ben Cao, or ***Illustrated Materia Medica:*** compiled by Su Song 苏颂 (1020-1101), a Confucian official, issued and printed in 1061, which records over 1,000 single medicinal formulas with over 900 illustrations. It is the first block-printed edition of illustrations of material medica.

经史证类备急本草

Jing Shi Zheng Lei Bei Ji Ben Cao, or ***Classic of Classified Materia Medica for Emergencies*:** compiled by Tang Shenwei 唐慎微 (1056-1093) in 1082, a Confucian physician, which summarizes achievements on materia medica of the former ages, includes records on materia medica from Confucian classics, historical records, philosophical writings, and miscellaneous works as well as the Buddhist and Taoist Scriptures. It includes 1,746 kinds of medicinal agents with directions for use and preparation, and many new prescriptions. It laid a solid foundation for the development of Chinese materia medica. Li Shizhen, a Confucian physician, took it as a chief source of his monumental work *Ben Cao Gang Mu*.

梦溪笔谈

Meng Xi Bi Tan, or ***Dream Pool Essays***: a writing consisting mainly of short sketches by Shen Kuo 沈括 (1031-1095), a politician and scientist of the Northern Song Dynasty finished in between 1086 and 1093. It includes what the author saw and heard in his life time as well as his personal understanding about these, involving various subjects like astronomy, mathematics, physics, chemistry, biology, geology, mateorology, medicine, agriculture, engineering, literature, history, music, painting, anthropology, archeology, linguistics, military affairs, law etc. One third of the space records, narrates and elucidates natural scientific knowledge, which reflects the scientific level of that time, and bears extremely high value. It is named as an encyclopedia of ancient China by Western scholars.

本草衍义

Ben Cao Yan Yi, or ***Augmented Materia Medica:*** compiled by Kou Zongshi 寇宗奭 (?-?), a Confucian official, in 1116, supplementing what *Jing Shi Zheng Lei Bei Ji Ben Cao* lacks such as some medicinal agents' actions and methods to differentiate similar ones. It includes 472 medicinal agents, and suggests that the dosage of a medicinal should vary according to age, constitution, and emergent or chronic condition.

朱子语类

Zhu Zi Yu Lei, or ***Excerpt of Analects of Zhu Xi***: a collection of questions and answers between Zhu Xi and his disciples compiled by Li Jingde 黎靖德 in 1263, printed and publised in 1270. Zhu Xi, or Chu His, 朱熹 (1130-1200), was a Confucian scholar of Song Dynasty, who became the leading figure and the most influential rationalist of Neo-Confucianism in China. His contribution to Chinese philosophy includes his assigning special significance to *The Analects of Confucius*, *The Mencius, The Great Learning,* and *The Doctrine of Mean*, "the Four Books", his emphasis on the investigation of things (*ge wu*), and the synthesis of all fundamental Confucian concepts.

通志

Tong Zhi, or ***Comprehensive History:*** a comprehensive history presented in a series of bibliographies by Zheng Qiao 郑樵 (1103-1162), a historian, thinker, and scientist of Southern Song Dynasty, finished in 1147.

Yuan Dynasty (1271-1368)

宋史

Song Shi, or ***The History of the Song Dynasty:*** the largest of the Twenty-Five Histories (dynastic histories from the remote antiquity till the Ming Dynasty) compiled in 1345 by officials of Yuan Dynasty (1271-1368) Tuotuo and Alutu.

Ming Dynasty (1368-1644)

针灸大全

Zhen Jiu Da Quan, or ***A Complete Book on Acupuncture and Moxibustion:*** compiled in 1439 by Xu Feng 徐凤 (?-?).

难经集注

Nan Jing Ji Zhu or ***A Collection of Annotations on The Classic of Difficult Issues:*** a collection of annotations on *The Classic of Difficult Issues* from Lu Guang 吕广 of the Three Kingdoms (220-265), Yang Xuancao 杨玄操 of the Tang Dynasty (618-907), Ding Deyong 丁德用, et al. of the Song Dynasty (960-1279) by Wang Jiusi 王九思 in 1505 of the Ming Dynasty (1384-1644), the extant earliest collection of annotations on *The Classic of Difficult Issues*. It has 5 volumes and 13 chapters.

本草纲目

Ben Cao Gang Mu, or ***The Compendium of Materia Medica:*** finished in 1578 by Li Shizhen 李时珍 (1518-1593), appraised as the "encyclopedia of China published in 1596", which not only makes great contribution to Chinese pharmacology, but also exerts far-reaching influences on pharmacology, botany, zoology, mineralogy, and chemistry of the whole world.

六科证治准绳

Liu Ke Zheng Zhi Zhun Sheng, or ***Standards of Diagnosis and Treatment in Six Branches of Medicine:*** a famous work with 120 volumes by Wang Kentang 王肯堂 (1549-1613), a Confucian official, which epitomized the achievements on medicine before its time and was highly appraised by medical practitioners afterwards.

类经

Lei Jing, or ***Classified Inner Classic:*** a famous work of comprehensive classified studies on *Huang Di Nei Jing* with 32 volumes, and one of the representative works by Zhang Jiebin 张介宾(1563-1640), also known as Zhang Jingyue 张景岳, a famous medical expert.

景岳全书

***Jingyue Quan Shu*, or *Jingyue's Complete Works*:** 64 volumes by Zhang Jiebin 张介宾(1563-1640), also known as Zhang Jingyue 张景岳, a famous medical expert.

Qing Dynasty (1644-1911)

绎史

Yi Shi: a historical record by Ma Xiao 马骕 (1621-1673), including five parts – Time Immemoria, Three Dynasties (Xia, Shang, and Western Zhou), Spring and Autumn, Warring States, and External Records.

张子正蒙注

Zhang Zi Zheng Meng Zhu, or ***Annotations on Zheng Meng by Zhang Tzu:*** one of the important philosophical works by Wang Fuzhi 王夫之 (1619-1692), a thinker and philosopher of his time who epitomized the thought of specific materialism of China. The author inherited and developed Zhang Zai's 张载 (1020-1077) thoughts of specific materialism by annotating his work "*Zheng Meng* 正蒙". Zhang Zai was a philosopher of the Northern Song Dynasty and one of the founding fathers of Neo-Confucianism.

本草崇原

Ben Cao Chong Yuan, or ***The Origin of Materia Medica:*** a monograph on materia medica with 3 volumes, which annotates *Shennong's Classic of Materia Medica,* by Zhang Zhicong 张志聪 (1616-1674). Based on the five circuit phases, six climatic factors, and waxing and waning between yin and yang, Zhang Zhicong founded the *Yao Qi* 药气 theory to expound actions of medicinals in details, which starts from the formation of properties and flavors, attributes of yin-yang and five-phases as well as shapes and colors of medicinals, and then is related to the machanism of curing an illness. His approach deeply influenced such medical experts as Xu Dachun 徐大椿 (1693-1771) and Chen Xiuyuan 陈修园 (1753-1823).

本草备要

***Ben Cao Bei Yao*, or *Essentials of Materia Medica*:** a clinical manual of materia medica and a door to Chinese medicine with 8 volumes and published in 1694 by Wang Ang 汪昂 (1615-1695). It mainly draws materials from *Ben Cao Gang Mu* or *The Compendium of Materia Medica* by Li Shizhen 李时珍 (1518-1593) published in 1596 and *Shen Nong Ben Cao Jing Shu* or *Commentaries on Shennong's Classic of Materia Medica* by Miu Xiyong 缪希雍 (1546-1627) published in 1625. It has exerted deep-going and far-reaching influences on Chinese medical majors of the later ages, for example, until 1963, it had been reprinted 107 times since its first publication.

画语录

Hua Yu Lu, or ***Arts of Painting:*** also known as *Shi Tao Hua Yu Lu* or *Ku Gua He Shang Hua Yu Lu,* a monograph on arts of painting by Shi Tao 石涛 (1630-1724), a painting wonder, whose paintings and achievements in Taoism, Buddhism, literature, and poetry exerted far-reaching and deep-going influences on the development of classical Chinese painting, and are appreciated by the people today.

康熙字典

Kang Xi Zi Dian, or ***The Kangxi Dictionary:*** a detailed dictionary of sinograms with far-reaching and deep-going influences on later generations finished in 1716 chiefly compiled by two ministers of Emperor Kangxi's reign Zhang Yushu 张玉书 (1642-1711) and Chen Tingjing 陈廷敬 (1639-1712).

古今图书集成

Gu Jin Tu Shu Ji Cheng, or ***Integration of Books from Past to Present:*** 10,000 volumes, the best and the most intact preserved classified book with the largest scale and richest materials ever extant in China compiled in 1706 by Cheng Menglei 陈梦雷 (1650-1641), a Confucian official, prefaced by Emperor Yongzheng 雍正 (1678-1735), the title of which was given by Emperor Kangxi 康熙 (1654-1722), among which 520 volumes are books on Chinese medicine.

医学源流论

Yi Xuen Yuan Liu Lun, or ***The Origin and Development of [Chinese] Medicine:*** A collection of 99 essays on Chinese medicine by Xu Dachun 徐大椿 (1693-1771) finished in 1757. It has 2 volumes: Vol. 1 one on the vessels, *zang fu* organs, pulse, illnesses, prescriptions and medicinals, and Vol. 2 on therapeutic methods, commentaries on medical books, clinical medicine and other topics. The book presents a lot of author's original creative ideas on Chinese medicine.

四库全书

Si Ku Quan Shu, or ***The Complete Library of the Four Branches of Literature:*** translated variously as *The Imperial Collection of Four Treasuries*, *The Complete Library in Four Branches of Literature*, or *The Complete Library of the Four Treasuries*, the largest collection of books in Chinese history and probably the most ambitious editorial enterprise in the history of the world, completed by 4,000 Confucian officials by Emperor Qianlong's order 乾隆 (1711-1799) in 1782 and comprising the four classical divisions of Chinese learning - classics, history, philosophy, and belle-letters.

说文释例

Shuo Wen Shi Li, or **Interpretations of Examples from *The Origin of Chinese Characters:*** a monograph on the stylistic rules and layout as well as philological rules of *The Origin of Chinese Characters* by Wang Jun 王筠 (1784-1854).

契文举例

Qi Wen Ju Li, or ***Examples of Oracle-Bone Inscriptions:*** the first work on philological studies on oracle scripts finished in 1904 by Sun Yirang 孙詒让 (1848-1908), a famous sinologist and educator.

Culture and Knowledge

Edited by Friedrich G. Wallner

Vol. 1 Friedrich G. Wallner: Structure and Relativity. 2005.

Vol. 2 Kurt Greiner: Therapie der Wissenschaft. Eine Einführung in die Methodik des Konstruktiven Realismus. 2005.

Vol. 3 Daniël Francois Malherbe Strauss: Paradigmen in Mathematik, Physik und Biologie und ihre philosophischen Wurzeln. Ins Deutsche übertragen von Martin J. Jandl. 2005.

Vol. 4 Friedrich G. Wallner: What Practitioners of TCM Should Know. A Philosophical Introduction for Medical Doctors. With a Supplement by *Kelvin Chan*. 2006.

Vol. 5 Kurt Greiner / Friedrich G. Wallner / Martin Gostentschnig (Hrsg.): Verfremdung – Strangification. Multidisziplinäre Beispiele der Anwendung und Fruchtbarkeit einer epistemologischen Methode. 2006.

Vol. 6 Kurt Greiner: Psychoanalytik als Wissenschaft des 21. Jahrhunderts. Ein konstruktivistischer Blick auf Struktur und Reflexionspotential einer polymorphen Kontextualisations-Technik. 2007.

Vol. 7 Kambiz Badie / Maryam Tayefeh Mahmoudi: Strangification: A New Paradigm in Knowledge Processing and Creation. 2007.

Vol. 8 Friedrich G. Wallner: Systemanalyse als Wissenschaftstheorie I: Von der Sprachlichkeit zur Kulturalität. Redigiert von Florian Schmidsberger und Kurt Greiner. 2008.

Vol. 9 Friedrich G. Wallner: Five Lectures on the Foundations of Chinese Medicine. Copyedited by Florian Schmidsberger. 2009.

Vol. 10 Friedrich G. Wallner / Gertrude Kubiena / Martin J. Jandl (eds.): Understanding Traditional Chinese Medicine. Consultant: Lena Springer. 2009.

Vol. 11 Fritz G. Wallner / Florian Schmidsberger / Franz Martin Wimmer (eds.): Intercultural Philosophy. New Aspects and Methods. 2010.

Vol. 12 Friedrich G. Wallner: Systemanalyse als Wissenschaftstheorie II: Kulturalismus als Perspektive der Philosophie im 21. Jahrhundert. 2010.

Vol. 13 Friedrich G. Wallner / Fengli Lan / Martin J. Jandl (eds.): The Way of Thinking in Chinese Medicine. Theory, Methodology and Structure of Chinese Medicine. 2010.

Vol. 14 Kurt Greiner / Martin J. Jandl / Friedrich G. Wallner (eds.): Aus dem Umfeld des Konstruktiven Realismus. Studien zu Psychotherapiewissenschaft, Neurokritik und Philosophie. 2010.

Vol. 15 Martin J. Jandl: Praxeologische Funktionalontologie. Eine Theorie des Wissens als Synthese von H. Dooyeweerd und R.B. Brandon. 2010.

Vol. 16 Friedrich G. Wallner: Systemanalyse als Wissenschaftstheorie III: Das Vorhaben einer kulturorientierten Wissenschaftstheorie in der Gegenwart. 2011.

Vol. 17 Friedrich G. Wallner / Fengli Lan / Martin J. Jandl (eds.): Chinese Medicine and Intercultural Philosophy. Theory, Methodology and Structure of Chinese Medicine. 2011.

Vol. 18 Gerhard Klünger (Hrsg.): Wörterbuch des Konstruktiven Realismus. Aus Vorlesungen, Seminaren und Werken von Friedrich G. Wallner. 2011.

Vol. 19 Fengli Lan / Friedrich G. Wallner / Claudia Wobovnik (eds.): Shen, Psychotherapy, and Acupuncture. Theory, Methodology and Structure of Chinese Medicine. 2011.

Vol. 20 Gerhard Klünger: Freiheit im Kontext der Wissenschaftskritik. 2012.

Vol. 21 Friedrich G. Wallner / Fengli Lan / Andreas Schulz (Hrsg.): Aspekte des Konstruktiven Realismus. 2012.

Vol. 22 Fengli Lan: Culture, Philosophy, and Chinese Medicine. Viennese Lectures. 2012.

www.peterlang.de